Digital Pathology: Records of Successful Implementations

Digital Pathology: Records of Successful Implementations

Catarina Eloy

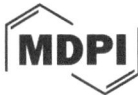

Basel • Beijing • Wuhan • Barcelona • Belgrade • Novi Sad • Cluj • Manchester

Catarina Eloy
Pathology Laboratory
IPATIMUP
Porto
Portugal

Editorial Office
MDPI AG
Grosspeteranlage 5
4052 Basel, Switzerland

This is a reprint of articles from the Special Issue published online in the open access journal *Diagnostics* (ISSN 2075-4418) (available at: www.mdpi.com/journal/diagnostics/special_issues/ Digital_Pathology_Successful_Implementations).

For citation purposes, cite each article independently as indicated on the article page online and using the guide below:

Lastname, A.A.; Lastname, B.B. Article Title. *Journal Name* **Year**, *Volume Number*, Page Range.

ISBN 978-3-7258-2038-2 (Hbk)
ISBN 978-3-7258-2037-5 (PDF)
https://doi.org/10.3390/books978-3-7258-2037-5

© 2024 by the authors. Articles in this book are Open Access and distributed under the Creative Commons Attribution (CC BY) license. The book as a whole is distributed by MDPI under the terms and conditions of the Creative Commons Attribution-NonCommercial-NoDerivs (CC BY-NC-ND) license (https://creativecommons.org/licenses/by-nc-nd/4.0/).

Contents

About the Editor vii

Preface ix

Catarina Eloy, João Vale, Mónica Curado, António Polónia, Sofia Campelos and Ana Caramelo et al.
Digital Pathology Workflow Implementation at IPATIMUP
Reprinted from: *Diagnostics* **2021**, *11*, 2111, doi:10.3390/diagnostics11112111 1

Filippo Fraggetta, Alessandro Caputo, Rosa Guglielmino, Maria Giovanna Pellegrino, Giampaolo Runza and Vincenzo L'Imperio
A Survival Guide for the Rapid Transition to a Fully Digital Workflow: The "Caltagirone Example"
Reprinted from: *Diagnostics* **2021**, *11*, 1916, doi:10.3390/diagnostics11101916 12

Jordi Temprana-Salvador, Pablo López-García, Josep Castellví Vives, Lluís de Haro, Eudald Ballesta and Matias Rojas Abusleme et al.
DigiPatICS: Digital Pathology Transformation of the Catalan Health Institute Network of 8 Hospitals—Planification, Implementation, and Preliminary Results
Reprinted from: *Diagnostics* **2022**, *12*, 852, doi:10.3390/diagnostics12040852 31

Diana Montezuma, Ana Monteiro, João Fraga, Liliana Ribeiro, Sofia Gonçalves and André Tavares et al.
Digital Pathology Implementation in Private Practice: Specific Challenges and Opportunities
Reprinted from: *Diagnostics* **2022**, *12*, 529, doi:10.3390/diagnostics12020529 52

Rachel N. Flach, Nina L. Fransen, Andreas F. P. Sonnen, Tri Q. Nguyen, Gerben E. Breimer and Mitko Veta et al.
Implementation of Artificial Intelligence in Diagnostic Practice as a Next Step after Going Digital: The UMC Utrecht Perspective
Reprinted from: *Diagnostics* **2022**, *12*, 1042, doi:10.3390/diagnostics12051042 62

Ankush U. Patel, Nada Shaker, Sambit Mohanty, Shivani Sharma, Shivam Gangal and Catarina Eloy et al.
Cultivating Clinical Clarity through Computer Vision: A Current Perspective on Whole Slide Imaging and Artificial Intelligence
Reprinted from: *Diagnostics* **2022**, *12*, 1778, doi:10.3390/diagnostics12081778 73

Sabyasachi Maity, Samal Nauhria, Narendra Nayak, Shreya Nauhria, Tamara Coffin and Jadzia Wray et al.
Virtual Versus Light Microscopy Usage among Students: A Systematic Review and Meta-Analytic Evidence in Medical Education
Reprinted from: *Diagnostics* **2023**, *13*, 558, doi:10.3390/diagnostics13030558 99

Angela Ishak, Mousa M. AlRawashdeh, Maria Meletiou-Mavrotheris and Ilias P. Nikas
Virtual Pathology Education in Medical Schools Worldwide during the COVID-19 Pandemic: Advantages, Challenges Faced, and Perspectives
Reprinted from: *Diagnostics* **2022**, *12*, 1578, doi:10.3390/diagnostics12071578 127

Athena Davri, Effrosyni Birbas, Theofilos Kanavos, Georgios Ntritsos, Nikolaos Giannakeas and Alexandros T. Tzallas et al.
Deep Learning on Histopathological Images for Colorectal Cancer Diagnosis: A Systematic Review
Reprinted from: *Diagnostics* **2022**, *12*, 837, doi:10.3390/diagnostics12040837 . . . . **141**

Filippo Fraggetta, Vincenzo L'Imperio, David Ameisen, Rita Carvalho, Sabine Leh and Tim-Rasmus Kiehl et al.
Best Practice Recommendations for the Implementation of a Digital Pathology Workflow in the Anatomic Pathology Laboratory by the European Society of Digital and Integrative Pathology (ESDIP)
Reprinted from: *Diagnostics* **2021**, *11*, 2167, doi:10.3390/diagnostics11112167 . . . . **173**

About the Editor

Catarina Eloy

Catarina Eloy is a Portuguese interventional pathologist, researcher and teacher devoted to the diagnosis and study of thyroid cancer. She graduated as pathologist in 2011, completed her PhD thesis on papillary thyroid carcinoma in 2012 at the Medical Faculty of Porto University, has been an Affiliated Professor of the Medical Faculty of Porto University since 2015 and published more than 100 manuscripts in indexed scientific journals. She has been the Head of the fully digital Pathology Laboratory of Ipatimup, Porto since 2013, and developed special interest in the modernization of the diagnostic processes, including digital and computational pathology.

Preface

Digital pathology workflow implementation remains challenging. In laboratories worldwide, there are growing examples of successful implementation and pathologists acknowledging the advantages of this new model of practicing pathology.

This Special Issue of *Diagnostics* is a collection of records of successful digital pathology implementation for primary diagnosis or secondary applications, that serve as an inspiration to those readers who are still skeptical about it. These records highlight the advantages of the use of whole slide images such as sharing and the image analysis, as well as the virtues of the digital workflow per se. The holistic approach of the digital workflow comprehends practical interventions in the laboratory workstations that are demonstrated in this Special Issue, as well as their respective monitorization, quality control and impact on clinical practice.

Catarina Eloy
Editor

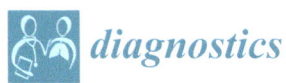

Article

Digital Pathology Workflow Implementation at IPATIMUP

Catarina Eloy [1,2,*], João Vale [1], Mónica Curado [1], António Polónia [1,2], Sofia Campelos [1], Ana Caramelo [1], Rui Sousa [1] and Manuel Sobrinho-Simões [1,2]

[1] Pathology Laboratory, Institute of Molecular Pathology and Immunology, University of Porto, 4200-135 Porto, Portugal; jvale@ipatimup.pt (J.V.); mcurado@ipatimup.pt (M.C.); antoniopolonia@yahoo.com (A.P.); sofia.campelos@gmail.com (S.C.); acaramelo@ipatimup.pt (A.C.); rsousa@ipatimup.pt (R.S.); ssimoes@ipatimup.pt (M.S.-S.)

[2] i3S—Instituto de Investigação e Inovação em Saúde & Pathology Department of Medical Faculty, University of Porto, 4200-135 Porto, Portugal

* Correspondence: catarinaeloy@hotmail.com

Abstract: The advantages of the digital methodology are well known. In this paper, we provide a detailed description of the process for the digital transformation of the pathology laboratory at IPATIMUP, the major modifications that operate throughout the processing pipeline, and the advantages of its implementation. The model of digital workflow implementation at IPATIMUP demonstrates that careful planning and adoption of simple measures related to time, space, and sample management can be adopted by any pathology laboratory to achieve higher quality and easy digital transformation.

Keywords: digital pathology; workflow; telepathology; implementation

1. Introduction

The Institute of Molecular Pathology and Immunology of the University of Porto (IPATIMUP) is a non-profit research institution with a pathology laboratory that is double accredited by the College of American Pathologists (CAP) and by NP EN ISO 15189 standards. It serves as a reference center for second opinions on difficult cases, biomarker identification, and training of pathologists and laboratory technicians. The experience with a telepathology project that started in 2013, and the wide use of scanned dark field images for fluorescent in situ hybridization tests, motivated the quest for digitization of the laboratory. Successful digital transformations of pathology workflow have been published in the literature [1–3]. The advantages of the digital methodology are well known and include time sparing workflows, as well as a reduction in costs [4,5].

The Food and Drug Administration (FDA) approval of the first scanning systems for primary diagnosis constitutes a relevant driver for the adoption of a digital workflow, representing general support of the regulatory institutions on the subject. The use of scanning systems other than those approved for clinical use by the regulatory institutions should be performed under strict surveillance by internal/external quality control programs [6].

In this paper, we describe the process for digital transformation of the pathology laboratory at IPATIMUP, including a detailed description of the modifications operated throughout the processing pipeline, as well as the advantages of its implementation.

2. Materials and Methods

The process for digital transformation of the laboratory started in 2016 when we decided to start preparing the staff and the respective structure. Pathologists and technicians underwent sessions of training and courses to understand the best way to start applying modifications to the laboratory, namely space and time, a new type of management, equipment renewal/acquisition, information technology infrastructure, and design of the validation of digital observation by the pathologist. The goal was to introduce whole slide images (WSIs) for diagnosis in all bright field tissue-related cases. Dark field fluorescent in situ hybridization (FISH) and immunofluorescence had already been achieved by a digital process since 2014 after the optimization of the D-Sight FLUO 2.0 scanner (Menarini Diagnostics®, Florence, Italy) for capture, matching of the fluorescent and haematoxylin and eosin (H&E) images, and semi-quantitative analysis, substituting an immunofluorescence microscope. At IPATIMUP, only routine cytology is left to be integrated in the digital workflow. The services provided by the pathology laboratory of IPATIMUP do not include, at the moment, autopsies or frozen sections.

We choose the Pannoramic®1000 (P1000) scanner (3DHISTECH Ltd.®, Budapest, Hungary) to obtain WSIs for primary and secondary diagnosis of all slides managed in the laboratory (100%), except for those of cytology, as mentioned above. Cytology slides that needed to undergo second revision in another institution or that were estimated to be consumed by molecular techniques were also scanned.

In July 2019, a P1000 scanner was installed in the center of the main laboratory surrounded by benches where specimen processing takes place. The scanning process, including quality control of the WSIs obtained was performed by trained technicians. All scanned slides were orderly incorporated in the file of the patient for microscopic observation after the functional integration of the scanner software with the laboratory information system (LIS) called SISPAT (JSalgado®, Porto, Portugal).

2.1. Digital Workflow

We describe the processing pipeline with emphasis on the major alterations introduced in the workflow of the pathology laboratory of IPATIMUP. For the successful implementation of these alterations, close interaction between technicians and pathologists was mandatory in order that the measures taken had no impact on the turn-a-round time or quality of the final product. Overall, there was an important investment in space contraction on the main laboratory area, since no important infrastructure interventions were done. The parallel benches were organized according to the flow of the sample, following a Lean approach, and allowing the insertion of a scanner station (Figure 1).

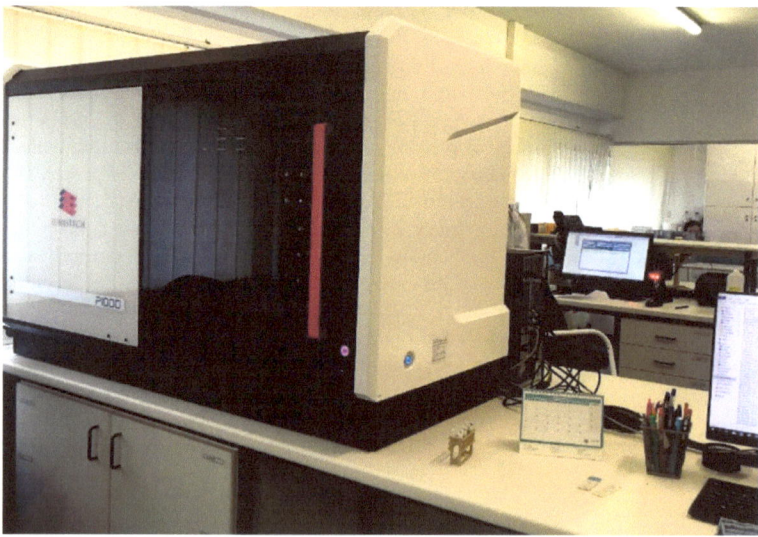

Figure 1. The scanner is located at the heart of the laboratory surrounded by benches where specimens processing takes place.

The scanner station was located in the confluent end of the histology and cytology lines, away from the paraffin-rich area (Figure 2). The location of the scanner within the main laboratorial area enabled a better communication process and fast management of samples. The disadvantages of having the scanner in the main laboratorial area were the increment in environmental noise produced by the instruments and the exposure of the scanner to potential particles produced during the entire process.

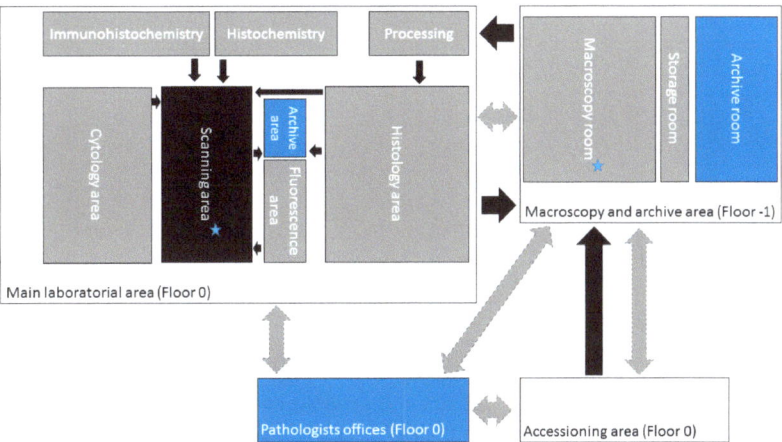

Figure 2. Schematic representation of the laboratory organization. The gray areas represent pre-scanner workstations, the black area represents the scanner workstation, and the blue areas represent the post-scanner segments. The archive area corresponds to a transitory paraffin block archive. The stars sign the bottleneck areas. The black arrows comprehend physical traffic of samples, and the gray arrows represent traffic of digital information.

The same contraction exercise was applied in the management of time. Since the number of technicians was not increased and the scanning process imposed additional time spent on the technical side, an effort was made to reduce lost time, redundant tasks, or uncoordinated efforts, increasing the overall efficacy of the laboratory. Specific goals related to the time for production of stained and unstained full rack slides were established to better manage the occupation of the scanner station.

During the preparation period of the laboratory, and before the scanner acquisition, importantly, we implemented a sample tracking system based on the LIS which facilitated mobile control of time and operator's intervention during the entire process. The tracking system was designed to use QR code readers at each station. Printed QR codes are part of the sample redundant identification in all phases of processing, from when the sample enters the institution until the report is signed out, including the physical and digital archives. This decision required the acquisition of computers or tablets for each workstation.

2.2. Sample Management and Macroscopic Examination

Good quality samples are easy to manage in the laboratory as compared with those with fixation problems that require additional time-consuming procedures to be suitable for diagnosis. To decrease the time required to manage problematic samples and to increase the quality of the image for diagnosis, an educational program was elaborated targeting nurses and physicians and highlighting the importance of controlling pre-analytic conditions. The administrative team was also trained to be able to identify problems with the packaging of samples in order to quickly promote their correct fixation by the technical team. The traffic of labeled samples with QR codes ran from the reception to the macroscopy room in scheduled batches and was performed to reduce people movements while keeping the macroscopy station as busy as possible.

After the QR code labeled samples were transferred to the macroscopy room, they were photographed using MacroPATH (Milestone Medical®, Bergamo, Italy), and fragments were collected to QR code printed cassettes (Figure 3). The photography system and cassette printer were connected with the LIS.

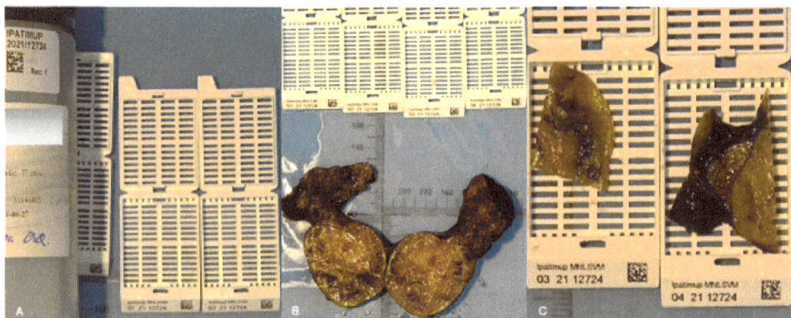

Figure 3. Containers with specimens are labeled with QR codes and photographed at arrival (**A**). Photographic documentation of the specimen is performed (**B**) as well as of the selected fragments inside the respective labeled cassettes (**C**).

The size of the fragments collected was adjusted to the area of the slide that was captured by the scanner, away from the borders. At this station, the cassettes were organized immediately in the processor racks separating the exams associated with the fast scanner (usually small biopsies) from those with a prolonged scanner time (usually large surgical specimens). These two types of exams were kept separated during the subsequent histology processing so they could be managed easily at the scanner workstation. Prioritization of urgent samples was also done at this station.

The inking of specimens was always adjusted. The colors selected to ink surgical margins were those best identified by the scanner, providing a clear image during WSI observation. Cellblocks and breast cancer biopsies (rich in adipose tissue, nearly transparent mainly after immunohistochemical stain) were also inked before processing so that the cores and the pellets of cells were automatically detected by the scanner.

2.3. Processing, Embedding, Cutting, Staining, and Mounting

During the aforementioned steps of specimen handling at the laboratory, traceability and records from each station were kept in the file of the patient at the LIS. Records of reagent changes and equipment performances were kept, granting the identification of causes for poor quality products.

In addition to improving space, time, and sample flow, we organized the histology pipeline into a continuous production of slides to scan. Embedding was now performed according to priorities, taking in consideration that fragments must be placed close to each other and in the center of the paraffin block to decrease the scanner area and avoid placing tissue in the non-scanned limits of the slide.

We improved the cutting station process by introducing updated microtomes that allowed a stable thickness of the tissue for an uneventful image capture. The confirmation of the paraffin block entry at the cutting station with the QR code reader ordered the print of the respective labeled slide, reducing the transcription errors, accelerating the identification, and transferring the QR code ID to the slide that would be read by the scanner.

The staining and mounting process was fully automatic and operated with the Tissue-Tek Prisma® Plus & Tissue-Tek Film® (Sakura®, Nagano, Japan) integrated system, following an optimal protocol with daily reviewed reagents and contaminant controls, to obtain the best and stable staining observed in WSI. The selection of the staining and mounting equipment took into consideration the compatibility of the racks with those of the scanner;

the scanner had been calibrated by the manufacturer according to the coverslip film used to adjust focus distance. Stained and mounted slides were dried in a 60 °C oven for 5 min to guarantee complete drying of the slides.

2.4. Scanning and Quality Control of WSIs

The glass slides were produced in racks, were orderly prioritized, and continuously arrived at the scanner station.

The scanner workstation consisted of a scanner and two computers. One was an Intel® Xeon Gold 5120 @ 2.20 GHz (Intel®, Santa Clara, CA, USA) processor, 96 GB of memory, a 240 GB SSD disk for 64-bit OS, 960 GB SSD for SWAP and a 2TB mechanical disk for local storage that gathered the WSIs, converted them using the 3DHISTECH Slide Converter, and then stored the slides in the 3DHISTECH CaseCenter server located at the building data center. The 3DHISTECH Slide Converter compressed all the WSI files by 80%. The connection to this server was performed by a non-dedicated 1 GB network that served all infrastructure. The CaseCenter server had an Intel® Xeon E3-1270 v6 (Intel®, Santa Clara, CA, USA) @ 3.80 GHz, 24 GB of RAM, 2x 240 GB SSD for 64-bit OS in RAID 1, and a 20TB volume of mechanical disk in RAID5. Through iSCSI, this server connected to the digital archive IBM FlashSystem 5000 with 220TB storage (that can scale up to 960TB to give extra volumes to the server) with distributed 6 RAID disk configuration. Another computer was used for WSI quality control operating in the patient files at the LIS.

At the scanner workstation, slides were transferred from the stainer racks to the scanner racks, according to the manufacturer's instructions. The racks were introduced in the P1000 position that required less movement of the scanner operative arm. After the scanning process using a 20× adapted protocol (0.25 µm pixel size), the WSIs were automatically transferred to the patient's file at the LIS and were available 30 s (average) after capture. Special protocols, such as those used in breast cancer biopsies and bright field in situ hybridization, used a 40× lens.

In the same station, all WSIs were opened by the technician and the WSI quality control process started. In each case, there was a verification of the matching of the identification, matching the number of fragments per slide in the WSI according to the photo of the slide captured by the scanner, and a verification of the focus and staining overall quality. If an irregularity was detected at this verification the technician, assigned for the quality control, recorded it at the LIS and ordered the return to the analytic phase where the error had occurred. In this situation, the original WSI was deleted to be substituted by the correct one. All WSIs used for diagnosis were archived and preserved for future consultation. If the case was ready for review by the pathologist, the technician released the file to enter the WSI in the diagnosis phase. The pathologist's assignment plan was determined daily, prior to the embedding phase.

Slides generated in the setting of complementary techniques, including histochemical stains, immunohistochemical stains, and bright field in situ hybridization were prepared following the aforementioned standards and following specific scanning protocols adjusted for each type of technique. Immunohistochemical slides required, after the washing step, extra dehydration and prolonged diaphanization to avoid drying artifacts and residues in the respective WSIs.

The complimentary technique slides all always included, in addition to the sample, a set of positive and negative controls (2–5 tissue cores) specific for the technique used in the slide (Figure 4). The production of traceable and reliable tissue microarray control sets required the construction of a quality regulated tissue control bank.

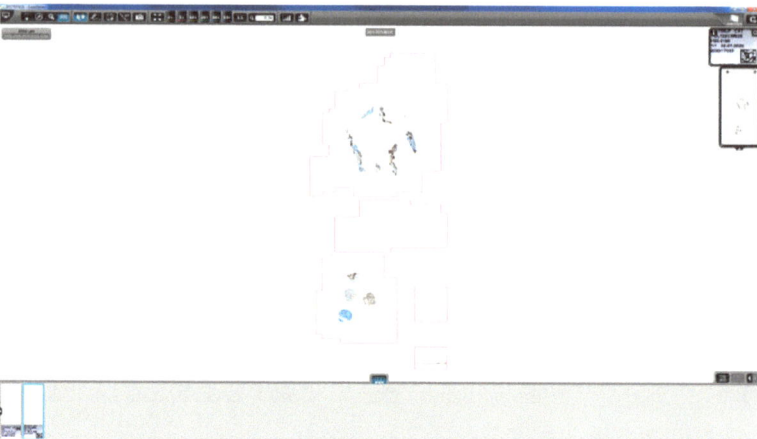

Figure 4. Print screen of a whole slide image representing an immunohistochemistry staining of a specimen together with the set of 5 control tissue microarrays for routine utilization.

2.5. WSI Review and Diagnosis

We targeted the environment at each pathologist's office for modifications, with the purpose of creating comfort/ergonomics for the pathologist who reviewed cases using a monitor. A larger desk with space to accommodate two monitors was installed and organized to allow wide-ranging movements of the mouse for navigation. Light regulation of the environment required the installation of blackout shutters on the windows, to be used on demand.

The workstation of the pathologist included one Dell Precision Tower 3620 equipped with an Intel® Core i7-6700 CPU (Intel®, Santa Clara, CA, USA) @ 3.40 GHz, 8 GB of RAM, ST500DM002-1SB10A ATA Disk with 466 GB and a NVIDIA QuADro M2000 (NVIDIA®, Santa Clara, CA, USA) with 4 GB. This workstation had two monitors one Sharp PN-K322BH (3840 × 2160 resolution in dots—QFHD, 32″) for slide analysis and one smaller monitor for regular tasks, i.e., a Dell (Dell®, Round Rock, TX, USA) P2417H (Full HD, 24″). The computer was connected to the LIS, CaseCenter, CaseViewer, and to other computers in the laboratory by a 1 GB network. Remote access to each workstation was available through a VPN connection that allowed the pathologist to work at a distance whenever it was required.

Management of all the information belonging to a case/patient was performed at the pathologist's workstation using only the LIS, including access to all clinical data, previous and simultaneous exams, and respective WSIs, pre-analytical data, analytical data including macroscopic description and photographs, WSIs of the current case (H&E and complimentary techniques if available), microscopic description and diagnosis templated, codification system, quality evaluation form, and sign out area, in addition to all the relevant information regarding deviations from the regular laboratory workflow.

The validation of the digital WSI observation for clinical use was performed using the CAP guidelines applied to each pathologist [6].

3. Results

The pathology laboratory of IPATIMUP designed a digital transformation of the workflow that started in 2016 with the introduction of pre- and post-scanner modifications. The scanner was installed in July 2019, the software functional integration with the LIS was achieved during October 2019, the quality control program was adapted during November 2019, and the validation for clinical use lasted until July 2020. During this validation process, a hybrid workflow was maintained, providing both glass slides and respective WSIs to the pathologists. Since July 2020, 8 out of 14 pathologists have been receiving WSIs for primary diagnosis instead of glass slides. The remaining 6 pathologists are not using WSIs because they are reviewing only cytology cases ($n = 1$); they are part of the telepathology project that includes mainly tele-macroscopy and is managed by a different source and software ($n = 2$) or they are reporting an average of less than 10 cases per month ($n = 3$). If we consider those pathologists that could use, in fact, WSIs for diagnosis, only 3 out of 11 pathologists were missing (27.3%), representing a percentage of adhesion to WSI of 72.7%. The laboratory activity encompasses about 40,000 paraffin blocks and 60,000 slides per year reflecting the management of nearly 25,000 cases per year. These numbers do not include those cases received from other institutions for second opinion and biomarkers evaluation. The slides produced or arriving from an external source that configure histology, cellblocks, histochemistry, immunohistochemistry, in situ hybridization (both bright and dark field), and direct immunofluorescence are all scanned. Table 1 summarizes the WSI bright field production of the 8 months operating fully digitally (from July 2020 to February 2021).

Table 1. WSI bright field results of the 8 months operating fully digitally.

	Month								
	July 2020	August 2020	September 2020	October 2020	November 2020	December 2020	January 2021	February 2021	Mean Value
Slides scanned (n)	7047	5818	8159	9099	7807	7135	6349	6004	7177
Cases scanned (n)	1688	1335	1814	1871	1697	1307	1290	1361	1545
Cases re-scanned (n; %) (by technique order)	30; 1.8	23; 1.7	31; 1.7	27; 1.4	5; 0.3	1; 0.1	5; 0.4	4; 0.3	16; 1.0
Cases with good image (%) (by pathologist order)	96.3	97.6	99.0	98.9	98.5	99.1	98.5	98.5	98.3
Cases with glass slides requested (%)	2.1	1.6	1.6	2.1	2.0	2.2	3.3	3.8	2.3

The average number of slides scanned per day is 326 with a total of 57,418 slides generated in 8 months.

The reasons for rescanning slides are poor focus or incomplete scanning of the fragments and/or difficulties associated with uneven thickness of the tissue. The most frequent cause of scanner failure is the misprinted QR code, thus, leading to failure to scan sections placed in the lower limits of the slide. The automation of the mounting process with restricted human manipulation of slides (wearing gloves), together with the lack of glass coverslip corners misaligned with the slides, enables clean preparations that are easy to adjust to the scanner racks.

The cases requesting glass slides for diagnosis include those illustrating breast or prostate cancer biopsies presenting suboptimal material for nuclear evaluation, cases suspicious for amyloid deposition with the need of polarized light technique after Congo Red staining and, mostly, intrinsically difficult cases. The preventive maintenance of the scanner (single scanner) that occurred in February (Table 1) justifies the increment in the number of cases needing glass slides during this month. We have no records of slide breakages so far, nor scanner mal functions due to poor handling by the technicians.

The average size of slides and respective time for scanner concerning the type of specimen is summarized in Table 2. Cellblock slides have always two sections, an average of 1400 megabytes in size, and take an average of 100 s to scan. The time to scan a 1.5×1.5 cm tissue sample is 51 s.

Table 2. Average sizes of slides and respective times for scanning concerning the type of specimen.

Type of Preparation		H&E	Histochemistry	Immunohistochemistry	Bright Field In Situ Hybridization
Type of Sample					
Small biopsy	Mean size (megabytes)	242	203	266	4767
	Mean time (seconds)	48	43	52	211
Large specimen	Mean size (megabytes)	1625	2046	1496	9930
	Mean time (seconds)	109	151	101	392

Validation of all types of preparations by each pathologist using the digital pathology model was achieved and approved after over 95% concordance rates (using the microscopic observation at the optical microscope for comparison purposes).

As a result of the measures operated in the workflow, we obtained the following results:

1. A 35% decrease in inadequate samples is recorded after the educational program targeting nurses and physicians to improve the quality of the pre-analytic conditions.
2. Case assignment is facilitated as it is recorded at the LIS.
3. Less than 24 h is needed from when a sample arrives at IPATIMUP until the respective (H&E) WSI is ready to review, allowing the establishment of a 48 h benchmark for turn-a-round time of all exams that do not need complementary techniques.
4. The quality of the laboratory product was not affected by the digital workflow implementation according to the registries in the internal quality control program of the laboratory.
5. The quality of the diagnosis produced in the laboratory was not affected by the digital workflow implementation, according to the results on the external quality control program.
6. During the COVID-19 pandemic lockdown, the pathologists keep working either at home or at the laboratory using WSIs to diagnose and to share cases, and asking for a second opinion using digital tools to annotate diagnostic specific questions. Flexibility in scheduling reviews is facilitated by the remote access; pathologists continued quality control activities at a distance, by observing WSIs for validation of techniques; technicians were able to do the quality control of WSIs for diagnosis at a distance.
7. Consultation of WSIs from previous or simultaneous exams from a patient is facilitated due to easy access to the digital image sparing time in retrieving glass slides from the physical archives.
8. To archive glass slides becomes easier since the slides travel from the scanner station to the physical archives in the proper order.
9. Costs with paper and printing were 25% reduced during the last year due to the transformation of paper records into digital ones, also offering the possibility of an ecological attitude welcomed by the team.
10. Sharing cases with other institutions for secondary observation using a digital link for WSIs of patients in 108 cases/629 slides during the first 6 months represents faster and cheaper communication, which also prevents loss of material and glass slide damage.
11. The digital workflow implementation brought new life to the research initiatives of the laboratory, as we had previously described [7].

4. Discussion

The digital transformation of the pathology laboratory at IPATIMUP is an example of successful implementation of the digital methodology for conducting pathology workflow at the tissue level (including cellblocks) for primary diagnosis. At IPATIMUP, only cytology is left to be integrated into the digital workflow. This is due to the very successful and intense production of smears after fine-needle aspiration that are difficult to manage in the WSI format. The WSIs of smears are time- and storage-consuming and usually do not reproduce the entire slide surface, leaving the limits of the slide left to be captured [8,9].

At IPATIMUP, we record a very low percentage of glass slide utilization (2.3% of cases) and the adoption of the WSI by the majority of pathologists (72.7%), indicating that pathologists trust the new methodology and understand its benefits. Pathologists must not be forced to accept this methodology change since it may compromise their diagnostic performance. The reasons for lack of acceptance may be related to expectations, habits, type of reported exams, and work conditions (speed of refresh, color calibration, and monitor quality) [2,10,11]. To prevent the lack of acceptance at our laboratory, we invested in creating comfort conditions at the office, individual participation in the validation process, laboratory informatic system (LIS)-centered operability, and diagnosis training under the new conditions during the extended hybrid workflow. Maintaining the possibility to revise the glass slides is advised since the sense of "no turning back" is avoided, and also because the reasons that triggered such requests may represent the need to optimize scanning protocols or situations in which technology needs to evolve (such as the use of polarized light for amyloid detection that is only available in some scanners) [3].

The technicians' trust in the digital methodology is also relevant to keep the team motivated, something that is measured by the low volume of rescanning (average 1%) and the high classification attributed to the slides by the pathologists at IPATIMUP (average 98.3% are good). The confidence of the technician in the laborious process of digital transformation may be threatened if a prolonged hybrid workflow is maintained, preventing the immediate collection of the benefits inherent to the new methodology.

The implementation of the abovementioned measures in the pre-scanner process, namely those related to the high performance automatic stainer and coverslipper compatible with the scanner, are those that motivate the low volume of rescanning, as also reported in the literature [1]. Furthermore, the scanner was calibrated by the manufacturer according to the film used in the automatic mounting to adjust focus distance.

The results, herein presented, suggest that the pre- and post-scanner segments of the workflow adaptations are, at least, as important as the choice of the scanner and can be an important cause of implementation failure.

Indirectly, digital transformation stimulates an increment in quality control measures such as the tracking system, improving safety, and stimulating the creation of validation habits and risk-oriented thinking. Specific features of the digital methodology that are related to increased quality and safety include the possibility of rapidly sharing cases for a second opinion at a distance, reducing the distance between people in adverse situations such as those experienced during the COVID-19 pandemic [12], and the possibility of archiving WSIs representative of glass slides requested by other institutions or destroyed by molecular techniques [1].

The time and space contraction measures operated at IPATIMUP, very much inspired in the Lean approach, are mainly without cost, improve workflow efficacy, and are useful for digital and non-digital laboratories. The digital pathology model implemented at IPATIMUP demonstrates that the turn-a-round time can be maintained after the digital transformation with the same amount of technical and medical staff, provided the workflow is carefully optimized. Differently, the overnight scanning process adopted by other laboratories may not be compatible with the preservation of the present turn-a-round time and occurs, in most instances, during an unsupervised period [1]. The adoption of simple measures at IPATIMUP such as mounting with film, drying the slides, and careful transfer of slides between racks, helped to prevent bad functioning of the scanner, loss of time, and additional costs.

Time and resource control measures include the identification of bottleneck stations where samples may accumulate. In our laboratory, the bottleneck stations are those of the macroscopy and scanner. At the macroscopy room, acceleration of the descriptions and documentation could only be achieved by the addition of a new technician, a measure that for now is not yet cost effective. At the scanner station, the benefit of having two scanners with low capacity instead of one with large capacity has been defended by some authors [1] and can benefit the general workflow since this possibility also represents the existence of a backup during malfunctioning or preventive maintenance intervention.

The most frequent reason associated with refusal to implement a digital pathology workflow is cost related [3]. In the digital pathology model implemented at IPATIMUP, the requested acquisitions were distributed in time, with the most relevant being related to the automatic strainer and coverslip, the scanner, and the digital archive. In addition, saving costs were possible due to a reduction in post office trades, as well as prints and paper representing an ecological attitude. In the future, the use of image analysis algorithms and the possibility of operating in a scalable economy, will certainly imbalance the costs.

The digital archive is a hot topic related to digital pathology with both positive and negative opinions about a permanent archive of WSIs [13]. We agree that the smaller the archive the better it is to manage and, in our laboratory, with relatively low volume, we may sustain a privileged position to easily achieve the digital transformation. Again, in line with the simple adopted measures described above, to use validated 20× scanning protocols, the concentration of the fragments at the embedding station, image compression balance, and the substitution of poorly focused WSIs by high quality ones may prevent unnecessary archive consumption.

The model of digital workflow implementation at IPATIMUP demonstrates that careful planning and adoption of simple measures related to time, space, and sample management may be adopted by any pathology laboratory to achieve higher quality and easy digital transformation. Without digital transformation, pathology laboratories will not be able to benefit from the advantages provided by the WSIs, namely the application of computational pathology tools that are transforming the way we integrate molecular pathology and tissue morphology [14].

Author Contributions: C.E. performed the study concept and design, as well as the literature review; J.V. provided acquisition, analysis, and interpretation of data; C.E., J.V., M.C., A.P., S.C., A.C. and R.S. contributed with writing and revision; M.S.-S. contributed with revision of the paper. All authors read and approved the final paper. All authors have read and agreed to the published version of the manuscript.

Funding: This research received no external funding.

Institutional Review Board Statement: The study was conducted according to the guidelines of the Declaration of Helsinki.

Informed Consent Statement: Not applicable.

Data Availability Statement: All data generated or analyzed during this study are included in this published article.

Acknowledgments: The authors thank Filippo Fraggetta for the constructive critics made on the contents of this document.

Conflicts of Interest: The authors declare no potential conflict of interest.

References

1. Fraggetta, F.; Garozzo, S.; Zannoni, G.F.; Pantanowitz, L.; Rossi, E.D. Routine Digital Pathology Workflow: The Catania Experience. *J. Pathol. Inform.* **2017**, *8*, 51. [CrossRef] [PubMed]
2. Retamero, J.A.; Aneiros-Fernandez, J.; Del Moral, R.G. Complete Digital Pathology for Routine Histopathology Diagnosis in a Multicenter Hospital Network. *Arch. Pathol Lab. Med.* **2020**, *144*, 221–228. [CrossRef] [PubMed]
3. Jahn, S.W.; Plass, M.; Moinfar, F. Digital Pathology: Advantages, Limitations and Emerging Perspectives. *J. Clin. Med.* **2020**, *9*, 3697. [CrossRef] [PubMed]
4. Baidoshvili, A.; Bucur, A.; van Leeuwen, J.; van der Laak, J.; Kluin, P.; van Diest, P.J. Evaluating the benefits of digital pathology implementation: Time savings in laboratory logistics. *Histopathology* **2018**, *73*, 784–794. [CrossRef] [PubMed]

5. Ho, J.; Ahlers, S.M.; Stratman, C.; Aridor, O.; Pantanowitz, L.; Fine, J.L.; Kuzmishin, J.A.; Montalto, M.C.; Parwani, A.V. Can digital pathology result in cost savings? A financial projection for digital pathology implementation at a large integrated health care organization. *J. Pathol. Inform.* **2014**, *5*, 33. [CrossRef] [PubMed]
6. Pantanowitz, L.; Sinard, J.H.; Henricks, W.H.; Fatheree, L.A.; Carter, A.B.; Contis, L.; Beckwith, B.A.; Evans, A.J.; Lal, A.; Parwani, A.V.; et al. Validating whole slide imaging for diagnostic purposes in pathology: Guideline from the College of American Pathologists Pathology and Laboratory Quality Center. *Arch. Pathol. Lab. Med.* **2013**, *137*, 1710–1722. [CrossRef] [PubMed]
7. Polonia, A.; Campelos, S.; Ribeiro, A.; Aymore, I.; Pinto, D.; Biskup-Fruzynska, M.; Veiga, R.S.; Canas-Marques, R.; Aresta, G.; Araujo, T.; et al. Artificial Intelligence Improves the Accuracy in Histologic Classification of Breast Lesions. *Am. J. Clin. Pathol.* **2021**, *155*, 527–536. [CrossRef] [PubMed]
8. Hanna, M.G.; Monaco, S.E.; Cuda, J.; Xing, J.; Ahmed, I.; Pantanowitz, L. Comparison of glass slides and various digital-slide modalities for cytopathology screening and interpretation. *Cancer Cytopathol.* **2017**, *125*, 701–709. [CrossRef] [PubMed]
9. Hanna, M.G.; Pantanowitz, L. Why is digital pathology in cytopathology lagging behind surgical pathology? *Cancer Cytopathol.* **2017**, *125*, 519–520. [CrossRef] [PubMed]
10. Jara-Lazaro, A.R.; Thamboo, T.P.; Teh, M.; Tan, P.H. Digital pathology: Exploring its applications in diagnostic surgical pathology practice. *Pathology* **2010**, *42*, 512–518. [CrossRef] [PubMed]
11. Griffin, J.; Treanor, D. Digital pathology in clinical use: Where are we now and what is holding us back? *Histopathology* **2017**, *70*, 134–145. [CrossRef] [PubMed]
12. Williams, B.; Fraggetta, F.; Hanna, M.; Huang, R.; Lennerz, J.; Salgado, R.; Sirintrapun, S.; Pantanowitz, L.; Parwani, A.; Zarella, M.; et al. The future of pathology: What can we learn from the COVID-19 pandemic? *J. Pathol. Inform.* **2020**, *11*, 15. [CrossRef] [PubMed]
13. Huisman, A.; Looijen, A.; van den Brink, S.M.; van Diest, P.J. Creation of a fully digital pathology slide archive by high-volume tissue slide scanning. *Hum. Pathol.* **2010**, *41*, 751–757. [CrossRef] [PubMed]
14. Vickovic, S.; Eraslan, G.; Salmen, F.; Klughammer, J.; Stenbeck, L.; Schapiro, D.; Aijo, T.; Bonneau, R.; Bergenstrahle, L.; Navarro, J.F.; et al. High-definition spatial transcriptomics for in situ tissue profiling. *Nat. Methods* **2019**, *16*, 987–990. [CrossRef] [PubMed]

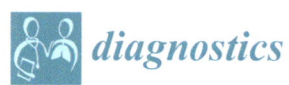

Article

A Survival Guide for the Rapid Transition to a Fully Digital Workflow: The "Caltagirone Example"

Filippo Fraggetta [1,*], Alessandro Caputo [2], Rosa Guglielmino [1], Maria Giovanna Pellegrino [3], Giampaolo Runza [4] and Vincenzo L'Imperio [5]

1. Pathology Unit, ASP Catania, "Gravina" Hospital, 95041 Caltagirone, Italy; rosa.guglielmino@aspct.it
2. Department of Medicine and Surgery, University of Salerno, 84121 Salerno, Italy; alessandro.caputo94@gmail.com
3. Health Care Management Unit, ASP Catania, "Gravina" Hospital, 95041 Caltagirone, Italy; mgiovanna.pellegrino@aspct.it
4. Superintendency Unit, ASP Catania, "Gravina" Hospital, 95041 Caltagirone, Italy; giampaolo.runza@aspct.it
5. Pathology, Department of Medicine and Surgery, ASST Monza, University of Milano-Bicocca, 20900 Monza, Italy; vincenzo.limperio@gmail.com
* Correspondence: filippofra@hotmail.com

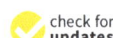

Citation: Fraggetta, F.; Caputo, A.; Guglielmino, R.; Pellegrino, M.G.; Runza, G.; L'Imperio, V. A Survival Guide for the Rapid Transition to a Fully Digital Workflow: The "Caltagirone Example". *Diagnostics* **2021**, *11*, 1916. https://doi.org/10.3390/diagnostics11101916

Academic Editor: Anna Crescenzi

Received: 13 September 2021
Accepted: 13 October 2021
Published: 16 October 2021

Publisher's Note: MDPI stays neutral with regard to jurisdictional claims in published maps and institutional affiliations.

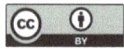

Copyright: © 2021 by the authors. Licensee MDPI, Basel, Switzerland. This article is an open access article distributed under the terms and conditions of the Creative Commons Attribution (CC BY) license (https://creativecommons.org/licenses/by/4.0/).

Abstract: Digital pathology for the routine assessment of cases for primary diagnosis has been implemented by few laboratories worldwide. The Gravina Hospital in Caltagirone (Sicily, Italy), which collects cases from 7 different hospitals distributed in the Catania area, converted the entire workflow to digital starting from 2019. Before the transition, the Caltagirone pathology laboratory was characterized by a non-tracked workflow, based on paper requests, hand-written blocks and slides, as well as manual assembling and delivering of the cases and glass slides to the pathologists. Moreover, the arrangement of the spaces and offices in the department was illogical and under-productive for the linearity of the workflow. For these reasons, an adequate 2D barcode system for tracking purposes, the redistribution of the spaces inside the laboratory and the implementation of the whole-slide imaging (WSI) technology based on a laboratory information system (LIS)-centric approach were adopted as a needed prerequisite to switch to a digital workflow. The adoption of a dedicated connection for transfer of clinical and administrative data between different software and interfaces using an internationally recognised standard (Health Level 7, HL7) in the pathology department further facilitated the transition, helping in the integration of the LIS with WSI scanners. As per previous reports, the components and devices chosen for the pathologists' workstations did not significantly impact on the WSI-based reporting phase in primary histological diagnosis. An analysis of all the steps of this transition has been made retrospectively to provide a useful "handy" guide to lead the digital transition of "analog", non-tracked pathology laboratories following the experience of the Caltagirone pathology department. Following the step-by-step instructions, the implementation of a paperless routine with more standardized and safe processes, the possibility to manage the priority of the cases and to implement artificial intelligence (AI) tools are no more an utopia for every "analog" pathology department.

Keywords: digital pathology; WSI; LIS; 2D-barcode; primary diagnosis

1. Introduction

A progressively increasing number of pathology departments are deploying, or planning to deploy, digital pathology systems for all or part of their diagnostic output [1–5]. Some authors already experienced the full transition to a digital workflow [6], eventually upgrading the scanning procedures at the magnification of 40× and even integrating artificial intelligence (AI) tools for the assessment of specific specimens (e.g., prostate biopsies) in routine practice [7]. Moreover, the employment of a secure virtual private network

(VPN) connection allowed pathologists to work off-site [8], significantly helping during the recent COVID-19 pandemic [9].

However, despite this revolutionary transition, real world data suggest that a fully digital approach to the histological workflow has been implemented in only a minority of pathology laboratories, in Italy as well as worldwide. Several reasons have been advocated to explain what is holding us to the traditional "analog" workflow [10]. Although some major benefits of the digital approach (e.g., safety, quality, efficiency, easy and equal access to expert pathologists/second opinions) are widely recognized, some points may still cause the reluctance of the pathology community, starting from the costs, the lack of validation data and the possible "threat" represented by this kind of implementation for the pathologists [11].

Moreover, the Food and Drug Administration (FDA) approved some but not all of the available scanning systems (Philips and Leica) for digital primary diagnosis. The current lack of approval for all the other devices (e.g., 3DHistech, Hamamatsu, Ventana, etc.) is further slowing down the transition, even in the United States where a widespread implementation of a fully digital workflow using WSI for primary diagnosis is still in progress.

All these components contribute to the generalized skepticism of the pathologists towards these innovative paradigms, at least partly explaining the slow implementation of digital pathology in routine. The adoption of the advocated workflow is further complicated by the substantial lack of an adequate tracking system based on linear or 2D barcodes in the majority of the laboratories, which could represent an obstacle to benefit from all the advantages of the digital transition [11].

Based on the previously reported "Catania" experience at the Cannizzaro Hospital [6], this paper shows the step-by-step process followed by the Pathology department of the Gravina Hospital in Caltagirone (Sicily, Italy) to switch from a non-tracked system to a fully digital workflow in a few months, fully embracing all the benefits of digital pathology.

This may exemplify a simple and efficient transition from the glass slides to the WSI, thanks to the logical implementations made in the Pathology Laboratory of Caltagirone, in which the introduction of slide scanners represents only the last intuitive step of a complete digital workflow. Our experience is reported to the benefit of the numerous laboratories planning or working to implement digital pathology (DP).

2. Materials and Methods

The Gravina Hospital represents the Pathology laboratory hub of the Azienda Sanitaria Provinciale (ASP) of Catania in Sicily (south of Italy), collecting specimens—mainly surgical and bioptic samples—from 7 different hospitals distributed in the Catania area (Figure 1). Starting from 2019, the pathology department of Caltagirone experienced a profound transformation that required about 4 months to switch from a non-tracked, "conventional" pathology workflow to a fully digital approach. Similar to the previous "Catania experience" [6], the entire workflow was converted into a digital one, but introducing some additional "digital" checkpoints through the different steps of the process.

To allow and facilitate this transition, the following implementations were needed:
1. Lean workflow and rearrangement of spaces and offices;
2. Implementation of the information technology infrastructure;
3. Implementation of the tracking system and checkpoint procedures;
4. Implementation of the automation;
5. Implementation of the scanning.

2.1. Lean Workflow and Rearrangement of Spaces and Offices

In order to achieve the best result of the digitization we first solved some logistic problems in the lab. Following the Lean approach philosophy [12,13], the spaces were rearranged: this started from a redistribution of the rooms in a linear manner based on the natural sequence of the sample processing steps. This significantly reduced the personnel and specimen transfers and optimized the working time through the arrangement of similar tasks (e.g., staining and scanning) in the same room and through the creation of inter-room communications. Thanks to a better distribution of the spaces, these modifications freed two rooms that were used to create the molecular section, previously absent in the lab partly due to the inefficient disposition of the spaces.

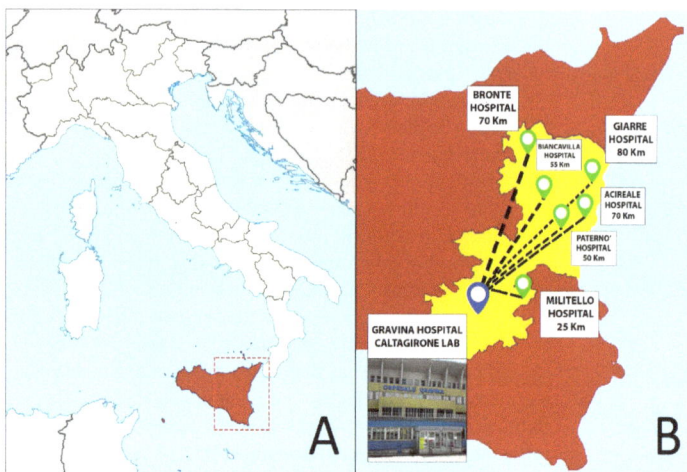

Figure 1. (**A**), Location of the Catania area in Sicily, south of Italy. (**B**), the different hospitals in the Catania territory referring to the Caltagirone pathology laboratory at Gravina Hospital.

2.2. Implementation of the Information Technology Infrastructure

Before the implementation of the digital workflow, a dedicated network as well as servers to store the images and the linked metadata were lacking in the lab. As a consequence, the spaces and offices were not equipped with the necessary access points for the network, and the different instruments used for the analog workflow were not interconnected through the laboratory information system (LIS). Thus, along with the adoption of a Lean approach to the workflow, we implemented the information technology infrastructure: this consisted in the creation of internet access points (network access) based on the position and type of instruments to be connected and a dedicated bandwidth of 100 Mbps.

The entire digital workflow switch has been centered on the implementation of an anatomic pathology LIS (AP-LIS), Pathox (version 13.22.0, Tesi Elettronica e Sistemi Informativi S.P.A., Milan, Italy), allowing the integration of the case/sample information from the accessioning to the reporting phases. The majority of the instruments present in the lab were integrated with the LIS using the 2D barcode system with interface exchanges handled through Health Level 7 (HL7) version 2.5 messages. Based on the previous experience [6], the integration took only a few days of work (including the implementation of the scanner which took 2 days). This is in contrast to other reported similar implementations that required more time to deploy [14,15]. Furthermore, the implementation of a secure VPN connection allowed the pathologists to access and report cases from home (Figure 2).

2.3. Implementation of the Tracking System and Checkpoint Procedures

The Lab lacked a proper tracking system and tissue blocks as well as glass slides were handwritten. Not all the steps of the workflow were appropriately tracked (i.e., gross examination, tissue processing and paraffin-embedding) and different/redundant paper sheets accompanied the workflow from the accessioning to the assembling and delivering of the glass slides for each phase. This "analog" workflow was abandoned in favor of a new paperless 2D-barcode tracking system, fully integrated with the LIS.

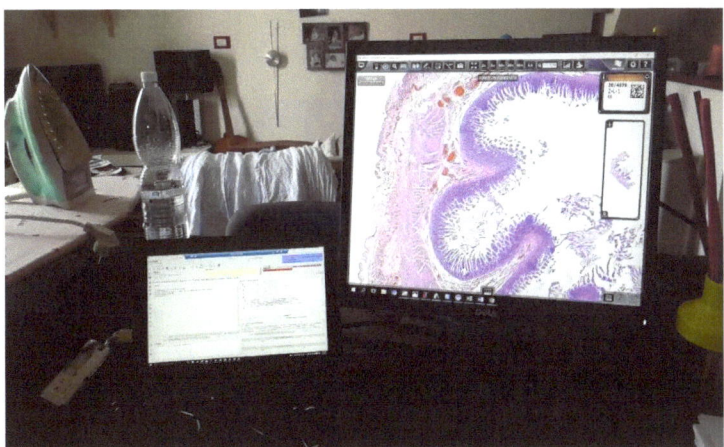

Figure 2. One of the "home-made" working stations used by pathologists for the off-site sign-out and reporting. The smaller monitor (on the left) has a sufficient size and resolution to run the LIS. The right display allows an adequate visualization of the WSI.

This new system was then implemented through the entire workflow, from accessioning to diagnosis. 2D barcodes were preferred to 1D ones because they are less space-demanding (fitting well on the tiny surface of both tissue blocks and glass slides), more easily applicable to the convex surfaces of tissue containers, and generally less prone to scanning issues. Moreover, we introduced laser printers for blocks in order to obtain a permanent mark of the barcode on the surfaces (See Grossing section of the Results). The implementation of the tracking system within the LIS gave us the possibility to monitor safely and efficiently every step of the workflow through the use of dashboards.

2.4. Implementation of the Automation

To promote the automation of the process following the Lean philosophy, some instrumental implementations were introduced in the laboratory, simplifying many laboratory procedures that were previously performed manually and in a repetitive manner (Table 1). All of these achievements were made possible mainly thanks to the HL7 connection and the widespread use of 2D barcodes. However, the prototype of automation was represented by the automatic assembling and delivering of the slides through the use of scanning systems together with the 2D barcode–based archiving of blocks and slides. Finally, the immunohistochemistry instrument (Autostainer Link 48, Agilent, Santa Clara, CA, USA) was completely interconnected with the LIS (Pathox) through the HL7 connection.

2.5. Imaging Technology

Since the main paradigm chosen for the digital workflow switch was based on the LIS-centric philosophy, this allowed a perfect integration of different scanning platforms independently from the vendor, the WSI formats (e.g., .tiff, .svs, .vms, .ndpi) and the provided platform for slides visualization. This change in the paradigm did not force the department to employ a specific scanner device, leading to choose a fast (35 s/slide) and high throughput (60 slides/h) scanner (Pannoramic 250 flash III, 3DHistech, Budapest, Hungary), with a load capacity of 300 slides and good performances with brightfield and darkfield applications. The digitization involved standard hematoxylin and eosin (H&E), special histochemical, immunohistochemical and immunofluorescence slides (for both conventional immunofluorescence and fluorescence in situ hybridization, FISH). For the frozen sections and intraoperative procedures, the Aperio LV1 IVD system (Leica Biosystem, Nussloch, Germany) was employed due to the ability to obtain live images from up to 4 slides with magnification up to $63\times$. Digitizing cytology slides was not undertaken due to the need for Z-stack image acquisition which increases scan time and file size [16]. The scanning system was operated by technicians who were trained to use these devices to support routine daily work. To further optimize the workflow, the scanning station was located in the same room where slides were stained, coverslipped, and prepared for archiviation (Stainer AUS 240, Bio-optica, Milan, Italy; Leica Coverslipper CV5030, Leica Biosystems, Nussloch, Germany). Regular maintenance was performed every month taking into account white/color balance and adjustment of the scanner focus.

Table 1. Automation introduced at every step of the workflow.

Phase	Automation Introduced
Accessioning	Adoption of order entry
	A4 flat scanner to digitize all the paper documents associated with the cases (i.e., endoscopic exams, clinical annotations, etc.)
Grossing	Introduction of a laser block printer at grossing
	Introduction of a camera device to take pictures at the grossing bench Possibility to capture the material in the block
Processing/embedding	Possibility of matching blocks produced at grossing with those sent to processing by using a real-time multi-barcode scanner
Sectioning	Possibility to capture the cut surface of the block for review purposes
	Automated printing of barcodes directly on glass slides rather than on labels
Staining	Automation of requests of histochemical and immunohistochemical stains, which are delivered directly to the stainer
Archiving	Improvement of the archiving of slides and blocks, whose position in the storage trays is random and tracked automatically by barcode scanning

After the scanning process, the slides were automatically assigned to the proper cases and "virtually" delivered to the pathologists [6]. The slides appeared in the "virtual tray" within the LIS and cases with scanning completed for all the slides belonging to them were considered ready to be reported.

Pathologists' workstations were composed of one computer with 2 monitors. Different computer devices have been implemented for the pathologists' workstations (Table 2), with central processor units (CPU) of different generations, different clock speed and vendors (Intel and AMD), random access memory (RAM) with different size (4 and 8 GB) as well as various video cards, mostly integrated.

Table 2. The different computer devices employed in the Caltagirone digital pathology lab for the pathologists' workstations. CPU, central processing unit; RAM, random-access memory; OS, operating system; W10, Windows 10 (Microsoft, Redmond, WA, USA).

CPU	Clock Speed	RAM	OS	Dedicated Video
AMD Ryzen 5Pro 2400 G	3.60 GHz	8 GB	W10 64 bit	none (CPU-integrated)
Intel Core i3-9100	3.60 GHz	8 GB	W10 64 bit	none (CPU-integrated)
Intel Core i7-8700	3.20 GHz	8 GB	W10 64 bit	none (CPU-integrated)
Intel Core i5-4590	3.30 GHz	8 GB	W10 64 bit	none (CPU-integrated)
Intel Core i3-2120	3.30 GHz	4 GB	W10 64 bit	none (CPU-integrated)
Intel Celeron 3865U	1.80 GHz	8 GB	W10 64 bit	none (CPU-integrated)

Two monitors with different roles have been connected to each computer, allowing the simultaneous evaluation of the case-page in the LIS and the respective WSI from different displays. As per manufacturer instructions, the employed LIS required a minimum of 17 inches monitor to run, and the department introduced devices with a range of

17–27 inches. On the other hand, the monitors dedicated to the visualization of the WSI were 24–27 inches in size (Table 3).

Table 3. Specifications of monitors used for WSI visualization.

Manufacturer	Size	Resolution	Type	Refresh Rate (Hz)
Hannstar	23.6 inch	1920 × 1080 pixels	LCD	60
Philips	27 inch	1920 × 1080 pixels	LED	75
Fujitsu	27 inch	2560 × 1440 pixels	LCD	60

WSIs were directly accessed from the AP-LIS. Specifically, a virtual slide tray was created and incorporated within the AP-LIS, as already described [6]. Accessioning of cases and real-time tracking of digital slides occurred directly from the AP-LIS. The creation of a single slide tray within the AP-LIS Pathox, displaying the macroimage (thumbnail) of several slides simultaneously, allowed the incorporation of WSI acquired from the Pannoramic 250 Flash III scanner, with the possibility to connect different scanners from different vendors (by using the image management system of the scanner as a simple middleware) without disrupting the end-user workflow. All images were saved on network-attached storage (96 TB Qnap NAS TVS-EC1280U-SAS-RP) using the dedicated 100 Mbps network connection. All the scanned slides are stored in the server as a digital database of WSIs, allowing a possible retrospective consultation directly from the AP-LIS. The eventual re-scan of a slide resulted in the overwriting of the previously scanned one, so that pathologists always had access to the most recent images. Validation of the WSIs for their use for primary histological diagnosis was made according to the CAP guidelines [17].

3. Results

In 2019, just before the advent of COVID19, the Caltagirone pathology department had a yearly workload of 8182 histological cases with a total of 42,245 corresponding slides. The entire activity of the laboratory has been modified starting from the limitations and issues related to the previous "analog" and non-tracked workflow, following different steps (checkpoints), as reported below. This allowed a complete transition towards a digital pathology approach, leading to the digital primary sign-out of all the cases through WSIs. Before the implementation of the digital workflow, no standard procedures and checkpoints were present along the different steps of sample processing. Addressing these deficiencies was mandatory for the full digital transition, in order to have a more efficient fully tracked and paperless workflow. Here we report the introduced checkpoints at every step of the specimen handling that should be followed to obtain a fully integrated system (Table 4).

3.1. Accessioning

Before: specimens were sent to the Pathology Lab of Caltagirone on specific days from different hospitals, accompanied by a request without an order entry. During the accessioning phase, a progressive number was created along with an additional internal paper (lab sheet), used later on as the working paper for the subsequent phases.

After: the creation of an appropriate checkpoint at this step allowed the laboratory personnel to complete these accessioning tasks in an unbiased way to minimize the risk of errors. To reach this aim we employed a combination of barcode printer and reader, as well as the introduction of a paper flat scanner (A4 format). These technologies helped in the univocal identification of the case/sample/patient from the accessioning phases (through the 2D barcode printer/reader), adopting an order entry that facilitates the tracking system fully integrated with the LIS. The implementation of the order entry gave us the possibility to monitor the upcoming material from the different hospitals. Moreover, the availability of scanned documentation linked to the case allowed the pathologist a rapid consultation of all the sources needed in a paperless way. By introducing these procedures (order entry and possibility to scan all the documents) the accessioning errors dropped from 6.3% to less than 0.5% of the cases, as expected [18,19].

Table 4. Different steps of specimen processing as they are performed before and after the implementation of digital pathology in the laboratory. DP, digital pathology; LIS, laboratory information system; WSI, whole slide image.

	Before DP Implementation	After DP Implementation
Accessioning checkpoint	Paper request with handwritten patient and specimen data	Order entry system, barcode identifying patient, case, and specimen container, information imported from the integrated hospital LIS with digital request (no more transcription errors)
	Manual check for correspondence between request paper and label on the specimen	Progressive number linked to the barcode generated and used for all sorts of assets generated for that case (tracking of the sample through its journey in the laboratory)
	Manual insertion of the case in the AP-LIS or (worse) new internal "working paper" generated to accompany the specimen in the different subsequent phases of the process (lab sheet)	The administrative will take a picture of the container and of the specimen and those photos will be attached to the case file (medico-legal registry)
	-	Documents attached to the specimen are scanned and attached to the case file (relevant information handy)
Grossing checkpoint	The grossing operator (e.g., pathologist) has the working paper (lab sheet) as the only reference to the case	Automatic access to the case by scanning the identification barcode on the sample container
	No pictures of the sample as it is when it arrives at the grossing room are taken.	Photographic documentation of different grossing steps (specimen in the container, during grossing and within the cassettes) guarantees the preservation of the case features and identification
	Manual transcription of macroscopic description of the sample by the pathologist or the assistant technician (dictation/transcription errors)	Direct dictation of the macroscopic description of the sample converted to text through voice recognition functions of the LIS
	Cassettes are labeled manually by the pathologist/technician	Cassettes are printed with the identification code of the sample to be tracked in further workstations
Sectioning checkpoint	The number transcribed by the grossing operator on the block is copied on the slide, possible source of errors	The code printed on the paraffin block may be scanned to open the case file through the integrated LIS preventing transcription errors
	The needed stain for each case is reported on the working paper (lab sheet) or indicated by the color of the cassette	The technician can check how many and which kind of slides are needed for each block directly on the LIS
	The generated slides are manually transcribed by the sectioning technician, no barcode is printed on the slide	For each paraffin block, one or more printed glass slides are generated through a dedicated printer, including the identification code
	After the sectioning phase, the block is archived and no pictures of the cut surface of the block are taken	After sectioning, each paraffin block may be photographed to assess whether all the material emerged on the glass slide/WSI
	The sectioning phase lack strict quality criteria, the presence of artifacts, folding, inappropriate coverslipping does not significantly impair the physical microscope visualization	Sectioning phase should follow high operative standards, reducing the risk of artifacts that can impair the scanning phase

3.2. Grossing

Before: cases were sent to the grossing room with the generated working paper. Here, the sample grossing was performed by a pathologist with the support of a technician and the macroscopic description was handwritten on the lab sheet, with obvious consequent transcription and interpretation errors. Moreover, since no barcodes were used and the cassettes/blocks generated during this phase were handwritten, the risk of possible subsequent errors was further amplified (Figure 3).

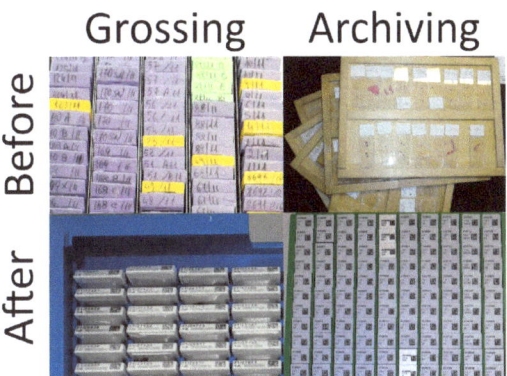

Figure 3. Comparison of some of the principal checkpoints before and after the implementation of DP tools. On the left, during the grossing phase the case identification number was handwritten on every cassette before the introduction of case-specific 2D-barcodes directly generated by the LIS and laser-printed on the cassettes. Similarly, hand-labeled glass slides were randomly returned to the technicians and manually archived (right). The introduction of WSI and scanner next to the staining instrument allowed the direct archiving of physical glass slides using the 2D barcodes.

After: the routine grossing practice radically changed starting from the introduction of a barcode reader, leading to univocal recall of the correct case in the LIS by the pathologist after scanning the specimen container. Moreover, a digital camera (MacroPATHOX, Tesi Elettronica e Sistemi Informativi S.P.A., Milan, Italy) and a BlocDoc (SPOT Imaging, Sterling Heights, MI, USA) instrument were introduced in the room. The camera is used to take pictures of the specimen as it is received (before any sectioning has taken place) and then additional pictures are taken after sectioning to document macroscopic features such as tumor size and depth of infiltration. The pictures can be marked up to identify where the samples have been taken. This allows connecting each block—and thus each WSI— to its original anatomic location. BlocDoc is used to document sampling: each cassette is photographed before its lid is closed [20]. This serves as the reference standard for each block, to be compared with the other pictures which are taken post-processing, post-microtome sectioning, as well as the slide macro and WSI pictures (Figure 4), and is of crucial importance for surgical and bioptic samples alike. This significantly reduced the risk of losing precious material, creating a back-up of information useful to cross-check the adequacy of the specimen in the subsequent steps. Furthermore, inconsistencies can be traced back to the specific moment in which they happened (Figure 4). Finally, the employment of a laser printer allowed the automatic production of barcoded cassettes, further reducing the rate of errors during the subsequent phases (Figure 3).

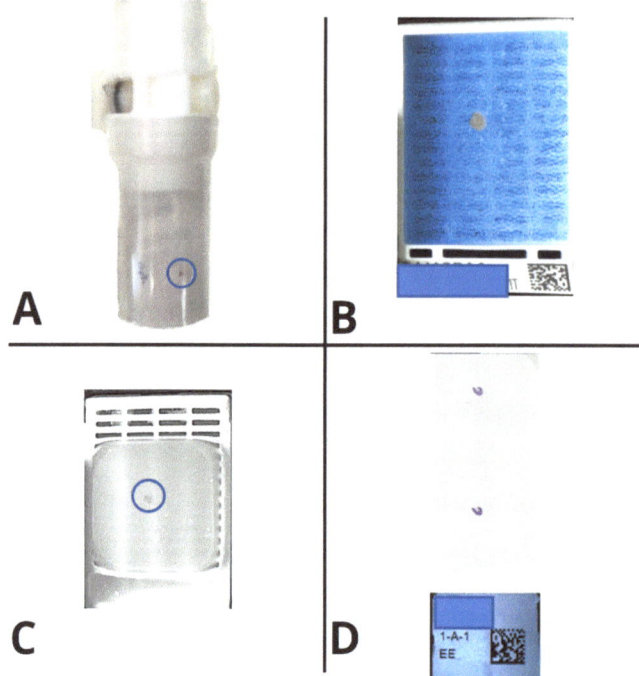

Figure 4. Digital pictures taken at each step of the life of the specimen and respective cassettes fully document the flow of tissue in the lab, allowing global traceability and high-resolution error tracking. (**A**) Specimen container as it is received; (**B**) Cassette at grossing, before closing its lid; (**C**) Surface of the FFPE block after microtome sectioning; (**D**) Macro picture of the glass slide after staining.

3.3. Processing

Before: cassettes containing the specimens were sent to the processing room, manually checking that all the cassettes generated during the grossing step are present in the rack that is going to be processed.

After: through the employment of barcode readers, the entire rack is scanned in one go (with a single picture) before it is processed and a check is performed to verify that all the produced cassettes are submitted to the subsequent phase, thanks to the integration with the LIS. The presence of a dedicated dashboard within the LIS, showing all the blocks produced during the current grossing session, allowed us to implement an automatic check. At the moment there are several instruments in the market capable of reading all the barcodes in short time matching the cassettes present in the rack with those produced at grossing. In the Caltagirone pathology lab, the implementation of MacroPATHOX allowed the scan of all the produced blocks directly from the rack (Figure 5), matching the material sent to the processing room with the specimens produced by the grossing operator.

3.4. Embedding

Before: technicians embedded all the material found inside the cassettes without the possibility to verify the integrity of the specimen after the grossing and processing phases, with the eventual risk of losing material along the workflow especially in cases characterized by multiple small fragments of tissue.

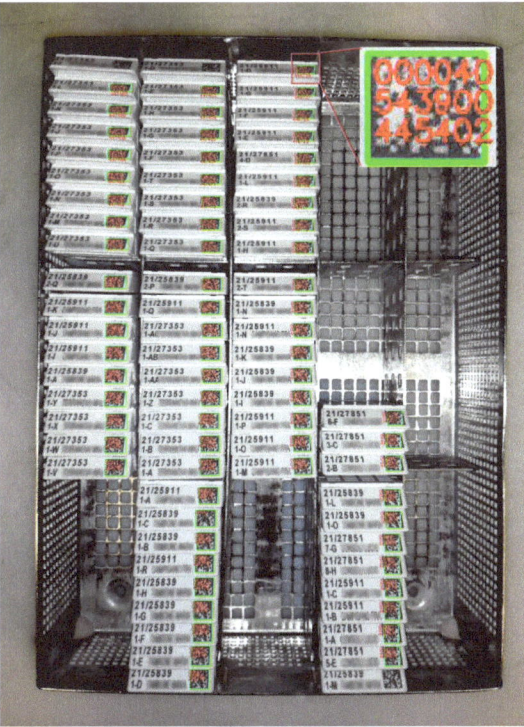

Figure 5. The reading process of barcodes directly from the rack containing the blocks during the processing phase after the digital transition. In the upper right inset the code extracted from the 2D barcode directly in the LIS.

After: this issue has been solved by the availability of photographic documentation obtained in the grossing room, directly available for consultation from the case page in the LIS by the technician who can compare what was submitted by the pathologist with what is actually present in the cassette at the embedding station. Moreover, a correct embedding may prevent poor-quality slides from being produced and thus reduce scanning errors. Large fragments tend to be hydrated and may have a size difficult to be fully captured by the scanner. The adjustment of the size of the sample fragments must start at the grossing station and be verified during embedding. Similarly, well-oriented tissue fragments, levelled and close to each other in the paraffin lead to a better-quality glass slide. Finally, the introduction of BlocDoc to capture the content of cassettes/blocks during the embedding phase can represent a further checkpoint step to control the workflow (Figure 6).

3.5. Sectioning

Before: blocks (handwritten) were consecutively positioned on the microtome, and sections were collected by the technicians with the corresponding number handwritten on the glass slide. However, this again exposes to possible risks of misidentification and case exchange that can be prevented by the introduction of appropriate checkpoints at this step of the workflow.

After: a barcode reader has been added to every microtome station, allowing the technician to automatically identify the case and block directly on the LIS. Moreover, thanks to a slide printer, every operator now has the possibility to produce as many glass slides as required by the specific case without potentially error-prone human interference (i.e., handwriting). Finally, after the sectioning phase the cut surface of the block can be captured with an appropriate device "BlocDoc" (SPOT Imaging, Sterling Heights, Detroit, MI, USA) to obtain archival documentation that can be useful for the pathologist to assess the integrity of the material reported on the final virtual slide (Figure 7). The subsequent manual archival of the blocks is now substituted by a fully automated system based on 2D barcodes (Figure 5).

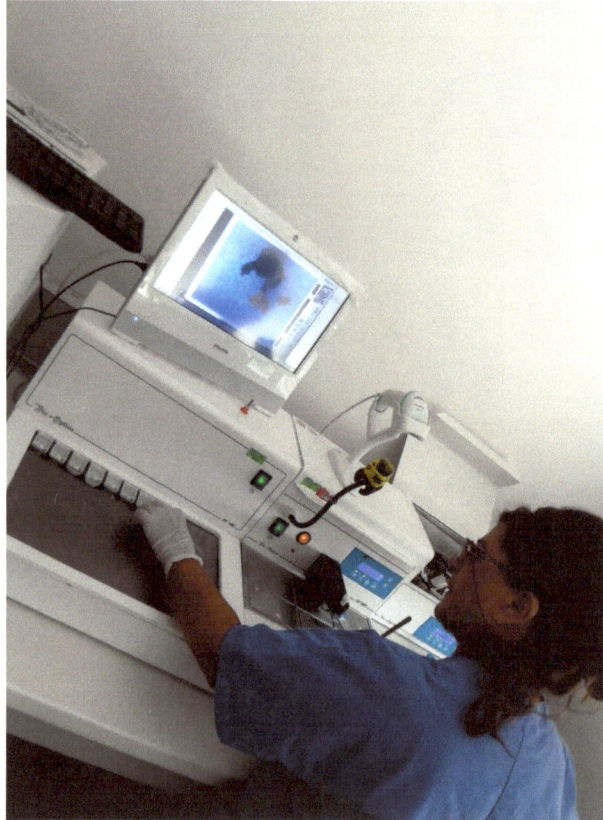

Figure 6. The BlocDoc at the embedding phase.

3.6. Staining and Scanning

Before: the staining was manually performed, glasses were assembled on trays and delivered to the pathologists together with the accompanying lab sheet generated at the accessioning. The employment of differently colored cassettes indicated the need to perform special stains, as well as different types of samples or level of urgency.

After: Slides from the sectioning room are unequivocally and individually identified through the employment of a barcode reader. Thanks to the full LIS integration, this allowed to obtain all the needed information regarding the required stains transmitted by the simple barcode scanning without the need of human interpretation (e.g., of the colors of the cassette). The staining process moved from manual to automated by introduction of an automatic stainer (Bio-Optica, Milan, Italy) and it now follows the highest qualitative standards to minimize interferences with the scanning phase (faint or darker staining, debris/precipitates). For this purpose, the implementation of daily internal controls and/or external quality control can help in the assessment of the quality of stained slides [21]. After air-drying, stained and coverslipped glass slides are loaded into scanner slide racks and scanned. Up to 300 slides can be loaded at a time; the scanner can operate continuously and more racks can be loaded while it is running. Since the workflow was organized in the production of small batches in order to obtain a continuous workflow, the scanner was loaded with glass slides just a few hours after staining (as soon as they were dry) with a limited use of the overnight batch scanning session. Implementation of continuous workflow within the laboratory (i.e., cutting, staining, and then immediate scanning before signout activity) allowed the laboratory to achieve complete slide creation and digitization of all the produced slides within the same day. We observed a scan failure rate of approximately 0.5%, mostly due to problems in the recognition of the 2D barcode printed on the slide, and occasionally due to network connectivity problems.

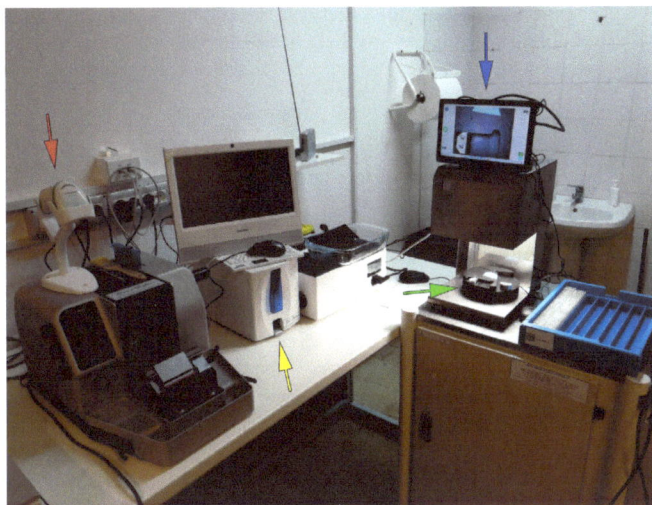

Figure 7. An example of a sectioning station. The technician can identify the block through a barcode reader (red arrow), entering the LIS page of the case and printing the related glass slides with a laser printer (yellow arrow). After sectioning, the technician can directly scan the cut surface positioning the block on the dedicated space in the BlocDoc instrument (green arrow), with the possibility to assess the preview of the obtained image (blue arrow).

3.7. Final Reporting and WSI Viewing

Before: pathologists assessed glass slides using a microscope. The final report was not written directly into the LIS but manually transcribed on the lab sheet originally generated at accessioning. The further requirements for the diagnosis (e.g., special stains, immunohistochemistry, additional recuts) were handwritten and personally delivered by the technicians through the creation of a new internal lab sheet. Since no administrative personnel was available, all the information reported on the lab sheets were personally typed inside the former LIS at the end of the day. The slides used to render the diagnoses were randomly returned to the technicians to be archived (Figure 3).

After: Today, the AP-LIS digitally presents a work list to the pathologist, as cases ready to be reported, urgent cases, cases waiting for additional cuts or additional staining, with clear indication of the presence of digital assets and/or pending status. Pathologists can then access each case from the work list and can open the respective virtual slides shown in the virtual tray with a double-click. WSIs appear on the dedicated monitor and are viewed using the original scanner viewing software. Moreover, the AP-LIS allows to make a direct and quick comparison with the gross specimen embedded in the paraffin block, thanks to the availability of BlocDoc (SPOT Imaging, Sterling Heights, Detroit, MI, USA) scans readily obtainable with a double-click on the tissue block entry in the "virtual tray".

Documents (digitized by the A4 flat scanner at the accessioning), and macroscopic images taken at the grossing were all available with a simple click. This allows fine-grained error tracking and global traceability. For example, if a fragment is missing in the WSI, the pathologist can examine the request form and pictures of each stage of the tissue processing (Figure 4) to identify exactly what went wrong. For example, the fragment might be present on the slide but missed by the scanner's tissue finder, or it may be embedded deep in the tissue block and require further sectioning to be analyzed. It may have been lost during processing, or it may have been missed at the grossing station, or it may not have been sent to the pathology lab at all (Figure 4). The pathologist can clearly identify what went wrong, when and where, without ever leaving his desk. Moreover, the final diagnosis could be rendered using the traditional narrative style or according to a well-defined synoptic report, optionally using guided checklists. A selection of images (gross or microscopic) can be included in the final report for clarity, directly from the LIS.

3.8. Archiving and Retrieval of Tissue Blocks

Before: After microtome sectioning, (handwritten) tissue blocks were manually and painstakingly reordered and archived consecutively by case number.

Retrieval of a block entailed identifying the correct drawer (by case number), then searching for the position in the drawer where the block should be, and hoping to find it there. In case of missing blocks (archival errors due to misreading of the handwritten label, or blocks retrieved and never re-archived) there was no way to know where the block was, who took it, or where it was last seen. This process was lengthy and error-prone. Frequently, the glass slides were delivered to the pathologists before the respective tissue blocks had been archived. If the pathologist requested a special stain, a painstaking search for the block in the archive as well as in the sectioning room would ensue, adding friction and delays.

After: After microtome sectioning, each block is immediately stored in a random spot in a dedicated rack, barcode facing up. At the end of the sectioning session, the rack is photographed by a dedicated scanner which, thanks to its integration with the LIS, automatically marks each block as archived and logs the rack number and the coordinates within the rack, as well as the operator, date, and time.

Retrieval is fully automated and computer-guided. The operator who wants to retrieve a block is guided by a handheld personal digital assistant (PDA) to the correct rack, and then to the position within the rack where he will find the block. Upon withdrawal of the block, the action is logged and timestamped, and the operator is responsible for re-archival of the block. If the block is not in the archive (e.g., being recut for additional stains), the system will indicate who has taken the block and is responsible for its rearchival.

3.9. Archiving and Retrieval of Glass Slides

Before: After staining, coverslipping and air-drying, the technician was responsible for assembly and delivery of the case to the pathologist. Only after rendering the diagnosis, the slides were collected by the technician who had to regroup them and archive them manually.

After: After staining, coverslipping and air-drying, the slides are placed in the scanner racks with no particular attention to order. After scanning, virtual slides are stored in a dedicated database with a storage capability of 96 TB, and glass slides are archived in a dedicated rack in a random order, in a manner similar to blocks. The rack is then scanned and archived. The LIS receives data about each slide (rack number, position within the rack, as well as date and time of the archival and responsible operator).

Retrieval is fully automated and computer-guided, similar to tissue blocks.

3.10. Intraoperative Diagnosis Using Hybrid Instrument

In the Caltagirone example, a particular hybrid instrument (Leica LV1, Leica Biosystem, Nussloch, Germany) was chosen for its better performance in the live streaming of frozen-section slides and was located in the same room where the intraoperative procedures were performed (grossing room). This is in line with the lean redistribution of the spaces and offices which had been performed before the fully digital instrumentation was installed in the lab, thus logically allocating the scanning tools next to the staining facility.

3.11. Molecular Pathology and Fluorescence

The rearrangement of the spaces and offices allowed the creation of an entire section of the laboratory dedicated to molecular pathology, previously absent in the department, introducing instrumentation for next-generation sequencing as well as for the "classic" genetic tests, such as real time PCR and FISH. The results of these exams were directly integrated in the case-page of the LIS, allowing the association of the standard histopathology report with the molecular characterization. Finally, the introduction of a scanner with optimal performances in darkfield applications (e.g., immunofluorescence), allowed the digitization of FISH samples that were directly associated to the case as any other WSI.

3.12. Computer-Aided Diagnosis (CAD) and Artificial Intelligence (AI) Tools

The deployment of the digital workflow gave the Caltagirone lab the opportunity to open the door to the third revolution in pathology, after the advent of IHC and genetics [22] through the introduction of artificial intelligence (AI) algorithms to aid the routine diagnostic assessment of cases. Although in a "futuristic" perspective some authors imagined a fully digital department in which all the cases/slides are presented to the pathologists after a first check performed by the AI algorithms, this has already been implemented in a first experience by one of the authors (FF) [6] and is now in the Caltagirone example an actual reality with a better concordance of diagnosis among pathologists when the AI tool Inify (Inify AI tool for prostate, Contextvision, Stockholm, Sweden) was used (92% vs. 98% concordance, personal data).

4. Discussion

In 2019 the Pathology department of Gravina Hospital in Caltagirone (Sicily, Italy) decided to start using digital slides for routine surgical pathology practice. The intent was to digitize all the histopathology glass slides, borrowing from the previous successful experience of Catania [6]. In this further example the digitization process was not merely limited to the "classic" paraffin block-derived slides (e.g., H&E, histochemical and immunohistochemical stains), extending the application to the fluorescence and frozen sections for intraoperative assessment as well. In the previous Catania experience the frozen sections were excluded from the scanning process due to logistic reasons and technical problems. To solve these issues, in the Caltagirone example a particular hybrid instrument (Leica LV1, Leica Biosystem, Nussloch, Germany) was chosen for its better performances in the live streaming of frozen slides and was located in the same room where the intraoperative procedures were performed (grossing room). This is in line with a lean redistribution of the spaces and offices which has been performed before the full digital instrumentation was installed in the lab, helping in the logical location of the scanning tools next to the staining facility.

As suggested by the guidelines [17], a specific period of time was dedicated to validate the WSI as a substitute for the glass slides. The digital pathology system was deployed primarily to support clinical diagnostic work. Additionally, the implementation of this system allowed the access to WSIs directly from the LIS even during multidisciplinary team meetings or tumor boards [23]. The ability to work remotely was also made possible by the implementation of a secure VPN connection.

The required training is far less than one might imagine. With computer-literate staff, training to use a new tool or machine does not take more than a short tutorial session (a few minutes to a few hours, depending on the tool) and 2–5 days to get used to it. Even for the most daunting things (e.g. the scanner, the LIS), complexity stems from the array of functions and settings, and not from the basic, everyday usage, which is surprisingly simple. The Caltagirone pathologists, as well as two of the authors (VL and AC) could proficiently load the scanner and launch a scanning job after a few minutes' training. Similarly, they could confidently use the LIS for all the everyday functions on day two.

There is no dedicated group of individuals for scanning, image storage and digital infrastructure management. Each technician and each pathologist is taught how to perform basic tasks (e.g., loading, launching, and unloading the scanner) and is expected to be able to perform them.Despite the absence of pathology residents and trainees due to the non-academic nature of the Gravina Hospital, the digital transition allowed us to share anecdotal and didactic cases with young pathologists belonging to different residency programs in the Italian territory. This aspect stresses the invaluable educational role of digital pathology [24,25], especially during the recent COVID19 pandemic [26].

However, to fully benefit from the advantages of the digital transition, the process should follow a strict optimization of the resources, namely time, space, people and instruments, creating the conditions for increased efficiency and consequently decreased costs. Just like digital pathology is only incidentally about the slide scanner, the digital transition is only secondarily a matter of instruments. The transition must start from a strong leadership moving the entire group, motivating all the people to be game-changers. The transition then goes through the people, changes mindsets, workflows, and finally converges on new instruments. The Lean approach is an example of a strategy that can facilitate the management of the staff for the maintenance of turn-around time, starting from the most appropriate arrangement of the space which allows a more linear workflow, the reduction of disorganized sample traffic and thus the realization of a less time-consuming diagnostic process. Although different guidelines have been dedicated to describe the different steps needed for the digital transition [17,27], they mainly focused on the validation of the WSI tool without additional recommendations for the optimization of the pre-analytical steps. As clearly shown by the Caltagirone example, the implementation of digital pathology cannot be performed without a solid base consisting in a fully tracked anatomic pathology workflow (e.g., using the order entry and 2D-barcodes), the adoption of the Lean approach (e.g., through the employment of different automation instruments) and a fully integrated system with the AP-LIS (Figure 8). This triad further allows the interoperability of the different devices employed in the laboratory, independently from the vendor or the software interface adopted by every specific instrument, as demonstrated by the implementation of a fast and high throughput scanner without any compatibility problem. Moreover, the customization of the LIS led to the association of WSI deriving from different devices in the same slide tray, demonstrating the high versatility of this approach.

We are currently working to validate WSI in gynecological liquid-based cytology (LBC) using a Pannoramic P1000 scanner (3DHistech). Recently, new instruments dedicated to digitizing the LBC have appeared in the market, with the possibility to run AI tools to support diagnosis. Even when cytology slides were examined using a conventional light microscope, in spite of the absence of the "final" part of the digital transition (the WSI), numerous improvements had spilled over to the workflow of cytology cases. For example, these cases are fully tracked by the LIS (i.e. no paper worksheets) and benefit from the linearity, efficiency, and order of the lab.

Another crucial point that should be addressed before the digital transition is represented by the need of a dedicated, high speed network in the anatomic pathology laboratory (100 Mbps in the Caltagirone example), to prevent possible network issues that can potentially impair each automated phase of the process, from accessioning to sign-out [28]. Moreover, the availability of a dedicated storage system with an adequate capacity to allow the archiving of WSI is of paramount importance. In the present experience, a database of 96 TB has been employed, without a significant impact on the overall costs of the digital transition. Recently, more advanced solutions have been developed. For example, using the RAID 6 technology (redundant array of independent disks, level 6), one can implement a local storage solution with redundancy and back-ups at much lower costs than similar cloud-based solutions (approximately 10,000.00 € for 100 TB).

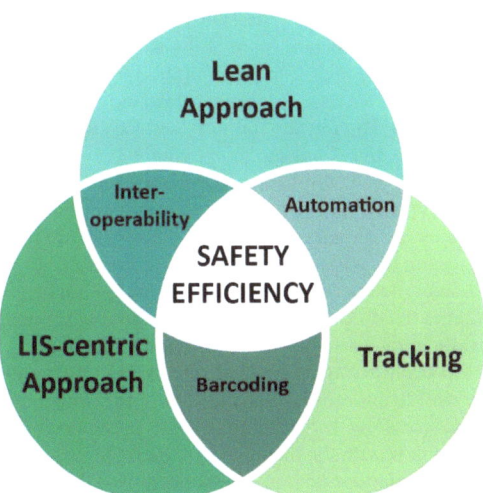

Figure 8. The importance and relationship of the main points required for the development of a reliable, sustainable and safe digital pathology workflow.

For the pathologists' workstation requirements, some guidelines proposed the minimum prerequisites that the computers and monitors should have to be employed in the WSI visualization for primary diagnosis [29]. Despite these recommendations, different subsequent reports demonstrated the feasibility of digital sign-out of the cases (even in off-site settings) independently from the workstation solution chosen by each pathologist [30] and with a wide variety of combination of CPUs (1.3–3.2 GHz), monitors (13.3 to 25 in) and browsers employed [31]. As a further demonstration of the relatively low technological requirements for digital sign-out, in Caltagirone the introduction of workstations with different technical specifications did not significantly impact on the final quality of the WSIs as well as on the end-user experience. This was valid for home working as well, thanks to the secure VPN connection. In this case home computers and non-medical-grade devices were used, without significant impact on the final histological diagnosis. Remote working for pathologists is still a young and underdeveloped concept, but the COVID pandemic helped boost its adoption. During the lockdowns, more than half of the cases were signed out remotely, effectively reducing on-site work to the bare minimum (i.e., grossing, intraoperative exams, and cytology). Incommensurable individual and social risks were avoided thanks to remote work.

The implementation of a digital workflow contributes to increase the efficiency and safety of the different processing phases, through the introduction of specific checkpoints at every step, allowing a more adequate quality control from the accessioning to the final reporting (Figure 4). In the present experience, only a minority of slides had scanning issues, most commonly due to focus problems or in the tissue finding algorithm. For example, abundant white adipose tissue (as can be seen in lipomas) can sometimes be ignored by the tissue finder, or some parts of the slide might be out of focus. Some authors advocate for a routine check of all WSIs by the technician before delivery. In our experience, these errors are rare (<5%), often affect very small parts of the slide, and rarely cause diagnostic problems. For these reasons, assigning the manual check of each WSI scan to the technicians would lead to a significant time-consuming process for less than 5% of rescan. As an alternative solution, in the proposed workflow the pathologists can eventually order, if needed, a rescan directly from the LIS (as it would happen for an additional stain or ancillary tests). Efforts are underway to automate this quality check phase [17–19]. Furthermore, tissue coverage can be checked by the pathologist by comparing the WSI to the slide macro image. In this setting, the recent introduction of a specific instrument, namely BlocDoc, for the detection of tissue inconsistencies, further allowed to increase the accuracy of the technicians' and pathologists' work. It has been estimated that the previous documentation time for the comparison of the physical glass slides and respective tissue blocks took around minutes or even hours for the pathologists and technicians. The introduction of BlocDoc allowed a significant reduction of the time required for this task thanks to the possibility of visualizing the tissue block scans directly from the pathologists' workstations rather than having to manually search and retrieve the tissue blocks themselves from the archive. The average turnaround time is significantly shortened by the digital transition. While apparently more time is required for each case (e.g., scanning the slides before delivering them generates a small delay compared with direct delivery to the pathologist), this is more than balanced by the savings in hands-on time (that is freed up for other tasks) and by the reduction of mistakes, variability and uncertainty in the tissue processing steps.

The completely agnostic approach to the digital pathology workflow is another important point to underline. We believe this is a strong point of our approach to implement the digital workflow. Interoperability is of paramount importance when implementing a digital workflow with the possibility to use WSI for primary histological diagnosis. Thanks to the use of a standard communication approach (i.e., HL7 communication standard) it will be possible not only to interface different machines (different printers for slides, blocks, labels, stainers, immunostainers, etc.) to the LIS, but also to integrate different scanners from different vendors.

The interoperability, together with the lean approach, gives to the path lab the possibility to implement the digital workflow in a very smooth way, without being tied to a single vendor. This is also in line with the possibility of a dynamic implementation of the automation or other things.

The dramatic changes of the Anatomic Pathology in Caltagirone significantly impacted even on the structural disposition of the instruments and offices. This eventually allowed us to re-allocate some spaces to new applications (e.g., obtaining the molecular pathology section previously absent in the lab), as well as significantly reducing the transfer of material and personnel around the laboratory, resulting in time- and cost-effectiveness.

This is further stressed by the relatively low impact of the different novelties introduced (e.g., laboratory reorganization, LIS, slide scanners, dedicated computers/screens, software, storage system. trained personnel) on the overall costs of the department. In Italy, it is customary to rent rather than buy instruments, so for example an expensive slide scanner impacts on the lab balance for only approximately 5000 €/month. The costs of storage have been discussed earlier, and regarding computers, we show that mid-level computers with ordinary monitors (500–600€ total) are adequate for WSI viewing and LIS operations.

Skepticism of technicians towards DP is often cited as a problem to overcome. We found that some features of the new workload are actually preferred by the technicians, if compared to the old workflow. Examples include having 2D barcodes printed directly onto blocks and slides with no need of handwriting, digitizing glass slides by simply loading a scanner with no need to assemble and deliver them, and archiving blocks and glass slides by using computers instead of wasting time to put everything in numerical order. This also demonstrates that the digital workflow corresponds to a decrease in workload for the technicians which is in contrast with the idea of additional workload.

Finally, the adoption of computer-aided diagnostic and artificial-intelligence tools is allowing the construction of a digital hub based in Caltagirone ("House of the Science") that will coordinate the widest renal pathology network in Italy, collecting cases from an already established nephropathology service in the North of the country that migrated all the routine renal biopsy diagnoses to WSI in 2014 [32]. This will further guarantee an equal access to the best diagnostic renal pathology services without the need to move patients, glass slides or paraffin blocks around Italy, additionally constructing a repository of non-neoplastic renal diseases that can serve as an educational atlas as well as a research database.

5. Conclusions

Based on the previous "Catania experience", the implementation of a fully digital workflow in the Gravina Hospital of Caltagirone was possible and easy to achieve in about 4 months. Following the step-by-step instructions, the implementation of a paperless routine with more standardized and safe processes, the possibility to manage the priority of the cases and to implement artificial intelligence (AI)-tools are no more an utopia for every "analogic" pathology department. Digitization of the slides is only the last step of the "digital workflow" that aims to achieve safety and efficiency for pathologists and patients. Our hope and vision is that ALL labs will switch to this digital workflow believing that this will become the standard of care in pathology, for a matter of ethics more than economics.

Author Contributions: F.F. performed study concept and design; V.L. and A.C. performed development of methodology and writing, review and revision of the paper; R.G. provided acquisition, analysis and interpretation of data; M.G.P. and G.R. provided technical and material support. All authors read and approved the final paper. All authors have read and agreed to the published version of the manuscript.

Funding: This research received no external funding.

Institutional Review Board Statement: Not applicable.

Informed Consent Statement: Not applicable.

Data Availability Statement: All data generated or analyzed during this study are included in the article.

Conflicts of Interest: Filippo Fraggetta is one of the inventors of "Sample imaging and imagery archiving for imagery comparison Merlo, P.T. et al. US patent 16/688/613 2020".

References

1. Thorstenson, S.; Molin, J.; Lundström, C. Implementation of Large-Scale Routine Diagnostics Using Whole Slide Imaging in Sweden: Digital Pathology Experiences 2006–2013. *J. Pathol. Inform.* **2014**, *5*, 14.
2. Stathonikos, N.; Veta, M.; Huisman, A.; van Diest, P.J. Going Fully Digital: Perspective of a Dutch Academic Pathology Lab. *J. Pathol. Inform.* **2013**, *4*, 15. [CrossRef] [PubMed]
3. Fraggetta, F.; Pantanowitz, L. Going Fully Digital: Utopia or Reality? *Pathological* **2018**, *110*, 1–2.
4. Al-Janabi, S.; Huisman, A.; Nap, M.; Clarijs, R.; van Diest, P.J. Whole Slide Images as a Platform for Initial Diagnostics in Histopathology in a Medium-Sized Routine Laboratory. *J. Clin. Pathol.* **2012**, *65*, 1107–1111. [CrossRef]
5. Snead, D.R.J.; Tsang, Y.-W.; Meskiri, A.; Kimani, P.K.; Crossman, R.; Rajpoot, N.M.; Blessing, E.; Chen, K.; Gopalakrishnan, K.; Matthews, P.; et al. Validation of Digital Pathology Imaging for Primary Histopathological Diagnosis. *Histopathology* **2016**, *68*, 1063–1072. [CrossRef]
6. Fraggetta, F.; Garozzo, S.; Zannoni, G.F.; Pantanowitz, L.; Rossi, E.D. Routine Digital Pathology Workflow: The Catania Experience. *J. Pathol. Inform.* **2017**, *8*, 51. [PubMed]
7. Fraggetta, F. Clinical-Grade Computational Pathology: Alea Iacta Est. *J. Pathol. Inform.* **2019**, *10*, 38. [CrossRef] [PubMed]
8. Williams, B.J.; Brettle, D.; Aslam, M.; Barrett, P.; Bryson, G.; Cross, S.; Snead, D.; Verrill, C.; Clarke, E.; Wright, A.; et al. Guidance for Remote Reporting of Digital Pathology Slides During Periods of Exceptional Service Pressure: An Emergency Response from the UK Royal College of Pathologists. *J. Pathol. Inform.* **2020**, *11*, 12. [CrossRef] [PubMed]
9. Browning, L.; Fryer, E.; Roskell, D.; White, K.; Colling, R.; Rittscher, J.; Verrill, C. Role of Digital Pathology in Diagnostic Histopathology in the Response to COVID-19: Results from a Survey of Experience in a UK Tertiary Referral Hospital. *J. Clin. Pathol.* **2021**, *74*, 129–132. [CrossRef]
10. Griffin, J.; Treanor, D. Digital Pathology in Clinical Use: Where Are We Now and What Is Holding Us Back? *Histopathology* **2017**, *70*, 134–145. [CrossRef]
11. Hanna, M.G.; Pantanowitz, L. Bar Coding and Tracking in Pathology. *Clin. Lab. Med.* **2016**, *36*, 13–30. [CrossRef]
12. Ho, J.; Kuzmishin, J.; Montalto, M.; Pantanowitz, L.; Parwani, A.; Stratman, C.; Ahlers, S.; Aridor, O.; Fine, J. Can Digital Pathology Result in Cost Savings? A Financial Projection for Digital Pathology Implementation at a Large Integrated Health Care Organization. *J. Pathol. Inform.* **2014**, *5*, 33. [CrossRef] [PubMed]
13. Hartman, D.J.; Pantanowitz, L.; McHugh, J.S.; Piccoli, A.L.; OLeary, M.J.; Lauro, G.R. Enterprise Implementation of Digital Pathology: Feasibility, Challenges, and Opportunities. *J. Digit. Imaging* **2017**, *30*, 555–560. [CrossRef]

14. Isaacs, M.; Lennerz, J.K.; Yates, S.; Clermont, W.; Rossi, J.; Pfeifer, J.D. Implementation of Whole Slide Imaging in Surgical Pathology: A Value Added Approach. *J. Pathol. Inform.* **2011**, *2*, 39. [PubMed]
15. Pantanowitz, L.; Guo, H.; Birsa, J.; Farahani, N.; Hartman, D.; Piccoli, A.; O'Leary, M.; McHugh, J.; Nyman, M.; Stratman, C.; et al. Digital Pathology and Anatomic Pathology Laboratory Information System Integration to Support Digital Pathology Sign-Out. *J. Pathol. Inform.* **2016**, *7*, 23. [CrossRef]
16. Hanna, M.G.; Monaco, S.E.; Cuda, J.; Xing, J.; Ahmed, I.; Pantanowitz, L. Comparison of Glass Slides and Various Digital-Slide Modalities for Cytopathology Screening and Interpretation. *Cancer Cytopathol.* **2017**, *125*, 701–709. [CrossRef]
17. Pantanowitz, L.; Sinard, J.H.; Henricks, W.H.; Fatheree, L.A.; Carter, A.B.; Contis, L.; Beckwith, B.A.; Evans, A.J.; Lal, A.; Parwani, A.V.; et al. Validating Whole Slide Imaging for Diagnostic Purposes in Pathology: Guideline from the College of American Pathologists Pathology and Laboratory Quality Center. *Arch. Pathol. Lab. Med.* **2013**, *137*, 1710–1722. [CrossRef] [PubMed]
18. Nakhleh, R.E.; Zarbo, R.J. Surgical Pathology Specimen Identification and Accessioning: A College of American Pathologists Q-Probes Study of 1 004 115 Cases from 417 Institutions. *Arch. Pathol. Lab. Med.* **1996**, *120*, 227–233. [PubMed]
19. Smith, M.L.; Wilkerson, T.; Grzybicki, D.M.; Raab, S.S. The Effect of a Lean Quality Improvement Implementation Program on Surgical Pathology Specimen Accessioning and Gross Preparation Error Frequency. *Am. J. Clin. Pathol.* **2012**, *138*, 367–373. [CrossRef] [PubMed]
20. L'Imperio, V.; Gibilisco, F.; Fraggetta, F. What Is Essential Is (no More) Invisible to the Eyes: The Introduction of Blocdoc in the Digital Pathology Workflow. *J. Pathol. Inform.* **2021**, *12*, 32.
21. Janowczyk, A.; Zuo, R.; Gilmore, H.; Feldman, M.; Madabhushi, A. HistoQC: An Open-Source Quality Control Tool for Digital Pathology Slides. *JCO Clin. Cancer Inform.* **2019**, *3*, 1–7. [CrossRef]
22. Salto-Tellez, M.; Maxwell, P.; Hamilton, P. Artificial Intelligence-the Third Revolution in Pathology. *Histopathology* **2019**, *74*, 372–376. [CrossRef]
23. Nofech-Mozes, S.; Jorden, T. Integration of Digital Pathology in Multidisciplinary Breast Site Group Rounds. *Diagn. Histopathol.* **2014**, *20*, 470–474. [CrossRef]
24. Boyce, B. Whole Slide Imaging: Uses and Limitations for Surgical Pathology and Teaching. *Biotech. Histochem.* **2015**, *90*, 321–330. [CrossRef]
25. Cheng, C.L.; Azhar, R.; Sng, S.H.A.; Chua, Y.Q.; Hwang, J.S.G.; Chin, J.P.F.; Seah, W.K.; Loke, J.C.L.; Ang, R.H.L.; Tan, P.H. Enabling Digital Pathology in the Diagnostic Setting: Navigating through the Implementation Journey in an Academic Medical Centre. *J. Clin. Pathol.* **2016**, *69*, 784–792. [CrossRef] [PubMed]
26. Hassell, L.A.; Peterson, J.; Pantanowitz, L. Pushed Across the Digital Divide: COVID-19 Accelerated Pathology Training onto a New Digital Learning Curve. *Acad. Pathol.* **2021**, *8*, 237428952199424. [CrossRef]
27. Available online: https://www.rcpath.org/uploads/assets/f465d1b3-797b-4297-b7fedc00b4d77e51/Best-practice-recommendations-for-implementing-digital-pathology.pdf (accessed on 26 May 2021).
28. Retamero, J.A.; Aneiros-Fernandez, J.; del Moral, R.G. Complete Digital Pathology for Routine Histopathology Diagnosis in a Multicenter Hospital Network. *Arch. Pathol. Lab. Med.* **2020**, *144*, 221–228. [CrossRef] [PubMed]
29. Hufnagl, P.; Zwönitzer, R.; Haroske, G. Guidelines Digital Pathology for Diagnosis on (and Reports Of) Digital Images Version 1.0 Bundesverband Deutscher Pathologen e.V. (Federal Association of German Pathologist). *Diagn. Pathol.* **2018**. [CrossRef]
30. Stathonikos, N.; van Varsseveld, N.C.; Vink, A.; van Dijk, M.R.; Nguyen, T.Q.; de Leng, W.W.J.; Lacle, M.M.; Goldschmeding, R.; Vreuls, C.P.H.; van Diest, P.J. Digital Pathology in the Time of Corona. *J. Clin. Pathol.* **2020**, *73*, 706–712. [CrossRef] [PubMed]
31. Hanna, M.G.; Reuter, V.E.; Ardon, O.; Kim, D.; Sirintrapun, S.J.; Schüffler, P.J.; Busam, K.J.; Sauter, J.L.; Brogi, E.; Tan, L.K.; et al. Validation of a Digital Pathology System Including Remote Review during the COVID-19 Pandemic. *Mod. Pathol.* **2020**, *33*, 2115–2127. [CrossRef]
32. L'Imperio, V.; Brambilla, V.; Cazzaniga, G.; Ferrario, F.; Nebuloni, M.; Pagni, F. Digital Pathology for the Routine Diagnosis of Renal Diseases: A Standard Model. *J. Nephrol.* **2020**, *34*, 681–688. [CrossRef] [PubMed]

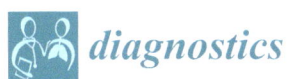

Article

DigiPatICS: Digital Pathology Transformation of the Catalan Health Institute Network of 8 Hospitals—Planification, Implementation, and Preliminary Results

Jordi Temprana-Salvador [1,*], Pablo López-García [2], Josep Castellví Vives [1], Lluís de Haro [2], Eudald Ballesta [2], Matias Rojas Abusleme [3], Miquel Arrufat [4], Ferran Marques [5], Josep R. Casas [5], Carlos Gallego [6], Laura Pons [7], José Luis Mate [7], Pedro Luis Fernández [7], Eugeni López-Bonet [8], Ramon Bosch [9], Salomé Martínez [10], Santiago Ramón y Cajal [1,†] and Xavier Matias-Guiu [11,12,†]

[1] Department of Pathology, Vall d'Hebron University Hospital, CIBERONC, 08035 Barcelona, Spain; joscastellvi@vhebron.net (J.C.V.); sramon@vhebron.net (S.R.y.C.)
[2] Functional Competence Center, Information Systems, Catalan Health Institute (Institut Català de la Salut), 08006 Barcelona, Spain; plopezg@gencat.cat (P.L.-G.); ldeharo@gencat.cat (L.d.H.); eballesta@gencat.cat (E.B.)
[3] Center for Telecommunications and Information Technology (Centre de Telecomunicacions i Tecnologies de la Informació, CTTI), Catalan Health Institute (Institut Català de la Salut), 08006 Barcelona, Spain; mrojasabusleme@gencat.cat
[4] Economic and Financial Management, Catalan Health Institute (Institut Català de la Salut), 08006 Barcelona, Spain; miquel.arrufat@gencat.cat
[5] Image Processing Group, Technical University of Catalonia (UPC), 08034 Barcelona, Spain; ferran.marques@upc.edu (F.M.); josep.ramon.casas@upc.edu (J.R.C.)
[6] Digital Medical Imaging System of Catalonia (SIMDCAT), TIC Salut, 08005 Barcelona, Spain; cgallego@ticsalutsocial.cat
[7] Department of Pathology, Germans Trias i Pujol University Hospital, 08916 Badalona, Spain; lponsmar.germanstrias@gencat.cat (L.P.); jlmate.germanstrias@gencat.cat (J.L.M.); plfernandez.germanstrias@gencat.cat (P.L.F.)
[8] Department of Pathology, Doctor Josep Trueta Hospital of Girona, 17007 Girona, Spain; elopezbonet.girona.ics@gencat.cat
[9] Department of Pathology, Verge de la Cinta Hospital of Tortosa, 43500 Tarragona, Spain; rbosch.ebre.ics@gencat.cat
[10] Department of Pathology, Joan XXIII University Hospital of Tarragona, 43005 Tarragona, Spain; mgonzalez.hj23.ics@gencat.cat
[11] Department of Pathology, Arnau de Vilanova University Hospital, 25198 Lleida, Spain; xmatias@bellvitgehospital.cat
[12] Department of Pathology, Bellvitge University Hospital, CIBERONC, 08907 Barcelona, Spain
* Correspondence: jtemprana@vhebron.net; Tel.: +34-93-274-68-09
† These authors contributed equally to this work.

Abstract: Complete digital pathology transformation for primary histopathological diagnosis is a challenging yet rewarding endeavor. Its advantages are clear with more efficient workflows, but there are many technical and functional difficulties to be faced. The Catalan Health Institute (ICS) has started its DigiPatICS project, aiming to deploy digital pathology in an integrative, holistic, and comprehensive way within a network of 8 hospitals, over 168 pathologists, and over 1 million slides each year. We describe the bidding process and the careful planning that was required, followed by swift implementation in stages. The purpose of the DigiPatICS project is to increase patient safety and quality of care, improving diagnosis and the efficiency of processes in the pathological anatomy departments of the ICS through process improvement, digital pathology, and artificial intelligence tools.

Keywords: digital pathology; computational pathology; artificial intelligence; deep learning; implementation; workflow; primary diagnosis; LIS; telepathology; network

1. Introduction

The Catalan Health Institute (Institut Català de la Salut, ICS) is the largest provider for the Catalan Health Service, the insurer of universal health coverage in Catalonia. It is the company with the most employees in Catalonia and the largest public company in Spain with almost 39,000 professionals who provide services to almost six million people throughout the territory [1]. The ICS manages 283 primary care teams, three large high-tech tertiary hospitals (Vall d'Hebron, Bellvitge, and Germans Trias), four regional reference hospitals (Arnau de Vilanova in Lleida, Joan XXIII in Tarragona, Josep Trueta in Girona, and Verge de la Cinta in Tortosa), and a regional hospital (Viladecans) (Figure 1). The ICS accounts for 7% of the Catalonian government budget with over 40 million primary visits and over 100,000 surgical interventions yearly.

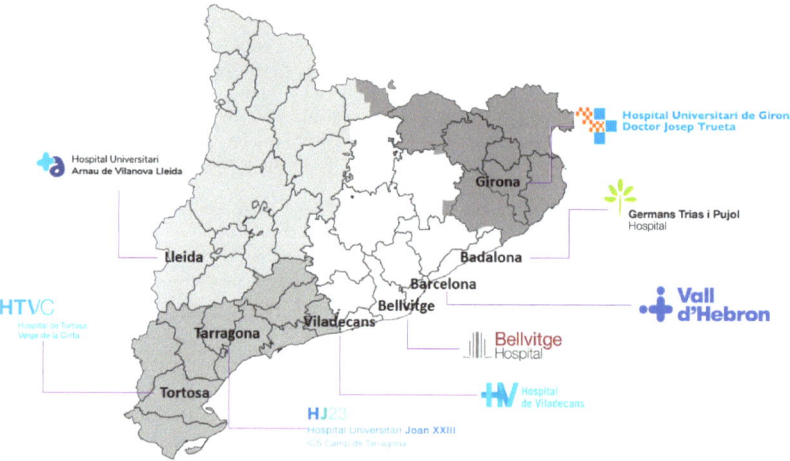

Figure 1. Map of Catalonia and the 8 ICS hospitals.

Some laboratories are beginning to deploy successfully digital pathology solutions for routine diagnosis which we believe will be a growing trend in the next few years [2–10]. In Catalonia, the DigiPatICS project plans to accomplish a complete digital pathology transformation of primary histopathological diagnosis for over 168 pathologists. Many groups have reported equivalency between digital pathology and conventional pathology [11–27].

With the DigiPatICS project, we aim to increase patient safety and quality of care, improving diagnosis and the efficiency of processes in Pathological Anatomy departments of the ICS through digital pathology and artificial intelligence (AI) tools [28]. With digital pathology, we aim for a network of eight hospitals to work as one in terms of case sharing and teaching, putting all our patients on equal footing. This transversal digital transformation will have an impact on the care of patients treated by all medical and surgical specialists.

First, we created a network between ICS centers. This helped us increase the reproducibility and quality of diagnoses, as well as offered greater equity and safety to patients. In turn, this network approach facilitated remote diagnosis, case sharing, subspecialization, and teaching for pathologists. In addition, we aimed for better working conditions, impacting the optimization of workflows, productivity, and, finally, turnaround times. We also intended to improve ergonomics and postural health, as well as to facilitate morphometric tools and the quantification of diagnostic and prognostic biomarkers to involve the optimization of time and a higher quality in diagnosis.

From a more technical point of view, the aim was to achieve a central digital repository of images on the network, thereby reducing the burden of slide file management and integrating medical imaging with SIMDCAT, a digital medical imaging system used in

Catalonia. It was also intended as a subproject to establish bidirectional communications with other locations, such as operating rooms.

The project included the development of artificial intelligence tools with machine learning and deep learning, taking advantage of the availability of whole slide images (WSIs) that were obtained after digitization. The objectives were to recognize tissue patterns, select tumor areas, and quantify them, among others. Hopefully, this use of artificial intelligence tools will contribute to improving the quality of diagnosis and the efficiency of processes.

2. Materials and Methods

DigiPatICS was created as a European Regional Development Fund (ERDF) project with European funds for the optimization of anatomopathological diagnosis in a network of public ICS hospitals in Catalonia through digitalization and artificial intelligence tools.

Subsequently, a market consultation was carried out, and, finally, it was tendered with the expedient CSE/CC00/1101202869/20/AMUP [29].

2.1. Planning, Scope, and Tender Process

A definition of needs was then carried out. We firmly believe meticulous planning is essential, taking into account all functional and technological requisites. Failing to detail such requirements can end in the failure of a digitization project, resulting in expensive scanners installed in pathology laboratories that are barely used. It is also important to highlight that going digital is not about acquiring pathology scanners; we focused our project on the purchase of a service with a shared risk with the bidder to achieve our objectives. Since this transformation was meant to be a one-way street with no possibility of going back to microscopes, all planning needed to included sufficient contingencies to avoid any kind of downtime for pathologists, as well as benefiting from the potential added value.

The purpose of the DigiPatICS project was to increase patient safety and quality of care, improving diagnosis and the efficiency of processes in pathological anatomy departments of the ICS using digital pathology and artificial intelligence tools.

In defining the scope, several questions arose:

- Do we want to save the whole slide images (WSIs) forever? Who will store them?
- Is our laboratory information system (LIS) ready?
- Do we want to (or have to) address pre-analytics?
- Do we want to address dark-field microscopy (direct fluorescence, FISH)?
- Do we want to digitize the macroscopic images?
- Do we need to update the hospital network?
- Do we need to update our pathologists' workstations?
- Do we want to share cases with the outside world?
- Is teaching important?
- Do we want artificial intelligence (AI) algorithms?
- Do we want to do telepathology?
- What do we do with cytology?
- Do we have money for everything?

Those concerns and how they were resolved will be addressed in the next pages, but we can already answer some of these. We did want to store all the WSIs forever and to use that repository to train our own artificial intelligence algorithms, which is clearly one of the great advantages of such a transformation. We also believed that this project must be an integral transformation, including routine histopathology, fluorescence, research, and macroscopic images. Tools for teaching and teleconsultation should be included, which meant having the option to share images outside our hospitals' secured LAN. We realized that our laboratory information system (LIS), preanalytics, network, and pathologist workstations all needed substantial upgrades to be able to undertake such a transformation [9].

What about cytology? Digitizing cytology, even if feasible [30–33], has some particularities: scanning times can be much longer than in histology (due to the need for more resolution, larger scan area, zero tolerance of out-of-focus areas, and Z-stacking). That means needing to install more scanners to be able to take on the same activity, and it impacts storage needs. Dark-field scanning (FISH) has similar issues, but there was a significant difference in the volume of slides to scan. Cytology involves a large number of samples to digitize in our hospitals (over 400,000 each year), which is not affordable currently in this project due to budgetary constraints.

The activity addressed in our project included all bright-field, routine histopathology, histochemistry, immunohistochemistry, direct immunofluorescence, ISH, and FISH slides. Cytology was scanned on an as-needed basis.

In Table 1, we summarize the total number of slides generated during 2019 at our eight hospitals broken down by type. To that number of over 1 million slides, an expected growth in activity of 10% to 15% must be added each year. In addition, some resources were reserved for research and non-strictly routine samples and were not accounted for in these numbers.

Table 1. Number of slides in 2019.

Routine Histopathology	814,573
Immunohistochemistry	186,453
Histochemistry	64,209
Direct Immunofluorescence	12,392
FISH	2695
CISH	1983
Total	**1,082,305**

Regarding the amount of personnel involved, DigiPatICS provided service to 107 pathologists, 7 biologists, 40 residents, and 14 observers, adding up to a total of 168 professionals working with digital diagnosis.

In the tender, all relevant aspects were taken into account for bidder evaluation, as shown in the following list:

Award criteria (*Total: 100 points*.)

- Automatic evaluation criteria. (*51 points*)
    - Economic valuation. (*40 points*)
        - Evaluation of the financial offer. (*30 points*)
        - Evaluation of the maintenance offer. (*10 points*)
    - Automatic technical evaluation. (*11 points*)
        - Quality management system. Certification of processes and algorithms. (*3 points*)
        - Process consulting. (*1 point*)
        - Image management platform adaptations. (*3 points*)
        - Storage for research slides. (*1 point*)
        - Short-term "hot" storage. (*3 points*)
- Criteria subject to judgment value. (*49 points*)
    - Scanners: deployment and image quality. (*17 points*)
    - Diagnostic viewer. (*8 points*)
    - Image management platform. (*4 points*)
    - Training module. (*2 points*)
    - Built-in tools and algorithms. (*3 points*)
    - Architecture and monitoring. (*1 point*)
    - Definitive storage in SIMDCAT. (*4 points*)
    - Integration of case information in a unified model. (*2 points*)

○ Server infrastructure requirements and DPCs. Coherence, management model, virtualization. (*2 points*)
○ Workstations. (*2 points*)
○ Artificial intelligence. (*3 points*)
○ Implementation and additional improvements. (*1 point*)

However, some aspects were considered very difficult to assess by evaluating their technical characteristics alone, and that is why three technical tests were defined for the scanner, viewer, and image management platform.

For the scanner test, a large sample of glass slides from the 8 hospitals was collected and fed to all the scanners offered by the 3 bidders for a week at 24 h a day. In the fastest scanner, over 10,000 glass slides were digitized. Real scanning speeds, jamming, incidents, etc. were recorded to ensure the reliability of the equipment (Figure 2).

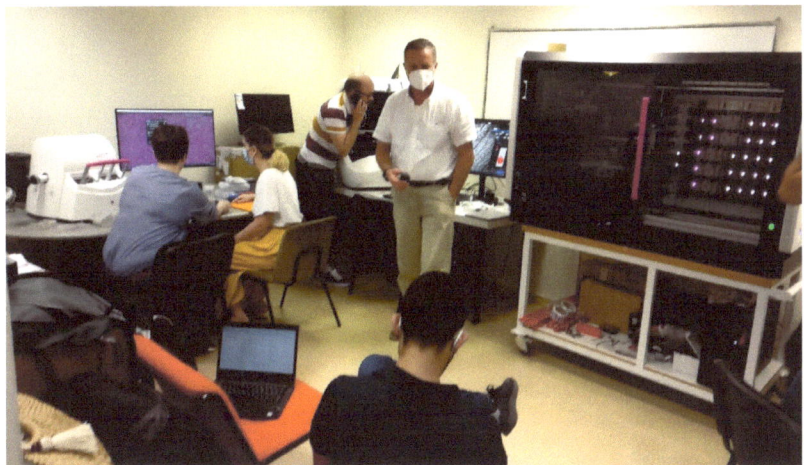

Figure 2. Testing room for test 1, showing the Palex 3DHISTECH team and equipment (PANNORAMIC SCAN II, PANNORAMIC 300 Flash DX, and PANNORAMIC 1000 Flash DX).

In the second and third tests, we brought together a group of pathologists from all the involved hospitals, along with IT experts, and they assessed the functionalities of the viewing software and the image management platform, as well as the image quality offered by the scanners using images scanned from ICS samples during the first technical test (Figure 3).

The contract file was definitively awarded by the decision of the Managing Director of the Catalan Health Institute (ICS) to the Palex Medical, S.A. 3DHISTECH Digital Pathology solution. This solution stood out for the proposal in the following main aspects:

- **Scanners:** Technical requirements, deployment requirements, and technical service requirements.
- **Image Management Platform:** Diagnostic Viewer, learning platform, and quantification modules.
- **Architecture:** SIMDCAT interaction (DICOM), unified image management model (for all slide types), infrastructure management, and coherence model.

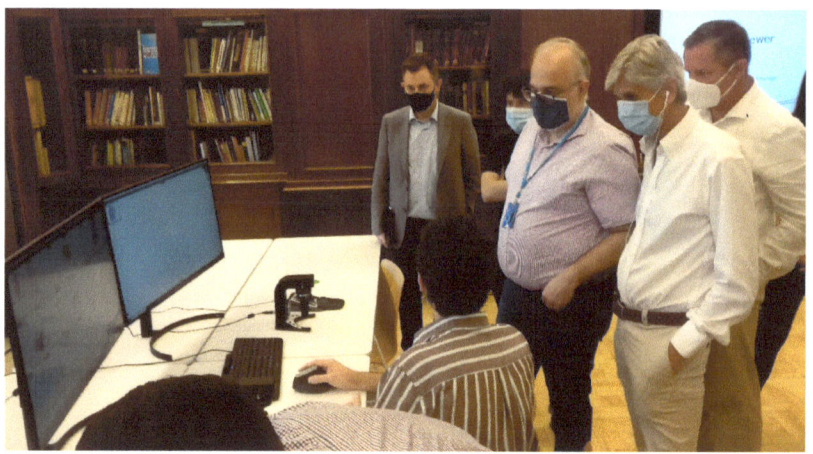

Figure 3. Testing room for tests 2–3, showing from left to right, Miquel Arrufat (ICS), Ramon Bosch (ICS), Pablo López-García (ICS), Josep Maria Argimon (ICS), and Tamás Regényi (3DHISTECH) with the Palex 3DHISTECH equipment (LG 32HL512D 8MP Diagnostic Monitor, Logitech MX Vertical Ergonomic Wireless Mouse, and 3DHISTECH SlideDriver).

2.2. Scanners and Technology for Obtaining Whole Slide Images (WSIs)

Twenty-four scanners were installed and integrated into the workflow of the eight hospitals. Different scanner models were deployed according to the needs of each institution. In Table 2, we summarize the number of each scanner type and the capabilities.

Table 2. Scanner deployment and capabilities summary.

Model	HT	DS	FL	IN	Z	S	N
PANNORAMIC 1000 Flash DX	✓	✓		✓	✓	1000	11
PANNORAMIC 300 Flash DX	✓		✓		✓	300	7
PANNORAMIC SCAN II			✓		✓	150	5
PANNORAMIC MIDI			✓		✓	12	1
Total							24

HT: high throughput capability; **DS**: double-width slide capability; **FL**: fluorescent scanning capability; **IN**: immersion scanning capability; **Z**: Z-stack scanning capability; **S**: slide capacity; **N**: number of deployed scanners; ✓: Capabilities available in each scanner.

The PANNORAMIC 1000 Flash DX (3DHISTECH Ltd., Budapest, Hungary) (P1000) is a large (154 × 100 × 91 cm) and heavy (270 kg) scanner, but it offers the largest slide capacity on the market at 1000 slides (using Leica slide racks, slide loading capacity could be further increased to 1200). It is the fastest whole-slide scanner on the market at up to 100 slides per hour and 2000 slides per day (at 40× resolution, 0.25 µm/pixel, single layer). The P1000 uses Sakura slide racks that seamlessly integrated with our laboratory workflow and allowed for priority slide handling and scanning in arbitrary order because it is flexible and automatic. It is also being used for double-width slides. Regarding image quality, it is able to scan at 0.25 µm/pixel, which is the 40× resolution equivalent (industry standard), and also at 0.12 µm/pixel, which is roughly the 80× resolution equivalent. Multilayer (Z-stack) and extended focus scanning are available, as well as automatic water immersion [34,35]. Furthermore, thanks to its AI-based software control, it is able to automatically rescan suboptimal slides, adding multilayer scanning if required. The P1000 are used for all bright-field and double-width slide related imaging.

The PANNORAMIC 300 Flash DX (3DHISTECH Ltd., Budapest, Hungary) (P300) is a fast bright-field and fluorescence scanner capable of high throughputs as a standalone machine in smaller institutions or serving as backup for P1000s in larger hospitals. It has the capacity for 300 slides, and its use is mainly for fluorescence, scanning FISH and direct immunofluorescence [36].

Both the PANNORAMIC SCAN II and the PANNORAMIC MIDI (3DHISTECH Ltd., Budapest, Hungary), with slide capacities of 150 and 12 slides, respectively, are mainly focused on fluorescence imaging but are still able to scan bright-field images, even though they are slower than their high-throughput counterparts [37].

2.3. Macroscopic Imaging

Regarding macroscopic imaging, 13 MacroPATH QX systems (Milestone Medical, Sorisole, Italy) were installed to obtain and incorporate gross imaging into the workflow. All the images were stored on the DigiPatICS servers and were fully integrated and available at the pathologist workstations for making diagnoses.

2.4. WSI Viewing: Hardware

To be able to view WSIs, 183 new workstations were installed (Table 3) for pathologists, residents, biologists, observers, and meeting rooms. Each pathologist workstation consisted of two 32-inch 4K UHD (3840 × 2160 pixel) diagnostic medical-grade FDA-approved monitors (LG 32HL512D) (Figure 4) that could be used indistinctly in flexible ways. Normal intended use is for a pathologist to have an LIS with all laboratory data, clinical data, and reporting available on one monitor, while on the other, a microscopic image is displayed. However, both monitors could be used for microscopic images, or both could be used for reporting, clinical data, bibliography, or other tasks. Biologist workstations were the same as those of the pathologists. Residents and observers shared the same workstations; however, they only consisted of one LG 32HL512D medical-grade monitor due to space constraints (the dual-monitor setup required over 150 cm of desk surface).

Table 3. Workstation and monitor deployment.

Equipment	N
Workstations	183
32″ 8MP Medical Monitor LG 32HL512D	286
55″ 4K UHD Monitor 55UH5F-B	6
4K UHD DICOM ProBeam LG Projector	7

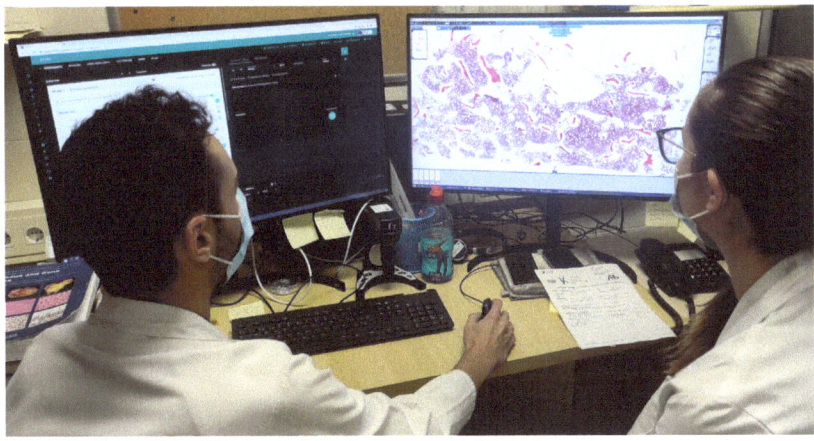

Figure 4. A pathologist in his office with a resident diagnosing with 2 LG 32HL512D 8MP diagnostic monitors.

Thirteen additional workstations with six 55-inch 4K UHD monitors and seven 4K UHD DICOM ProBeam LG projectors were installed in small and medium meeting rooms for teaching and clinical sessions as a replacement for multi-head microscopes (Figure 5).

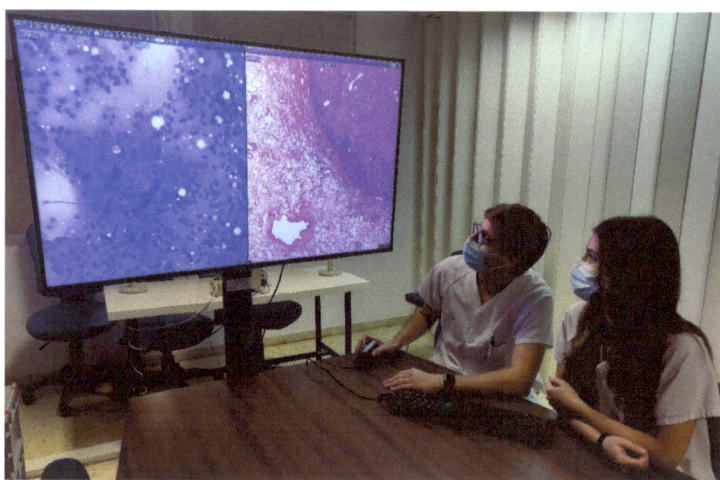

Figure 5. Residents diagnosing using a 55-inch 4K UHD monitor (55UH5F-B).

Each workstation was comprised of an Intel Core i5-9600K processor (Intel Corporation, Santa Clara, CA, USA), 16 Gb RAM, 512 Gb SSD, and an RTX 2060 graphics card (Nvidia Corporation, Santa Clara, CA, USA). All workstations were the same for easier maintenance, compatibility, and interchangeability of workplaces. Each workstation also contained a Logitech BRIO 4K UHD webcam (Logitech International, Lausanne, Switzerland) and a Jabra Evolve 40 headset with a microphone (GN Group, Ballerup, Denmark). Both the webcam and microphone aimed to facilitate networking between pathologists from the same hospital, from different hospitals within the ICS, or even with professionals outside our network.

Furthermore, each workstation contained a Logitech MX Vertical Ergonomic Wireless Mouse (Logitech International, Lausanne, Switzerland), since vertical mice seem to put less strain on the wrist and demonstrate better ratings than conventional mice [38]. Each pathologist could also choose between two other ergonomic devices: a Kensington Expert Mouse Wireless Trackball® (Kensington Computer Products Group, Redwood Shores, CA, USA) and a SlideDriver (3DHISTECH Ltd., Budapest, Hungary) (Figure 6). All devices were supported by our viewing software. The SlideDriver offers microscope-like navigation on digital slides for those who prefer a traditional method. Most of our pathologists and residents selected the SlideDriver as their input device (80% approximately).

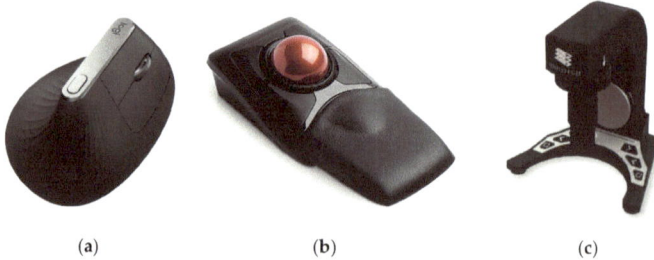

(a)   (b)   (c)

Figure 6. Ergonomic devices: (**a**) Logitech MX Vertical Ergonomic Wireless Mouse; (**b**) Kensington Expert Mouse Wireless Trackball®; (**c**) SlideDriver.

2.5. WSI Viewing: Software

The diagnostic viewer used for all digital images was ClinicalViewer (3DHISTECH Ltd., Budapest, Hungary). It uses streaming technology to avoid downloading WSIs for diagnosis. It is capable of opening bright-field, fluorescence, double-slide, Z-stack, and macroscopic photography, etc. It also includes many positively valued features, such as the possibility of viewing and navigating up to nine automatically synchronized images at once. It also has IVD support and quantification algorithms, as well as some more standard tools, such as free rotation, free zoom, annotation, measuring, and object counting tools (Figure 7).

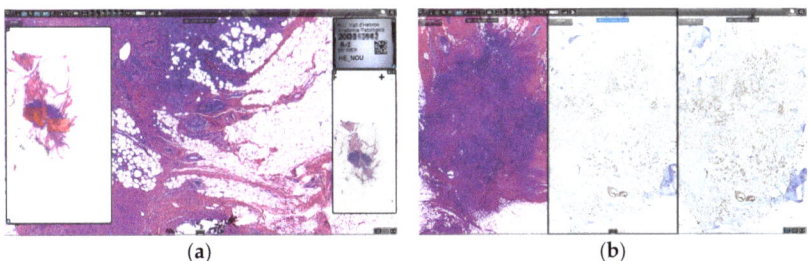

(a) (b)

Figure 7. ClinicalViewer: (**a**) slide with navigation panel; and (**b**) three auto-aligned slides.

The software also had a telepathology option available and a module to create training courses. Possessing all the WSI viewing needs, including fluorescence, integrated into one software system (one viewer) facilitated pathologist ergonomics and also enabled simplifying the technological model with fewer integrations required.

2.6. ETPAT: Our Laboratory Information System (LIS)

The evolution of information systems in the last ten years has been meteoric. It has changed the paradigms for accessing and possessing the necessary information at each point of contact a patient has with a health system.

At the Catalan Health Institute (ICS) and within the ARGOS project, we have spent 15 years directing information towards users and clinical care, and we have progressively moved from the initial free texts to structured information. The ARGOS project started in 2006. It is a project to integrate in a transversal and transparent way all the information systems involved in clinical assistance to the citizens of the Catalan Health Institute and its eight hospitals, including the hospital information system, nursing, pharmacy, clinical analysis laboratory, pathology laboratory, and critical care units. Currently, ARGOS is the priority information system in Catalonia and is present in 23 hospitals of the Catalan public health network.

The SALUT4D project began in 2020 and is the evolution of clinical workstations within the ARGOS project. Its objective is to provide the necessary information at each moment of care to different professionals. It is based on four dimensions seeking to present the necessary data at each point of care:

1. Where am I? Scope of work: emergencies, hospitalization, ambulatory consultation, operating room, etc.;
2. Who am I? Nurse, surgeon, internist, psychologist, etc.;
3. Whom do I attend? A patient with hypertension, diabetes, bronchitis, etc.;
4. How do I attend to it? With a computer, tablet, smartphone, etc.

The system presents the information that a professional needs clearly and orderly. The system is based on a clinical dictionary with more than 40,000 variables stored in a MongoDB-type database called the Global Variables Repository (RGV). This repository contains data from all sources: laboratory, pathological anatomy, radiology, vital sign monitors, pharmacy, etc.

To construct this platform, created and designed for and by the ICS, HTML5 technology, SAP® ISH® (Information System Hospital), and SAP® ISHMed® (SAP SE, Walldorf, Germany) were used. The system connects directly with the Shared Clinical History of Catalonia (HC3) and provides access to information on all public hospitals and all primary care facilities in a fully integrated manner.

The work methodology was based on requirements submitted by over three hundred health professionals who continuously provided their contributions. Through AGILE methodologies, the new clinical workstation was progressively built.

The new station is already in operation at the eight ICS hospitals and will gradually come into operation in twenty-three sections of the ARGOS system throughout 2022.

In order to incorporate the peculiarities of the new, fully digital workflow, a new LIS for our pathology laboratories named ETPAT was developed. It was deemed necessary to develop and improve pathologist workstations to provide them with tools that allow the integration of information from all sources and electronic records available. ETPAT has a fully integrative approach to all processes occurring in our pathology labs, from electronic requests from clinicians to pathology reports, with full traceability of all steps involved at the laboratory. Moreover, it enables the optimization of paper management as much as possible. This software was based on HTML5 and was prepared for 32-inch 4K UHD monitors, taking advantage of the hardware on hand (Figure 8).

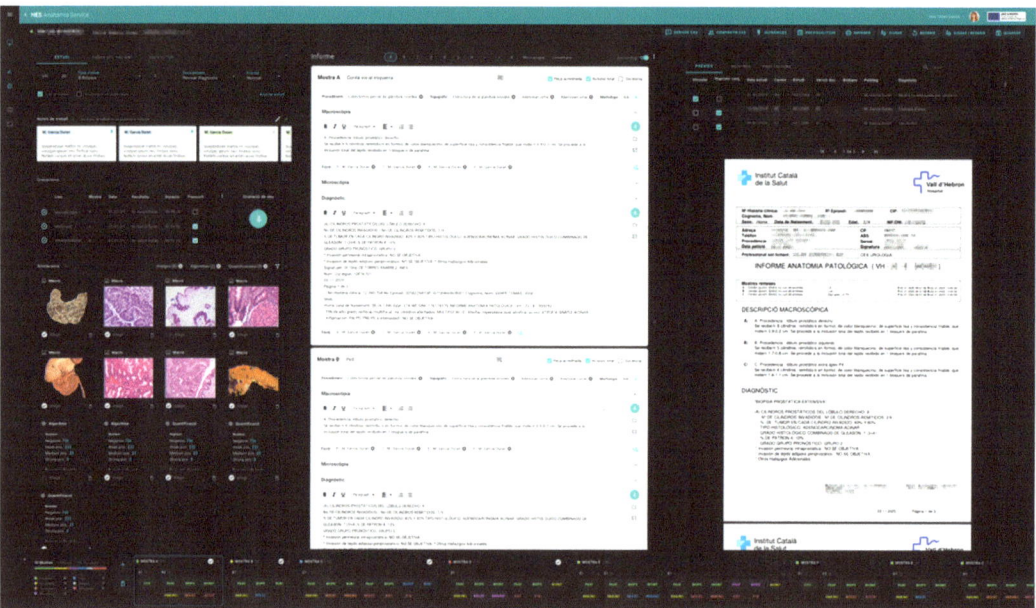

Figure 8. ETPAT screenshot (our proprietary LIS).

One of the most relevant aspects was the unification of workflow for all ICS laboratories, which should be able to work seamlessly as a network, or even as one big institution. The catalogs of techniques and sample types were also more coherent. All traceability data was integrated and convenient, and we were able to collect information on who carried out each phase of the diagnostic process to allow the correct attribution of costs and activities.

This new LIS is clearly ready for the digital workflow of macroscopic and microscopic images and was fully integrated with the image management platform. In addition, the management of second opinions and case consultations was incorporated.

2.7. Network Needs, Local Area Network (LAN), and Wide Area Network (WAN)

The main source for generating information by volume of data was the scanners (in the order of around 2 petabytes yearly), which were located across the different centers included in the scope of the project.

The systems were connected to a 10 Gbps network between the scanners and the local storage data processing center (DPC). The same criteria applied to the artificial intelligence platform.

The network requirements for the DigiPatICS project were high, since access to the images needed to be instantaneous, as it was on a microscope. Images were accessed via streaming, but a large bandwidth was still required, making it necessary to adapt cabling and infrastructure, as well as switches, routers, and other telecommunications equipment. Each workstation required a 300 Mbps connection to the DPC to be able to stream the WSIs, but to ensure performance, the connection was established at 1 Gbps. MacroPATHs required a 100 Mbps connection.

Adjustments were made to the WAN infrastructure to ensure that communications between the central repository and the centers were capable, on one hand, of transferring daily information to the central DPC and, on the other hand, of allowing consultation between hospitals and their corresponding DPCs. This WAN needed to support an approximate flow of 6 TB each night for the DigiPatICS project activity alone.

To achieve these goals, both the Department of Health and Catsalut public institutions recognized this need and facilitated the creation of a dedicated network to support the data traffic requirements mentioned and response times for data recovery.

2.8. On-Premise Data Processing Centers (DPCs)

The project proposal was to provide a good user experience to all users of the image management platform, as well as to facilitate their work, optimize performance times, and reduce the time invested in obtaining a correct diagnosis. That is why we considered infrastructure to be a fundamental technological pillar in this project that needed to be sized based on performance, scalability, and reliability criteria without excessively oversizing the system or implementing complex architectures that would create greater difficulties in maintenance. For the project, the deployment of its own infrastructure was carried out, but at the same time, it was integrated transversally across the health ecosystem.

A common structure was used at all centers that only changed in terms of local storage dimensioning, adapting to the number of slides estimated per center. In this way, we made infrastructure maintenance easier. All the DPCs were provided with the energy and cooling requirements necessary for correct operation of the various systems, as well as redundant systems in terms of communications, servers, storage, and a secondary DPC in case of disaster recovery.

The system at each center was designed to have a high-availability configuration, meaning, in the event of a disaster in one of the elements of the system, it would be capable of continuing to offer service with minimum downtime, or even without interruption, depending on the source of the problem.

The high-availability elements implemented were:

- A host server cluster under VMware vSphere in an active-passive configuration;
- Disk storage configured in RAID;
- Mirrored disk arrays with asynchronous replication.

The various redundant elements of the high-availability scenario were located in a DPC or complementary technical room that was not the main DPC in order to minimize the impact of any possible disaster on the main DPC. Artificial intelligence equipment was excluded from this high-availability policy.

At each center, a virtualization infrastructure was deployed, consisting of a set of two identical servers under a VMware vSphere infrastructure. This allowed the system to have the capacity to maintain service quality in an event where it was necessary to activate a contingency scenario (disaster recovery) in a matter of a few minutes. These servers were HPE ProLiant DL325 models dimensioned with AMD EPYC processors that offered the necessary computing capacity for all DICOM image integration, storage management, and processing operations that were carried out continuously. They also served as a virtualization platform for the controller structure of the AI cluster.

As for storage, MSA 1050 cabinets were chosen and presented to the host servers through iSCSI controllers. These storage cabinets contained a battery of SSD disks intended exclusively for virtual machine operating system disks. For medical image storage, a pool of rotational HDD disks was deployed. This decision was made based on the following factors:

- Once the medical image was generated, it was not modified (writing on the disc only one time);
- Access was completed in blocks through streaming (reduced reading rate);
- Each center had its own local storage (limited number of simultaneous writes).

For all these reasons, the increase in cost of deploying SSD technology for image storage was not justified for the required performance.

The same storage technology was used in all the centers, including the central DPC, with only capacity varying as a factor of the number of digitized images estimated per center. The total storage capacity between the eight hospitals was approximately 500 TB, which allowed short-term storage of up to 75 days for images.

The deployed server and storage infrastructure had the activation of the HPE IRS service, which automatically opened a ticket to the manufacturer in the event of a hardware component failure, guaranteeing proper functioning of the infrastructure.

The entire server infrastructure was backed by a backup policy based on Veeam Backup that was integrated into existing control panels in each center in order to facilitate maintenance tasks.

Within the scope of this project, integration with SIMDCAT was included for the publication of images as a form of definitive storage. Publishing to SIMDCAT was asynchronous under a queue management system that published the images as soon as they became ready. As the publication to SIMDCAT was continuous, the need to make a backup copy of all the scanned images outside the same disk array cluster was not considered, delegating the backup function to the same SIMDCAT. If the need arose to retrieve one or more images, a small application was implemented that allowed downloading these images from SIMDCAT and placing them back in local storage. Only in the event of a major disaster would the procedure be the same as indicated above; however, there may be a minimal number of scanned images that would not have had the opportunity to be published in SIMDCAT due to the asynchronous nature of the publication process. In such a case, the images would be rescanned.

2.9. SIMDCAT and DICOM

SIMDCAT is the Digital Medical Image System of Catalonia. It is currently the unified system used by the network of entities called SISCAT (Comprehensive Health System of the Public Utility of Catalonia) to preserve digital medical images and provide services and digital resources based on the same software architecture using cloud services and to make information accessible from various electronic medical records. The system is used by approximately 450 Catalan health centers and by all SISCAT professionals to securely collect and share digital medical images generated by the centers. SIMDCAT was the definitive repository of this project in which the images and associated data were stored. SIMDCAT was set up in 2018 to provide the public health system with a secure and technologically advanced environment in which to store and share digital medical image services.

The project to develop in SIMDCAT a specific environment for pathological anatomy medical images presented multiple benefits for agents of the Catalan health system. Professionals in this specialty were provided with a network work environment based on cloud technology, and the anatomopathological diagnosis process was optimized so that medical images were immediately and safely available to professionals. As for patients, the quality of care was improved, and their safety was increased.

Finally, the sustainability of resources and costs of health information systems was promoted by providing a common and shared system for all providers.

SIMDCAT's cloud-based technology is focused on the use of DICOM as a standard in the storage and distribution of medical objects. The capacity of standard DICOM beyond radiology has been demonstrated in recent years, where PACS image storage systems have evolved into the VNA (Vendor Neutral Archive); SIMDCAT constitutes a VNA that allows the management of medical objects using the DICOM standard as a reference framework. In the case of pathology, the DICOM 145 extension is adopted; this extension facilitates the storage and distribution of medical objects independent of the device that generates the information. SIMDCAT adopts DICOM 145 natively, incorporating the pyramidal treatment of images, thus facilitating navigation through an image. SIMDCAT also adopts the DICOM 122 extension that reflects the representative data model of pathology.

SIMDCAT manages the information in a private cloud model with a high-redundancy system to guarantee the availability of the information. Saving the information in different storage systems using data object technology, this model allows growth according to the needs of the system, optimizing available resources in addition to freeing hospitals from the custody and distribution of information.

2.10. Artificial Intelligence and the Polytechnic University of Catalonia–BarcelonaTech (UPC)

It is now recognized that artificial intelligence represents a turning point for society that is at least as significant as the Industrial Revolution. The ICS aims to be an autonomous and primary player in the creation of artificial intelligence algorithms to avoid dependance on a commercial solution. Therefore, we wished to set up an artificial intelligence platform tailored to the needs of the ICS. This platform was developed with free software and needed to be modeled to accommodate other artificial intelligence projects in addition to DigiPatICS.

Currently, the ICS has signed a collaboration agreement with the Image Processing Group (GPI) of the Polytechnic University of Catalonia–BarcelonaTECH (UPC) (imatge.upc.edu) for the development of artificial intelligence tools and platforms within the healthcare field, specifically in the field of medical imaging. The group belongs to the Intelligent Data Science and Artificial Intelligence Research Center (IDEAI), which is a hub created at the UPC in 2017 for the development of artificial intelligence. GPI has extensive experience in image processing and the development of artificial intelligence algorithms with a long history in the healthcare field.

GPI develops computer vision and deep learning (DL) tools to tackle WSI analysis tasks in DigiPatICS for stains, such as H&E, HER2, KI67, RE, and RP, as well as other immunohistochemical stains. DL technology that relies on instance and semantic segmentation architectures has the potential to provide high-quality results when properly trained. GPI has also introduced strategies, such as:

Dataset annotation: As the training database was limited in the first stage, a more classical computer vision strategy relying on morphological algorithms and machine learning (ML) tools produced proposals easier to validate by annotators and generated the ground truth needed to avoid limiting the performances of DL approaches.

Integration of AI algorithms: Integration into specialist workflow was facilitated by combining the systematic processing of a large number of WSIs with on-demand assessment by pathologists for improving the systematic results or for obtaining specific quantifications:

1. Nightly batch processing and inference on the WSIs yielded raw results, such as segmentation confidences and classification probabilities, as well as potential segmentation masks;
2. The results were integrated into 3DHISTECH ClinicalViewer using a specific plug-in and offered to the pathologists upon request when examining the slides;
3. The pathologists could select or deselect regions in the WSI to visualize and quantify the results or to fine-tune inference results (classification and segmentation) using sliders;

4. Pathologists could also select specific areas for further online analysis on inference servers to be performed during the session with the viewer at their workstations.

Pathologists in the analysis loop: The strategy in Point 3 allowed not only flexible interaction for online and on-demand analysis, but also for recovering information about pathologists by selecting specific regions of interest and tuning inference results for reports. This information represents invaluable data and comments to further improve the annotated datasets.

Training in the ICS development servers: A specific committee formed by AI specialists and clinicians periodically reviewed the comments and data produced by pathologists using the viewer. This committee decided on the feedback and data and set strategies for incremental training and improvement of the DL network architecture involved with continuously improving the inference results.

The former strategies facilitated the usage of AI tools in the daily work of pathologists, as well as productivity.

As mentioned, all images were stored in a central repository, SIMDCAT, where they were available for AI training after dissociation. AI training was performed in this central repository, where a large number of whole slide images were readily at hand. GPI researchers did not have direct access to sensitive clinical data, and datasets and whole slide images always remained within the ICS infrastructure. In fact, it should be noted that the entire circuit in production moved through an isolated dedicated network in an intranet environment, and the training environment was in a separate VLAN and intranet infrastructure. Once the inference algorithms were trained, they were run on-premise at each hospital DPC. In no case was the information transferred to external DPCs.

3. Results

The digital pathology transformation envisioned in the DigiPatICS project involved great changes in most of the steps of workflow in our pathology laboratories. As mentioned above, all the processes were integrated in our LIS ETPAT.

3.1. Laboratory Workflow, Traceability, and Barcode Generation

All incoming samples, biopsies, cytologies, autopsies, and even molecular requests are accompanied by an e-request generated in our electronic health record system by the clinicians who input all the necessary clinical data.

At the time of registration, the request receives an identification number that is labeled with a datamatrix-type barcode. Each sample container is also labeled with a unique datamatrix-type barcode. The barcode structure is as follows, maintaining logical hierarchy, as seen in Figure 9. The case or request barcode includes the institution, the year, the sample type, and the case number (i.e., VH22B051337, for Vall d'Hebron, year 2022, biopsy number 51,337). When labeling a container, the container ID is appended (i.e., VH22B051337A for container A). When a cassette is required, a datamatrix-type barcode is also printed with the number of the paraffin block appended (i.e., VH22B051337A014 for block 14). For glass slides, whether they come from paraffin block sections or are cytologies, another number is appended, representing the slide number (i.e., VH22B051337A014001 for histological section 1). The full ID is printed and appears in a datamatrix-type barcode in each slide.

Most of our laboratory equipment, including scanners, is able to read these barcodes and is integrated with our LIS, providing automatic checkpoints for many steps of processing.

The first checkpoint is when the sample is received with the labeling of the containers, as described previously. It is a manual step completed by technicians, but in the new LIS, the process was simplified so it was closer to optimal. The next step, grossing, was also improved: MacroPATHs were installed inside the pathology fume hoods, and computers with the LIS were placed next to them. Pathologists, residents, or technicians could print the cassettes, capture gross examination pictures, and dictate or type the macroscopic description in a convenient and fully digital way. Pictures of cassette contents are obtained and are available for verification in the next laboratory steps. After filling a cassette with tissue, the barcode is scanned for the first checkpoint of the paraffin block. The next checkpoint is when the cassette enters the tissue processor, and a technician reads the barcodes using a handheld device. Unfortunately, this step remained manual because our tissue processors could not read barcodes. We hope this will change in the future.

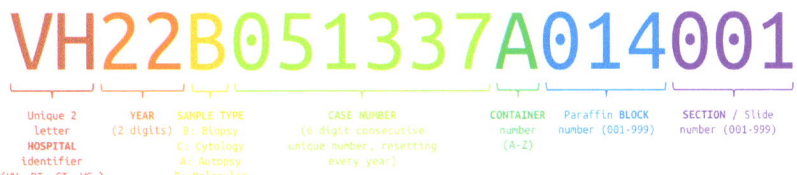

Figure 9. Barcode anatomy.

Each embedding station had a computer with a barcode reader within reach. A technician read the barcode of the paraffin block, and the LIS displayed the tissue type and the confection notes (if present) and provided access to macroscopic images for verification, while, in fact, creating another checkpoint.

The next checkpoint is clearly when sectioning. Every microtome station had a barcode reader, a slide label printer, and a computer with the LIS. When scanning the paraffin block, the LIS displayed the tissue type and other information on that block, such as how many and which slides must be obtained from it. At the same time, it printed the slide labels automatically, which include the datamatrix barcode described previously. This automation reduced the human error of manual workflow [3].

At this point, the automatic part started. In most hospitals, Sakura Tissue-Tek Prisma Plus and Tissue-Tek Film (Sakura Finetek Europe B.V., Alphen aan den Rijn, The Netherlands) were used. After sectioning, a technician loaded the slides in the Sakura racks. Then, the racks were stained, coverslipped with film, dried, and scanned using P1000s. Routine slides did not have to be treated individually until archiving because all the equipment used the same racks. In terms of traceability, an automatic checkpoint was recorded by Sakura Tissue-Tek Film, which was integrated with our LIS, and the final checkpoint was notified by a 3DHISTECH P1000 when the slide was scanned.

Using the same Sakura racks for all equipment enabled us to optimize technician slide handling time and reduced errors. Immunohistochemistry and histochemistry used the same Tissue-Tek Film, so checkpoints stayed the same. In cases of double slides, the steps needed to be conducted manually, but their volume was negligible compared to routine histology, where workflow optimization was key.

In some hospitals, other automatic stainers were used, such as VENTANA HE 600 (Roche, Basel, Switzerland). Integration was possible, but an extra step of transferring the slides from HE 600 trays to the scanner rack was needed.

Subprocesses, such as slide allocation and delivery to pathologists, did not exist anymore, since the digital workflow did not require such manual steps.

Regarding the destruction of containers, a new system was implemented. A tablet with the LIS, along with a handheld datamatrix barcode reader, was used to scan the containers. If the containers were ready for elimination, a confirmation message appeared, and a checkpoint was created.

The whole workflow was designed for optimization and security. We aimed to reduce the time technicians spent on worthless tasks, allowing them to focus on what was important and increase their satisfaction in the workplace. Also, the checkpoints enabled a better awareness of sample status by all personnel and an obvious increase in safety.

It is also worth mentioning that the transformation was carried out simultaneously as a radical change with all the pathologists in the same center starting digital work at the same time. The alternative of making a gradual change implied many more difficulties by having to maintain two circuits (old and new) in the same laboratory. This measure was taken considering the possible reluctance and skepticism of the staff, which would be lessened if they could quickly see an optimization of circuits despite initial incidents. No benefits of a gradual approach were seen by the authors if all the infrastructure was in place.

Regarding validation of WSIs for use in primary diagnosis, the digital pathology solution provided all necessary legal certifications, but it still was tested and validated previously by many pathologists using all types of preparations. The solution was also tested in the scanner and viewer technical tests during the bidding process. When the pathologists started working with digital slides, all of them could compare digital slides with glass slides until their grade of confidence was enough. No specific period of time or amount of resources was dedicated for this purpose; it was a matter of obtaining enough comfort for the pathologists in their routine workflow. A continuous validation of tissue detection was performed in every single case, since the pathologists had available the captured image of the slide next to the slide overview, as seen in Figure 7a, and were thus certain there was no tissue missing on the WSI.

Furthermore, all the pathology departments involved in DigiPatICS were certified or accredited for ISO 9001 or ISO 15189. Because the ISO 15189 standard confirms technical competence of the laboratory and ensures reliability of test results, a continuous validation strategy was recommended following CAP recommendations [39,40].

The initial reticence on the part of a couple pathologists could not be reversed despite several talks and explanations to try to make them partners in the transforming project. However, these reluctances completely disappeared after a few days of working in the digital flow without the need for any external intervention. The advantages of the new technology were obvious and sufficient on their own.

3.2. Scanning

Being able to scan slides and obtain WSIs are perhaps the obvious concerns of any digital pathology project, but, as mentioned, these are not the only relevant points.

It was essential that the scanners did not stop due to jamming, so the glass slides needed to be optimal. This implied possessing a decent glass or film coverslip; either could work as long as the quality of the histological slide was good. Labels also needed to fit perfectly within the boundaries of the glass slide. Anything that protruded could cause jamming. Slides needed to be fully dried, and under no circumstance could be dripping glue [20].

Furthermore, we considered crucial for the workflow the presence of automatic scanning with two objectives and, therefore, two resolutions, $40\times$ (0.25 µm/pixel) and $80\times$ (0.12 µm/pixel), to cover all possible needs. The scanners used different scanning profiles ($40\times$ or $80\times$, Z-stack, etc.) depending on the sample and the stain type indicated by our LIS (ETPAT). The process was fully automatic. It was also possible to select profiles manually or tweak some settings, but manual parameterization was not used for high-throughput routine scanning. Routine scanner loading needed to be as easy, fast, and straightforward as possible for the laboratory technicians. In order to have the automatic profile feature in addition to automatic tissue detection obtained by an AI algorithm in the scanner control software, it was very important to scan slides at a suitable resolution.

The second concern regarding scanners was their deployment. Correct dimensioning is essential to address daily routine activity. Individual scanning speed or capacity is very important, but less relevant than the deployment of equipment meeting the needs of the center. In the event of a breakdown or maintenance, the remaining equipment must be able to compensate. Scanner deployment must also take into account the expected growth of activity (in our case, 10–15% annually). Scanners must not create bottlenecks in the workflow, and going fully digital cannot involve a delay in turnaround time. In our daily routine, scanning occurred right after the slides were dried, and the first WSIs were available during the morning. The scanners were continuously loaded until the end of the technician shift for each institution (in some cases 16:00, and 21:00 in others), and the scanners were supposed to finish scanning overnight, around 2:00–3:00 a.m. in our institutions producing more slides, thus having time until 8:00 a.m. to accommodate this expected increase in activity before the pathologists started diagnosing. This workflow guaranteed no delay in turnaround time, even after adding steps to the conventional system, by completing slide production and digitation of all slides within the same day. The remaining advantages of digital pathology should optimize our routines and reduce diagnostic and reporting times.

Another aspect considered was where to physically locate the scanners. The location needed to be convenient for technicians within their workflow so that the new steps were not disruptive. Scanners were located near a stainer or coverslipper or next to a glass slide archive whenever possible.

Fluorescence workflow was taken into account to try to keep the slides cool and to preserve them from light.

3.3. Monitors

The need for a high-quality monitor is indisputable, although recommendations for ideal screen size and resolution have changed over time. Currently, a size between 24 and 32 inches with a high resolution is considered necessary, and the trend is probably upwards. A larger monitor, such as the ones we used, with a smaller pixel size allows for a greater field of vision, avoiding displacement through digital preparation. However, this means that objects appear smaller when the original maximum magnification is reached and that it requires more bandwidth to stream the image [41–43].

It is also important to take into account color fidelity (the panel can be calibrated), lighting (no backlight bleed), contrast, pixel size, pixel density, brightness, color space (sRGB, Adobe RGB), color depth, etc. However, a good monitor is not going to make up for poor digital preparation. A high-quality monitor is important to guarantee image fidelity and ergonomics, as well as to avoid visual fatigue for the user (Figure 10).

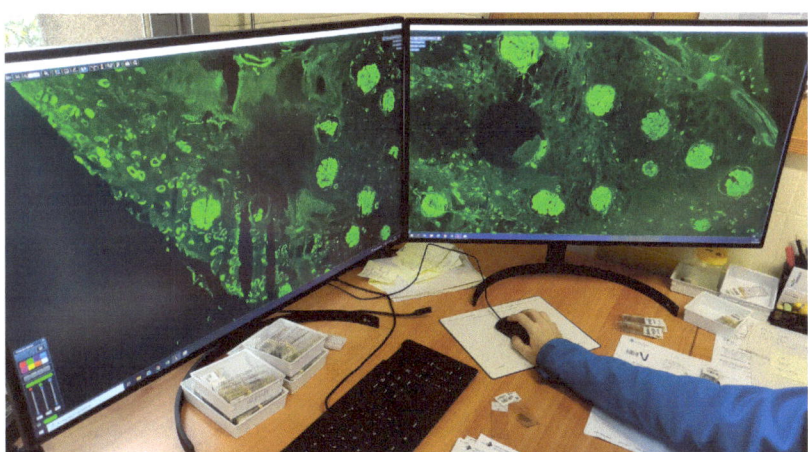

Figure 10. Fluorescence seen in a totally integrated fashion on two 32-inch LG 32HL512D 8MP diagnostic monitors.

3.4. Teaching, Telepathology, and Networking

Many of the planned advantages of this project, such as networking between ICS hospitals, having a teaching platform, and being able to teleconsult cases with external pathologists, although not available right now, were binding in the contract and will be implemented in the following months [44]. The system will have an on-demand function to publish studies to an Internet environment with previously anonymized data to allow the sharing of images.

4. Discussion

The DigiPatICS project, as a transformation of the Catalan Health Institute Network of eight hospitals, represented an important technological, organizational, and functional challenge.

We incorporated digital pathology and artificial intelligence in pathology departments with an organizational change that modified work dynamics, as seen in the previous paragraphs. This change responded to current and future challenges with the aim of improving quality, efficiency, effectiveness, equity, speed, systematization, and reproducibility of diagnoses. These improvements affected other disciplines and increased patient safety with the following benefits: improvement of diagnostic conditions by incorporating the digitalization of preparations with maximum guarantees of traceability while minimizing material losses and identification errors; and improvement of workflow, productivity, and turnaround times. Moreover, there was also improvement in working conditions in terms of ergonomics. The viewers also provided tools for morphometry and quantification of diagnostic and prognostic biomarkers and facilitated the digital access of preparations from previous patient examinations without interrupting the diagnostic process [4,7].

In the near future, we will enable access to images for decision making between pathology departments and other facilities (operating rooms, interventional examination rooms, transplantation, or clinical committees) using bidirectional communication. Also, the images will be available for clinical sessions, tumor boards, and pre- and postgraduate teaching. Being able to store pathology images digitally also reduces the workload for management of histological preparation files. Ergonomics, workflow improvement, and convenience of access to historical slides also encourage research.

Successfully exchanging whole slide images and artificial intelligence algorithms between institutions had the following implications: We improved the reproducibility of diagnoses, both in terms of interpretation and in the way they are reflected in medical reports, ensuring system-wide equity and fairness. We encouraged an optimal exchange of information between hospitals, establishing second-opinion strategies according to clinical practice guidelines that immediately benefitted patients. Thus, we also encouraged the movement of patients between hospitals in a coordinated way, avoiding the physical movement of biological material with fewer delays and courier costs and ensuring preservation. Lastly, we aimed to make more efficient use of the existing critical mass in terms of prevalent, complex, infrequent, and difficult diseases and guaranteeing equity between hospitals, regardless of size and geographical location, with the end-goal of organizing references for pathologies and territories.

From a technological standpoint, innovation also occurred. We stored all images using DICOM standards in SIMDCAT, a unified system used by the SISCAT network of entities to preserve digital medical images, provide digital services and resources based on the same software architecture, and make digital medical images accessible. This repository can be used independently by different viewers and is also independent of the scanning system. The transformation of the laboratory information system and all IT infrastructure is key in this type of project.

In addition, from the technological point of view, we aimed to achieve an improvement in algorithms for the quantification of immunohistochemical biomarkers and for the assessment of in situ hybridization. In the future, we hope to develop artificial intelligence algorithms with machine learning and deep learning in order to recognize patterns and segment tumor areas. We need to look for tools that help pathologists do their jobs with AI algorithms developed by our researchers. We produced an image repository large enough for this aim. Artificial intelligence optimizes the reproducibility of diagnoses. The boom in artificial intelligence will involve very significant changes in the way pathologists work in the coming years.

All things considered, it is important to seek a digital pathology system and, therefore, a manufacturer and a distributor that adapt to the real needs of each particular case. In the DigiPatICS project, we looked for a complete holistic solution for our pathology departments. As shown, it was very difficult to compare products according to data sheets exclusively, and it was very laborious to define a digital pathology project for all technical and functional implications.

The growing enthusiasm for digital pathology and the new possibilities artificial intelligence offers indicate an emerging revolution in pathology that will change our way of working. However, for broad adoption, an integrative approach of digital pathology across clinicians, pathologists, laboratory information systems, viewers, hardware, research, and teaching is imperative. Digital pathology must simplify our workflows and not add complexity. Vast repositories of diagnosed images will allow us to make great strides in this direction. With our solution meeting these needs, we hope to inspire other pathologists and to provide useful guidance for their successful digital transformations.

5. Conclusions

The DigiPatICS project aimed to deploy digital pathology in an integrative, holistic, and comprehensive way within a network of 8 hospitals, incorporating 168 pathologists and over 1 million slides each year. After careful planning, implementation was carried out simultaneously for all the pathologists in each institution. A digital pathology system needed to be integrated with all health information systems, including electronic medical records. Teleconsultation, teaching platforms, fluorescence, and cytology were taken into account. The digital transformation of a pathology department represented a technological, organizational, and functional challenge. It provided an effective and safe diagnostic tool with clear benefits for diagnosis quality and patient safety.

Author Contributions: Conceptualization, P.L.-G. and J.T.-S.; methodology, P.L.-G., J.T.-S., L.d.H. and E.B.; writing—original draft preparation, J.T.-S.; writing—review and editing, P.L.-G., J.T.-S., L.d.H., E.B., M.R.A., J.C.V., F.M., J.R.C., C.G. and X.M.-G.; supervision, L.d.H., E.B., M.A., J.C.V., M.R.A., E.L.-B., P.L.F., J.L.M., L.P., R.B., S.M., S.R.y.C. and X.M.-G.; project administration, L.d.H., E.B. and M.A.; funding acquisition, L.d.H., M.A., S.R.y.C. and X.M.-G. All authors have read and agreed to the published version of the manuscript.

Funding: This project was funded by European Regional Development Funds, Programa operatiu FEDER de Catalunya 2014–2020 and SA18-014623 DIGIPATICS. UPC activity in this project was partially supported by PID2020-116907RB-I00 and funded by MCIN/AEI/10.13039/501100011033.

Institutional Review Board Statement: Not applicable.

Informed Consent Statement: Not applicable.

Data Availability Statement: All data generated or analyzed during this study are included in the article.

Acknowledgments: The authors thank over 250 people who were directly involved in making the DigiPatICS project a reality, including pathology laboratory teams, administration teams, artificial intelligence teams, network and IT teams, the SIMDCAT integration team, technical support, infrastructure teams, programmers, and logistics teams.

Conflicts of Interest: The authors declare no conflict of interest.

References

1. El ICS. Available online: http://ics.gencat.cat/es/lics/ (accessed on 25 December 2021).
2. Schüffler, P.J.; Geneslaw, L.; Yarlagadda, D.V.K.; Hanna, M.G.; Samboy, J.; Stamelos, E.; Vanderbilt, C.; Philip, J.; Jean, M.-H.; Corsale, L.; et al. Integrated Digital Pathology at Scale: A Solution for Clinical Diagnostics and Cancer Research at a Large Academic Medical Center. *J. Am. Med. Inform. Assoc.* **2021**, *28*, 1874–1884. [CrossRef] [PubMed]
3. Fraggetta, F.; Caputo, A.; Guglielmino, R.; Pellegrino, M.G.; Runza, G.; L'Imperio, V. A Survival Guide for the Rapid Transition to a Fully Digital Workflow: The "Caltagirone Example". *Diagnostics* **2021**, *11*, 1916. [CrossRef] [PubMed]

4. Eloy, C.; Vale, J.; Curado, M.; Polónia, A.; Campelos, S.; Caramelo, A.; Sousa, R.; Sobrinho-Simões, M. Digital Pathology Workflow Implementation at IPATIMUP. *Diagnostics* **2021**, *11*, 2111. [CrossRef] [PubMed]
5. Retamero, J.A.; Aneiros-Fernandez, J.; Del Moral, R.G. Complete Digital Pathology for Routine Histopathology Diagnosis in a Multicenter Hospital Network. *Arch. Pathol. Lab. Med.* **2020**, *144*, 221–228. [CrossRef] [PubMed]
6. Hanna, M.G.; Pantanowitz, L.; Evans, A.J. Overview of Contemporary Guidelines in Digital Pathology: What Is Available in 2015 and What Still Needs to Be Addressed? *J. Clin. Pathol.* **2015**, *68*, 499–505. [CrossRef]
7. Eloy, C.; Bychkov, A.; Pantanowitz, L.; Fraggetta, F.; Bui, M.M.; Fukuoka, J.; Zerbe, N.; Hassell, L.; Parwani, A. DPA–ESDIP–JSDP Task Force for Worldwide Adoption of Digital Pathology. *J. Pathol. Inform.* **2021**, *12*, 51. [CrossRef]
8. Fraggetta, F.; L'Imperio, V.; Ameisen, D.; Carvalho, R.; Leh, S.; Kiehl, T.-R.; Serbanescu, M.; Racoceanu, D.; Della Mea, V.; Polonia, A.; et al. Best Practice Recommendations for the Implementation of a Digital Pathology Workflow in the Anatomic Pathology Laboratory by the European Society of Digital and Integrative Pathology (ESDIP). *Diagnostics* **2021**, *11*, 2167. [CrossRef]
9. Chong, T.; Palma-Diaz, M.F.; Fisher, C.; Gui, D.; Ostrzega, N.L.; Sempa, G.; Sisk, A.E.; Valasek, M.; Wang, B.Y.; Zuckerman, J.; et al. The California Telepathology Service: UCLA's Experience in Deploying a Regional Digital Pathology Subspecialty Consultation Network. *J. Pathol. Inform.* **2019**, *10*, 31. [CrossRef]
10. Williams, B.J.; Treanor, D. Practical Guide to Training and Validation for Primary Diagnosis with Digital Pathology. *J. Clin. Pathol.* **2020**, *73*, 418–422. [CrossRef]
11. Mukhopadhyay, S.; Feldman, M.D.; Abels, E.; Ashfaq, R.; Beltaifa, S.; Cacciabeve, N.G.; Cathro, H.P.; Cheng, L.; Cooper, K.; Dickey, G.E.; et al. Whole Slide Imaging Versus Microscopy for Primary Diagnosis in Surgical Pathology. *Am. J. Surg. Pathol.* **2018**, *42*, 39–52. [CrossRef]
12. Borowsky, A.D.; Glassy, E.F.; Wallace, W.D.; Kallichanda, N.S.; Behling, C.A.; Miller, D.V.; Oswal, H.N.; Feddersen, R.M.; Bakhtar, O.R.; Mendoza, A.E.; et al. Digital Whole Slide Imaging Compared with Light Microscopy for Primary Diagnosis in Surgical Pathology: A Multicenter, Double-Blinded, Randomized Study of 2045 Cases. *Arch. Pathol. Lab. Med.* **2020**, *144*, 1245–1253. [CrossRef]
13. Montezuma, D.; Monteiro, A.; Fraga, J.; Ribeiro, L.; Gonçalves, S.; Tavares, A.; Monteiro, J.; Macedo-Pinto, I. Digital Pathology Implementation in Private Practice: Specific Challenges and Opportunities. *Diagnostics* **2022**, *12*, 529. [CrossRef]
14. Girolami, I.; Pantanowitz, L.; Marletta, S.; Brunelli, M.; Mescoli, C.; Parisi, A.; Barresi, V.; Parwani, A.; Neil, D.; Scarpa, A.; et al. Diagnostic Concordance between Whole Slide Imaging and Conventional Light Microscopy in Cytopathology: A Systematic Review. *Cancer Cytopathol.* **2020**, *128*, 17–28. [CrossRef]
15. Goacher, E.; Randell, R.; Williams, B.; Treanor, D. The Diagnostic Concordance of Whole Slide Imaging and Light Microscopy: A Systematic Review. *Arch. Pathol. Lab. Med.* **2016**, *141*, 151–161. [CrossRef]
16. Houghton, J.P.; Ervine, A.J.; Kenny, S.L.; Kelly, P.J.; Napier, S.S.; McCluggage, W.G.; Walsh, M.Y.; Hamilton, P.W. Concordance between Digital Pathology and Light Microscopy in General Surgical Pathology: A Pilot Study of 100 Cases. *J. Clin. Pathol.* **2014**, *67*, 1052–1055. [CrossRef]
17. Elmore, J.G.; Longton, G.M.; Pepe, M.S.; Carney, P.A.; Nelson, H.D.; Allison, K.H.; Geller, B.M.; Onega, T.; Tosteson, A.N.A.; Mercan, E.; et al. A Randomized Study Comparing Digital Imaging to Traditional Glass Slide Microscopy for Breast Biopsy and Cancer Diagnosis. *J. Pathol. Inform.* **2017**, *8*, 12. [CrossRef]
18. Tabata, K.; Mori, I.; Sasaki, T.; Itoh, T.; Shiraishi, T.; Yoshimi, N.; Maeda, I.; Harada, O.; Taniyama, K.; Taniyama, D.; et al. Whole-Slide Imaging at Primary Pathological Diagnosis: Validation of Whole-Slide Imaging-Based Primary Pathological Diagnosis at Twelve Japanese Academic Institutes. *Pathol. Int.* **2017**, *67*, 547–554. [CrossRef]
19. Williams, B.J.; Bottoms, D.; Treanor, D. Future-Proofing Pathology: The Case for Clinical Adoption of Digital Pathology. *J. Clin. Pathol.* **2017**, *70*, 1010–1018. [CrossRef]
20. García-Rojo, M.; De Mena, D.; Muriel-Cueto, P.; Atienza-Cuevas, L.; Domínguez-Gómez, M.; Bueno, G. New European Union Regulations Related to Whole Slide Image Scanners and Image Analysis Software. *J. Pathol. Inform.* **2019**, *10*, 2. [CrossRef]
21. Pantanowitz, L.; Sharma, A.; Carter, A.B.; Kurc, T.; Sussman, A.; Saltz, J. Twenty Years of Digital Pathology: An Overview of the Road Travelled, What Is on the Horizon, and the Emergence of Vendor-Neutral Archives. *J. Pathol. Inform.* **2018**, *9*, 40. [CrossRef]
22. Ho, J.; Ahlers, S.M.; Stratman, C.; Aridor, O.; Pantanowitz, L.; Fine, J.L.; Kuzmishin, J.A.; Montalto, M.C.; Parwani, A.V. Can Digital Pathology Result In Cost Savings? A Financial Projection For Digital Pathology Implementation at a Large Integrated Health Care Organization. *J. Pathol. Inform.* **2014**, *5*, 33. [CrossRef] [PubMed]
23. Aeffner, F.; Zarella, M.D.; Buchbinder, N.; Bui, M.M.; Goodman, M.R.; Hartman, D.J.; Lujan, G.M.; Molani, M.A.; Parwani, A.V.; Lillard, K.; et al. Introduction to Digital Image Analysis in Whole-Slide Imaging: A White Paper from the Digital Pathology Association. *J. Pathol. Inform.* **2019**, *10*, 9. [CrossRef] [PubMed]
24. Abels, E.; Pantanowitz, L.; Aeffner, F.; Zarella, M.D.; van der Laak, J.; Bui, M.M.; Vemuri, V.N.; Parwani, A.V.; Gibbs, J.; Agosto-Arroyo, E.; et al. Computational Pathology Definitions, Best Practices, and Recommendations for Regulatory Guidance: A White Paper from the Digital Pathology Association. *J. Pathol.* **2019**, *249*, 286–294. [CrossRef] [PubMed]
25. Araújo, A.L.D.; Arboleda, L.P.A.; Palmier, N.R.; Fonsêca, J.M.; de Pauli Paglioni, M.; Gomes-Silva, W.; Ribeiro, A.C.P.; Brandão, T.B.; Simonato, L.E.; Speight, P.M.; et al. The Performance of Digital Microscopy for Primary Diagnosis in Human Pathology: A Systematic Review. *Virchows Arch.* **2019**, *474*, 269–287. [CrossRef] [PubMed]

26. Hanna, M.G.; Reuter, V.E.; Ardon, O.; Kim, D.; Sirintrapun, S.J.; Schüffler, P.J.; Busam, K.J.; Sauter, J.L.; Brogi, E.; Tan, L.K.; et al. Validation of a Digital Pathology System Including Remote Review during the COVID-19 Pandemic. *Mod. Pathol.* **2020**, *33*, 2115–2127. [CrossRef]
27. Alassiri, A.; Almutrafi, A.; Alsufiani, F.; Al, N.A.; Al, S.A.; Musleh, H.; Aziz, M.; Khalbuss, W. Whole Slide Imaging Compared with Light Microscopy for Primary Diagnosis in Surgical Neuropathology: A Validation Study. *Ann. Saudi Med.* **2020**, *40*, 36–41. [CrossRef]
28. Rojo, M.G. Artificial intelligence in Pathological Anatomy. *Rev. Esp. Patol.* **2019**, *52*, 205–207. [CrossRef]
29. Anuncios de Licitación | Licitaciones | Perfiles de Contratante | Plataforma Electrónica de Contratación Pública. Available online: https://contractaciopublica.gencat.cat/ecofin_pscp/AppJava/es_ES/notice.pscp?mode=full&idDoc=63997703&reqCode=viewCn (accessed on 25 December 2021).
30. Capitanio, A.; Dina, R.E.; Treanor, D. Digital Cytology: A Short Review of Technical and Methodological Approaches and Applications. *Cytopathology* **2018**, *29*, 317–325. [CrossRef]
31. Pantanowitz, L.; Parwani, A.V.; Khalbuss, W.E. Digital Imaging for Cytopathology: Are We There Yet? *Cytopathology* **2011**, *22*, 73–74. [CrossRef]
32. Van Es, S.L.; White, V.; Ross, J.; Greaves, J.; Gay, S.; Holzhauser, D.; Badrick, T. Digital Cytopathology: A Constant Evolution (Comments on Capitanio, A.; Dina, R.E.; and Treanor, D. Digital Cytology: A Short Review of Technical and Methodological Approaches and Applications). *Cytopathology* **2018**, *30*, 262–263. [CrossRef]
33. Eccher, A.; Girolami, I. Current State of Whole Slide Imaging Use in Cytopathology: Pros and Pitfalls. *Cytopathology* **2020**, *31*, 372–378. [CrossRef] [PubMed]
34. PANNORAMIC®1000 RX. Available online: https://www.3dhistech.com/wp-content/uploads/2021/09/p1000-rx-brochure-v7-final.pdf (accessed on 25 December 2021).
35. 3DHISTECH Ltd. PANNORAMIC®1000. Available online: https://www.3dhistech.com/research/pannoramic-digital-slide-scanners/pannoramic-1000/ (accessed on 25 December 2021).
36. 3DHISTECH Ltd. PANNORAMIC 250 Flash III. Available online: https://www.3dhistech.com/research/pannoramic-digital-slide-scanners/pannoramic-250-flash-iii/ (accessed on 25 December 2021).
37. PANNORAMIC®Slide Scanners. Available online: https://www.3dhistech.com/wp-content/uploads/2020/06/br-sc-102019--1.pdf (accessed on 25 December 2021).
38. Alcaraz Mateos, E.; Caballero-Alemán, F.; Albarracín-Ferrer, M.; Cárceles-Moreno, F.; Hernández-Gómez, R.; Hernández-Kakauridze, S.; Hernández-Sabater, L.; Jiménez-Zafra, I.; López-Alacid, A.; Moreno-Salmerón, C.; et al. Research on Devices for Handling Whole Slide Images on Pathology Workstations. An Ergonomic Outlook. *Diagn. Pathol.* **2016**, *2*, 2016. [CrossRef]
39. Pantanowitz, L.; Sinard, J.H.; Henricks, W.H.; Fatheree, L.A.; Carter, A.B.; Contis, L.; Beckwith, B.A.; Evans, A.J.; Lal, A.; Parwani, A.V. Validating Whole Slide Imaging for Diagnostic Purposes in Pathology: Guideline from the College of American Pathologists Pathology and Laboratory Quality Center. *Arch. Pathol. Lab. Med.* **2013**, *137*, 1710–1722. [CrossRef] [PubMed]
40. Williams, B.J.; Knowles, C.; Treanor, D. Maintaining Quality Diagnosis with Digital Pathology: A Practical Guide to ISO 15189 Accreditation. *J. Clin. Pathol.* **2019**, *72*, 663–668. [CrossRef]
41. Rojo, M.G.; Bueno, G. Analysis of the Impact of High-Resolution Monitors in Digital Pathology. *J. Pathol. Inform.* **2015**, *6*, 57.
42. Marchessoux, C.; Dufour, A.N.; Espig, K.; Monaco, S.; Palekar, A.; Pantanowitz, L. Comparison Display Resolution On User Impact For Digital Pathology. *Diagn. Pathol.* **2016**, *1*. [CrossRef]
43. Randell, R.; Ambepitiya, T.; Mello-Thoms, C.; Ruddle, R.A.; Brettle, D.; Thomas, R.G.; Treanor, D. Effect of Display Resolution on Time to Diagnosis with Virtual Pathology Slides in a Systematic Search Task. *J. Digit. Imaging* **2015**, *28*, 68–76. [CrossRef]
44. Wilbur, D.C.; Madi, K.; Colvin, R.B.; Duncan, L.M.; Faquin, W.C.; Ferry, J.A.; Frosch, M.P.; Houser, S.L.; Kradin, R.L.; Lauwers, G.Y.; et al. Whole-Slide Imaging Digital Pathology as a Platform for Teleconsultation: A Pilot Study Using Paired Subspecialist Correlations. *Arch. Pathol. Lab. Med.* **2009**, *133*, 1949–1953. [CrossRef]

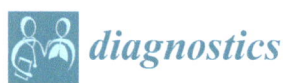 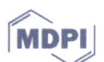

Article

Digital Pathology Implementation in Private Practice: Specific Challenges and Opportunities

Diana Montezuma [1,2,3,*], Ana Monteiro [1], João Fraga [4], Liliana Ribeiro [1], Sofia Gonçalves [1], André Tavares [1], João Monteiro [1] and Isabel Macedo-Pinto [1]

1. IMP Diagnostics, Edifício Trade Center do Bom Sucesso, 61, Sala 809, 4150-146 Porto, Portugal; ana.monteiro@impdiagnostics.com (A.M.); liliana.ribeiro@impdiagnostics.com (L.R.); sofia.goncalves@impdiagnostics.com (S.G.); andre.tavares@impdiagnostics.com (A.T.); joao.monteiro@impdiagnostics.com (J.M.); isabel.macedo.pinto@impdiagnostics.com (I.M.-P.)
2. Cancer Biology & Epigenetics Group, Research Center of IPO Porto (CI-IPOP)/RISE@CI-IPOP (Health Research Network), Portuguese Oncology Institute of Porto (IPO Porto)/Porto Comprehensive Cancer Center (Porto.CCC), R. Dr. António Bernardino de Almeida, 4200-072 Porto, Portugal
3. Doctoral Programme in Medical Sciences, School of Medicine & Biomedical Sciences, University of Porto (ICBAS-UP), Rua Jorge Viterbo Ferreira 228, 4050-513 Porto, Portugal
4. Department of Pathology, Portuguese Oncology Institute of Porto (IPO Porto), R. Dr. António Bernardino de Almeida, 4200-072 Porto, Portugal; joao.fraga89@hotmail.com
* Correspondence: diana.felizardo@impdiagnostics.com

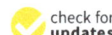

Citation: Montezuma, D.; Monteiro, A.; Fraga, J.; Ribeiro, L.; Gonçalves, S.; Tavares, A.; Monteiro, J.; Macedo-Pinto, I. Digital Pathology Implementation in Private Practice: Specific Challenges and Opportunities. *Diagnostics* **2022**, *12*, 529. https://doi.org/10.3390/diagnostics12020529

Academic Editor: Catarina Eloy

Received: 19 January 2022
Accepted: 16 February 2022
Published: 18 February 2022

Publisher's Note: MDPI stays neutral with regard to jurisdictional claims in published maps and institutional affiliations.

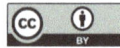

Copyright: © 2022 by the authors. Licensee MDPI, Basel, Switzerland. This article is an open access article distributed under the terms and conditions of the Creative Commons Attribution (CC BY) license (https://creativecommons.org/licenses/by/4.0/).

Abstract: Digital pathology (DP) is being deployed in many pathology laboratories, but most reported experiences refer to public health facilities. In this paper, we report our experience in DP transition at a high-volume private laboratory, addressing the main challenges in DP implementation in a private practice setting and how to overcome these issues. We started our implementation in 2020 and we are currently scanning 100% of our histology cases. Pre-existing sample tracking infrastructure facilitated this process. We are currently using two high-capacity scanners (Aperio GT450DX) to digitize all histology slides at 40×. Aperio eSlide Manager WebViewer viewing software is bidirectionally linked with the laboratory information system. Scanning error rate, during the test phase, was 2.1% (errors detected by the scanners) and 3.5% (manual quality control). Pre-scanning phase optimizations and vendor feedback and collaboration were crucial to improve WSI quality and are ongoing processes. Regarding pathologists' validation, we followed the Royal College of Pathologists recommendations for DP implementation (adapted to our practice). Although private sector implementation of DP is not without its challenges, it will ultimately benefit from DP safety and quality-associated features. Furthermore, DP deployment lays the foundation for artificial intelligence tools integration, which will ultimately contribute to improving patient care.

Keywords: digital pathology; WSI; LIS; artificial intelligence; routine diagnosis

1. Introduction

Digital pathology (DP) is gaining momentum worldwide as an innovative technology associated with improved laboratory efficiency and productivity. A progressive growth in DP deployment in many laboratories across the globe is taking place, but, in spite of this, real world data indicate that a fully digital transition has been accomplished in only a minority of pathology departments [1–3]. Moreover, most of the successful implementations reported in the literature concern public health laboratories and hospitals [1,4–8]. The reasons for low DP adoption in private practice laboratories are mostly related to the initial high costs of implementation, necessary workflow adjustments and pathologists' receptivity. This is counterbalanced with future prospects of laboratory expenses reduction [8,9], easy remote access to cases and simple web-based case consultation by expert colleagues and improved data security [10,11]. In addition, already available digital tools to assist diagnosis (such as easy measuring, pinpointing or annotating relevant areas, etc.)

can facilitate some pathologists' tasks. Furthermore, the possibility to digitize glass slides enables the advent of artificial intelligence (AI) tools in pathology, which will be key in aiding pathologists in analysing and interpreting high-volume data [12]. The use of AI in pathology has clear potential, as recently demonstrated by the recent US Food and Drug Administration (FDA) approval of Paige Prostate, an AI-based pathology product for in vitro diagnostic use in detecting prostate cancer in biopsies [13]. Moreover, state-of-the-art AI approaches can be used for advanced tasks, including survival and therapy response prediction, which, if rigorously validated, can enhance clinical decision-making in the future [14]. Herein, we outline the roadmap of our implementation and address the specific hurdles of DP deployment in a private setting. We suggest how to overcome these issues so as to fully benefit from all the advantages and opportunities of DP.

2. Materials and Methods

2.1. Our Laboratory

IMP Diagnostics is composed of two laboratories, a central headquarters, based in Porto, and a Lisbon facility. It is a high-volume laboratory, having handled, in 2021, around 215,000 cases. These corresponded to 108,478 histology cases, 90,482 cytology samples and 18,085 molecular tests. The histology cases corresponded to a total of 296,814 slides (H&Es and immunostains). We receive cases not only from Portugal but also from other countries, namely Angola, Cape Verde Islands and Mozambique. There are currently 20 pathologists (4 full-time) and two dermatologists (with dermatopathology subspecialisation) working at our institution. We are a comprehensive private laboratory and not only provide pathology diagnostic services, but we also have a Research and Development (R&D) department, currently focusing on computational pathology projects.

2.2. Information Technology Infrastructure and Tracking System

Our Laboratory Information System (LIS) and sample tracking software are from GestPath (Esblada Medical, Barcelona, Spain). GestPath is a pathological anatomy process management system that digitizes all workflows, covering all areas and users of the service. Our lab already had an integrated 2D-barcode based tracking system, since 2016, which is mandatory for fully DP implementation. This enables adequate sample tracking in every step of the workflow. Patient requests and information arrive to the laboratory in two ways: paper request or direct digital link with the clinic/hospital. Regarding the paper requests, we scan these in order to make them available to consult from the LIS in the near future.

2.3. Imaging, Server and Storage Technology

We have two Aperio GT450DX Scanners by Leica Biosystems. These scanners each have a 450-slide capacity and enable brightfield applications and digitizing at $40\times$ equivalent resolution (0.26 µm/pixel). The scanning in our laboratory includes standard H&E and special histochemical and immunohistochemical stains. We do not digitize immunofluorescence or cytology slides. The Image Managing System (IMS) we use is the Aperio eSlide Manager WebViewer viewing software by Leica Biosystems. Our DP server is a ProLiant DL380 Gen10, with $2\times$ CPU Intel Xeon Silver 4208 CPU-2.10 GHz and 64 GB RAM, running Aperio eSlide Manager virtualized using 16 vCPU and 32 GB of RAM. Our data storage is from NetApp FAS2700 Series (FAS2750) and has 600 TB raw capacity plus 9.7 TB Flash Cache. We have 1 Gigabit per second (Gbps) internal and external client networks and the connection between the server and our internal network is 10 Gbps. Additionally, we have acquired a $2\times$ CPU Intel DL Boost, $4\times$ NVIDIA Tesla Volta V100, 384 GB RAM server for research purposes. For now, we are storing all the digitized slides (as well as the corresponding physical slides) and we do not apply any compression to the files. Regarding the glass slides, we follow the Best Practices Manual of Anatomical Pathology (defined in Portuguese law) and store them for at least 10 years (if malignant) or ≥ 5 years (other conditions). All tissue blocks are stored for 10 years at least. To date there are no rules in

Portuguese law regarding the storage of digital pathology images, but we are expecting to keep in line with physical storage.

2.4. Pathologists' Workstations

We currently have eight available workstations in the Porto laboratory. Most pathologists work part time, so all of them have access to the workstations during their work period. We mainly have two types of workstations (with some variations):

1. Workstation HP Z2 G5 Tower, Intel i7-10700, 16 GB RAM, 512 GB SSD; Radeon Pro W5500 graphic card; Monitor HP Z24N G3 24" (for reporting on LIS) and LG Clinical Monitor LED IPS 27" 16:9 8MP 4K 27HJ712C (for WSI viewing);
2. HP ProOne 600 AIO, Intel Core i5-9500, 8 GB RAM, 256 GB SSD; Intel UHD Graphics 630 graphic card; LCD wide screen FHD IPS 21,5" (for reporting on LIS) and LG Clinical Monitor LED IPS 27" 16:9 8MP 4K 27HJ712C (for WSI viewing).

2.5. LIS and IMS Integration

To allow for this integration, an initial step of requirements definition and vendor negotiation was undertaken. Bidirectional communication between LIS and IMS was implemented allowing the continuous exchange of information between the two systems. Communication between the LIS and the IMS is performed by means of a Health Level 7 messaging protocol. As pathologists are expected to mostly open the case images through the LIS, icons were created on the LIS screen to open the associated paper requests (if available), to call up the specific case images on the IMS. The worklist enables the pathologists to recognize completely digitized cases from only partially digitized ones (there is a specific icon which appears transparent in pending cases and that turns opaque when the case is completely digitized). In addition, an option for pathologists to request re-digitization or physical glass slides retrieval when needed is also being created.

2.6. Quality Control

As a way to test the DP system, before full implementation, we took advantage of our R&D department's simultaneous AI project in colorectal cancer samples [15] and we evaluated the quality of 2963 digitized slides (1664 archive cases and 1299 routine cases). We divided the errors by those detected by the scanners and those detected in the subsequent pathology QC check. The quality control (QC) was performed by pathologists and biomedical scientists first by scanning the entire WSI at low magnification (4–10×) and then zooming in at 40× in multiple areas.

2.7. Validation

It is recommended that pathologists go through a training and validation process to ensure adequate transition to DP. This process is not unsubstantial as it requires pathologists to familiarize themselves with a different workflow, learn to handle new software and diagnose from an on-screen image. We followed an adapted version of the Royal College Guidelines, consisting of two phases [16]. As many of our pathologists see more than one diagnostic area, for phase 1 of the validation process, we opted for a mixed initial archive validation set (15 to 20 cases) with a representation of the most commonly described pitfalls in analogue to DP transition [17]. These case sets were elaborated in a personalized manner to each pathologist or small group of pathologists with 2 to 3 diagnostic areas. Then, the pathologists started to assess their routine workflow digitally, checking the corresponding glass slides before case sign-out (validation phase 2). This takes a variable amount of time, according to each pathologist, as it depends on self-assessment, and it is the pathologist's decision when to start to analyse digitized cases only.

3. Results

3.1. Implementation Track, Challenges and Opportunities

Although we can pinpoint the kick-off of our implementation to the scanners installation (23 September 2020), the process began much earlier, around 2018, from the initial idea, to planning the project's feasibility, raising funds and assembling a team (Figure 1). Scanner installation was followed by an in-house assessment of our requirements for IT integration and initial vendor negotiation, with the LIS–IMS integration kick-off starting in January 2021. The integration process then took around 5 to 6 months to be fully completed. Concomitantly, an initial test scanning phase was undertaken (digitizing 2963 slides, 44% archive material and 56% routine), followed by the incremental digitization of the routine workload. We have opted to begin by scanning single subspecialty areas and then scaling up to full digitization; around 110,000 histology slides have been digitized so far. The median scan time during the test phase was 98 s per slide, and the median size file was 1077 megabytes (MB). After the test phase, we optimized fragment placement within the slide (closer positioning of the fragments enabling narrower areas for digitization) and median scanning times and file size improved (74 s/slide and 792 MB median file dimension). In July 2021, we started pathologists' validation, which is still ongoing, and by January 2022, we reached 100% histology digitization. Our implementation track is further discussed in the next section.

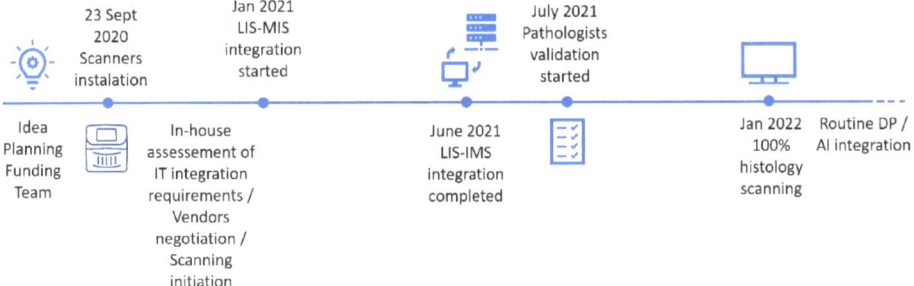

Figure 1. Digital implementation track timeline. DP, Digital Pathology; IMS, Image Managing System; LIS, Laboratory Information System.

The main challenges encountered in DP implementation in our private practice were the high initial investment, difficulty to reorganize the lab workflow to include the scanning steps and little time availability of pathologists to engage in the initial learning phase. Moreover, although DP deployment in the private setting has its challenges, it also shows opportunities: easier and faster case delivery to the pathologists (which is extremely relevant for us, as we have two Porto buildings, as well as two laboratories in different cities, and physical slides need to be transported between sites); simpler case sharing between colleagues located in different places; and enabling working from home (for example, we have recently been able to hire a pathologist that is located in a different city, since he can easily work remotely). At this time, we still perform manual case distribution to subspecialized pathologists, but DP can also enable using computer-aided solutions, namely, to perform automatic case distribution. As we are a private laboratory with a Research and Development Unit, conducting studies in AI solutions for pathology, implementing DP was paramount. This may also be the case for other institutions/departments with an interest in investigation and development in this field. The main challenges and opportunities are outlined in Table 1 and are further addressed in the Discussion section.

Table 1. Challenges and opportunities in DP deployment in private practice.

Challenges
<ul><li>High investment in initial deployment and development.</li><li>Necessity for workflow adjustments in the technical laboratory.</li><li>Time constraints in case turnaround time in the private setting make initial learning phase more difficult for pathologists.</li><li>Software and hardware glitches and malfunction are more prone to happen, comparing with conventional microscopy.</li></ul>
Opportunities
<ul><li>Easy and fast delivery of cases to pathologists.</li><li>Diminishes the need for physical slide transport (namely across different laboratories).</li><li>Facilitates case sharing between colleagues in different locations.</li><li>Enables easy case consultation by experts in other locations.</li><li>Allows working from home and a more flexible schedule.</li><li>Possibility to hire pathologists at different locations of the laboratory.</li><li>Essential for AI and DP Research and Development projects.</li><li>Will enable the use of Computer Aided Solutions in routine work.</li></ul>

3.2. Quality Control

Common errors detected by the scanner included an inability to read the QR code on the slide and image quality issues and tilted slides (the scanner detects slides incorrectly inserted in the rack). Rarely, internal errors were signalized when the scanner was unable to pull out the slide from the rack or insert it back in, causing the scanning process to stop. During our test phase, 46 out of 2172 WSIs, in which this information was available, showed an error detected by the scanners (2.1%), with "skipped barcode" being the most common (25 cases). Regarding the other error types presented by the scanners: 14 "low image quality" cases (14/46 cases); 3 "tilted slide" (3/46 slides); 2 "no tissue" (2 cases, in which a minute fragment was not detected by the scanner); and 2 "internal errors". In the ensuing manual pathology QC, the most commonly encountered issues were out of focus areas (which could vary between only focal areas to extensive ones), striping (horizontal stripes are seen across the image) and stitch error/mismatch (most WSI scanners capture contiguous images from the glass slide as patches and these sub-images are then put together to create the WSI. Sometimes this process can result in misalignment between the image patches or visible striping). In Figure 2, examples of errors detected during pathology QC are shown: 545 of 2963 WSIs had issues detected by the pathology QC (18.4%), but the majority of these corresponded to only small out-of-focus areas (440; 80.7%), with no probable impact in case diagnosis. As such, more relevant issues were seen in 105 slides (3.5% of all the analysed slides). Most of these (70 slides) were cases with apparent pre-scanning hitches, such as bubbles or folds. So, regarding slides in pristine conditions, only 35 presented significant errors detected on path QC. An additional detected issue corresponded to cases of duplicate or non-read slides that were only detected during pathology QC, with no warning message from the scanner (59 cases, 2%).

3.3. Validation

We started the validation process in July 2021, first with only one pathologist to allow for team and system verification and adjustments without disrupting routine workflow. We then scaled the validation process to small groups of pathologists at a time. We decided to start with the Porto headquarters laboratory, and only after will we start Lisbon's pathologists' validation process. Regarding phase 1 of the validation process, it has taken longer than predicted: around one to two months. For pathologists who have already initiated validation, most are in the final stage: routine observation of scanned slides and confrontation with corresponding glass slides before case sign-out. In our experience, the most commonly reported difficulties have been difficulty to discriminate H. pylori in gastric biopsy samples, nuclear detail assessment and mitosis counting. Granulomas and fungi detection were also considered potential pitfalls.

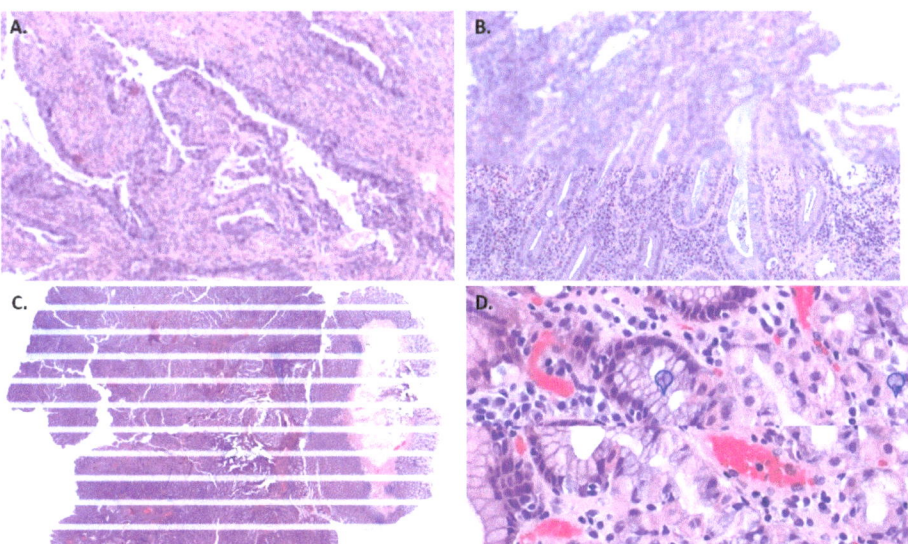

Figure 2. Errors detected in pathology quality control. (**A**). Out of focus. (**B**). Out of focus horizontal band. (**C**). Striping; (**D**). Stitch error/mismatch.

4. Discussion

4.1. Implementation Track, Challenges and Opportunities

In Figure 1, we describe our implementation path. One major issue in private settings is the ability to fund such a high-stake investment. In our case, as our implementation is part of a wider innovation project, part of our deployment (circa 70%) was financed by the European Regional Development Fund through an Operational Programme for Competitiveness and Internationalization. Applying for external funding may help other institutions in the process of DP deployment. Although DP is described as cost-efficient, leading to time savings in workflow and costs reduction [8,18,19], there should be no doubt that implementing DP represents a significant initial expense, as well as ongoing costs. Importantly, the possibility of future integration with AI solutions and operating in a scalable economy will introduce additional value [20,21]. In our case particularly, since we have laboratories in different locations, further relevant savings are expected due to the decreased transport of slides/blocks between cities. Regarding our implementation timeline, we were caught in the COVID pandemic and, although this emphasized the value of easy remote access to the lab, it has negatively impacted our deployment, and some phases took longer than anticipated. After the scanners installation, and before the official IT integration request was made, it was necessary to first define our system requirements in-house and to negotiate our options with the vendors, which took around 2 to 3 months. The integration process between the LIS and IMS then took approximately 5 to 6 months, being concluded in June 2021. Since the LIS provider did not have prior experience of integration with our IMS vendor, it had to be customized and built from scratch. Another issue in this process was the fact that the visualization software was not fully optimized for the 4 K monitors and, as such, we had to lower monitor resolution to improve performance. This precluded taking full advantage of the 40× high quality digitization and it is still being addressed with vendors (it is expected to be fixed in the new version of the software). As stated by Stathonikos N. et al., the process towards digital implementation is, at times, a "rocky road" and, as such, some issues during this undertaking are to be expected [6]. Importantly, turnaround time for case sign-out in private practice is highly constrained, so the most difficult step of the process was probably to initiate full capacity digitization (achieved in January 2022), since we had to adjust our workflow to limit the delay caused by adding the scanning step to the process. The way to improve this was to maintain a sustained flow, loading both scanners continuously, and also to optimize pre-scanning bottleneck steps. We opted for an incremental rollout for DP, firstly just scanning subspecialty areas and then scaling up to full digitization. This gave us more time to address possible constraints and difficulties. We also tried to diminish cases to be digitized overnight, since if a significant error occurred, there would not be a way to fix it timely. As such, we currently digitize almost all slides during the day, leaving only small batches, if needed, at night. Each laboratory must estimate its needs before deciding which equipment to acquire. Being a high-volume facility, we need to scan a large volume of slides daily (around 1000 slides on average), so our choice of having two high throughput scanners was crucial. After the initial test phase, we also optimized fragment placement within the slide (closer positioning enabling narrower areas for digitization) and the average scanning time and slide file size diminished. Regardless, these values are just a pointer, and will be different across different labs, as they vary according to the sample types: slides with more material (surgical specimens or dispersed biopsy fragments in the slide) will result, as expected, in longer scanning times and heavier file sizes.

4.2. Quality Control

Most articles addressing digital QC report a low scanning error rate, usually around 1–1.5%%, and, at most, less than 5% [1,7,9,22]. However, most studies only report the errors detected by the scanner and not by visual assessment of WSI image quality. Different labs report different ways to perform pathology QC: from checking all WSIs [5], to a percentage of cases, or even not performing a WSI QC, since it takes a significant amount of time for technicians to execute and can be considered unnecessary if the error rate is negligible [1]. In our experience, significant focus errors were encountered in 3.5% WSIs during the manual pathology QC in the test phase. On further review, we realized that many of these slides had some pre-scanning issues, such as bubbles, folds, excess mounting medium, etc. Thus, it is extremely important to optimize pre-analytical steps. First of all, to ensure adequate slide labelling; in our lab the slides are engraved with the QR codes, which leads to less scanning errors (most of the registered "skipped barcode" cases happened in archive slides, with stick on labels). Another important step is to ensure the slides have correctly aligned coverslips and are free of excessive mounting media. We use an automated equipment (HistoCore SPECTRA ST, Leica Biosystems) to obtain consistent staining and coverslipping. Regardless, sometimes we still have small bubbles appearing or excess mounting medium and addressing this issue has been a continuous process with the vendor. Some authors advocate the use of film coverslippers to minimize these problems [7,20]. Other important aspects to tackle are to make sure slides are clean by waiting until slides are fully dry before loading them into the scanner, and to ensure that slides are placed flat into the scanner rack. Regarding duplicate and non-read cases (which occurred in 2% of analysed cases), it was found to be a random event, in which the scanner did not recognize a rack and would process it twice (duplicating the slides) or, alternatively, would not scan it. This happened in two test batches and has occurred again, randomly, and, unfortunately, not so uncommonly, during the routine implementation phase, requiring multiple technical interventions by the vendor until the problem was finally solved. Lastly, we would recommend choosing the scanner location wisely. For a lean streamline, locate the scanners in a way that allows for a continuous workflow within the technical laboratory. Additionally, make sure scanners are placed on a flat surface, with as little vibration as possible. A missed issue when we started implementing DP in our laboratory was that one of the scanners was placed between two joint tables, causing some instability and probably contributing to scanning disturbances. After the initial test phase, we decided to register all scanner detected errors and to perform occasional pathology QC in a percentage of cases (about 5–10% of the daily workflow, randomly selected), as a way to address any issues and to give feedback to vendors if significant errors happened. Despite this, we continue to adjust our quality control necessities as implementation proceeds, as it requires a balance between necessity and time availability to perform it. Additionally, our LIS system will allow the pathologists to request the re-digitization of any slide they consider low quality. The analysis of these reported cases will give us a best estimation of the true impact of scanning errors on diagnosis. We expect to be in line with other studies that state that re-scanning requests are infrequent and do not impact global turnaround time [22], but we must emphasize that the initial deployment phase has shown more quality issues than anticipated.

4.3. Validation

As previously stated, phase 1 of the validation process has taken pathologists longer than predicted: around one to two months. The fact that many pathologists work in the laboratory only part time, alongside a significant workload, made it difficult to evaluate the archive slide boxes and it was carried out over a gradual period of time. In fact, one of the biggest issues in deploying DP in a private laboratory is that many pathologists work only part time and the turnaround time for case sign-out is highly constrained. So, during the adjustment period, when a two-track observation (analogue and digital) is necessary, the pathologist's efficiency can be negatively impacted (having to see the same case twice). This is a practical handicap of DP implementation in a private setting. One way to ease this during phase 2 of validation was that pathologists only had to assess a percentage of daily workload in both digital and glass slides, at their own pace. Additionally, realizing the added value DP can represent once it is fully implemented (such as possibility to work remotely, simplicity in second opinion requests, available digital tools to assist diagnosis and, in the near future, AI driven solutions) has facilitated the pathologists' engagement to this initial validation phase. Furthermore, many pathologists report an easy and relatively fast learning curve, and, as such, the two-track period can be shortened and cause less disruption [23]. Even so, we have decided to maintain the parallel analogue and digital workflows for a period of about one year, in accordance with other implementation reports [4–6], to allow a smooth transition to routine use of DP. Moreover, as advised in the Royal College Guidelines [16,17], it will be up to each pathologist to decide when to abandon glass slides in favour of WSI visualization. Of note is that the two-track workflow, although allowing the pathologist to gain more confidence in DP, precludes all users from taking full advantage of DP benefits, since there is no immediate reduction in time spent and workload related to assembling and delivering glass slides to the pathologists [24]. Other laboratories must be aware of this when deciding their validation procedure. As previously stated, the most common reported difficulties have been difficulty to discriminate H. pylori in gastric biopsies (even when using immunostains, since the focus may be suboptimal in the surface area where most of the bacilli are observed); assessing nuclear detail and counting mitosis. Granulomas and fungi were also more difficult to see on digital versus conventional slides. These findings are in line with other literature reports [5,6,17]. We expect further practice and plan additional improvements to the visualization software that will diminish these issues, as it is currently necessary to check the corresponding physical slides in doubtful cases. Furthermore, future coupled computer-aided solutions have the potential to be noninferior or even superior to conventional microscopy regarding some of these issues: automatic counting mitosis or assessment of the presence of microorganisms, for example, could potentially be performed by robust AI algorithms, solving these current challenges.

5. Conclusions

We are currently digitizing 100% of our histology slides and pathologists are performing the validation process for routine diagnosis using WSIs. DP implementation in a private setting is not without its challenges and has specific difficulties that are important to draw attention to, namely the high costs of its deployment and the pathologists' low time availability to engage in the initial learning phase. Scanning device selection should be based on planned use and budget and care should also be given to LIS–WSI integration and archive requirements. Despite this, we believe the benefits of DP in the long run will far exceed the initial handicaps in its deployment. DP provides lower costs associated with slides assembly, retrieval and transport; facilitates remote work and case consultation (enabling, for example, to hire pathologists from distant locations); and the use of digital tools to ease many diagnostic tasks. DP's potential for improvement in patient safety, work quality and efficiency is, in itself, a sufficient argument for its widespread implementation [25]. The European Society of Digital and Integrative Pathology (ESDIP) has recently provided consensus-based recommendations for the implementation of a DP workflow for the Pathology Laboratory in a practical document that can further assist other practices to successfully deploy DP in Europe [26]. Additionally, future implementation of AI-based solutions will provide many advantages over traditional pathology, namely generating highly precise and consistent readouts that can assist pathologists in their daily decisions. After all, is there any pathologist who will not be happy to automate PD-L1 counting? We hope that DP implementation is seen in a holistic approach, as described by Betmouni S. [2], considering not only technology and pathology laboratories, but also the broad healthcare team and patients as potential beneficiaries.

Author Contributions: D.M. and I.M.-P. defined study concept and design; D.M. wrote the manuscript: original draft preparation, review, and editing; I.M.-P., A.M. reviewed and edited the manuscript; J.F. data acquisition; A.T. provided the IT technical information for the article; J.M., S.G. and L.R. provided technical support and performed data acquisition. All authors read and approved the final paper. All authors have read and agreed to the published version of the manuscript.

Funding: This work is financed by the ERDF—European Regional Development Fund through the Operational Programme for Competitiveness and Internationalization—COMPETE 2020 Programme within project POCI-01-0247-FEDER-045413.

Institutional Review Board Statement: Not applicable.

Informed Consent Statement: Not applicable.

Data Availability Statement: Not applicable.

Conflicts of Interest: The authors declare no conflict of interest.

References

1. Fraggetta, F.; Caputo, A.; Guglielmino, R.; Pellegrino, M.G.; Runza, G.; L'Imperio, V.A. Survival Guide for the Rapid Transition to a Fully Digital Workflow: The "Caltagirone Example". *Diagnostics* **2021**, *11*, 1916. [CrossRef] [PubMed]
2. Betmouni, S. Diagnostic digital pathology implementation: Learning from the digital health experience. *Digit. Health* **2021**, *7*, 20552076211020240. [CrossRef] [PubMed]
3. Schüffler, P.J.; Geneslaw, L.; Yarlagadda, D.V.K.; Hanna, M.G.; Samboy, J.; Stamelos, E.; Vanderbilt, C.; Philip, J.; Jean, M.H.; Corsale, L.; et al. Integrated digital pathology at scale: A solution for clinical diagnostics and cancer research at a large academic medical center. *J. Am. Med. Inform. Assoc.* **2021**, *28*, 1874–1884. [CrossRef] [PubMed]
4. Fraggetta, F.; Garozzo, S.; Zannoni, G.F.; Pantanowitz, L.; Rossi, E.D. Routine Digital Pathology Workflow: The Catania Experience. *J. Patho.l Inform.* **2017**, *8*, 51.
5. Stathonikos, N.; Nguyen, T.Q.; Spoto, C.P.; Verdaasdonk MA, M.; van Diest, P.J. Being fully digital: Perspective of a Dutch academic pathology laboratory. *Histopathology* **2019**, *75*, 621–635. [CrossRef] [PubMed]
6. Stathonikos, N.; Nguyen, T.Q.; van Diest, P.J. Rocky road to digital diagnostics: Implementation issues and exhilarating experiences. *J. Clin. Pathol.* **2021**, *74*, 415–420. [CrossRef]
7. Retamero, J.A.; Aneiros-Fernandez, J.; Del Moral, R.G. Complete Digital Pathology for Routine Histopathology Diagnosis in a Multicenter Hospital Network. *Arch. Pathol. Lab. Med.* **2020**, *144*, 221–228. [CrossRef] [PubMed]
8. Hanna, M.G.; Reuter, V.E.; Samboy, J.; England, C.; Corsale, L.; Fine, S.W.; Agaram, N.P.; Stamelos, E.; Yagi, Y.; Hameed, M.; et al. Implementation of Digital Pathology Offers Clinical and Operational Increase in Efficiency and Cost Savings. *Arch. Pathol. Lab. Med.* **2019**, *143*, 1545–1555. [CrossRef]
9. Quigley, J.C.; Lujan, G.; Hartman, D.; Parwani, A.; Roehmholdt, B.; Van Meter, B.; Ardon, O.; Hanna, M.G.; Kelly, D.; Sowards, C.; et al. Dissecting the Business Case for Adoption and Implementation of Digital Pathology: A White Paper from the Digital Pathology Association. *J. Pathol. Inform.* **2021**, *12*, 17. [CrossRef]

10. Jahn, S.W.; Plass, M.; Moinfar, F. Digital Pathology: Advantages, Limitations and Emerging Perspectives. *J. Clin. Med.* **2020**, *9*, 3697. [CrossRef]
11. Pallua, J.D.; Brunner, A.; Zelger, B.; Schirmer, M.; Haybaeck, J. The future of pathology is digital. *Pathol. Res. Pract.* **2020**, *216*, 153040. [CrossRef] [PubMed]
12. Bera, K.; Schalper, K.A.; Rimm, D.L.; Velcheti, V.; Madabhushi, A. Artificial intelligence in digital pathology—New tools for diagnosis and precision oncology. *Nat. Rev. Clin. Oncol.* **2019**, *16*, 703–715. [CrossRef] [PubMed]
13. Food and Drug Administration. Available online: https://www.accessdata.fda.gov/cdrh_docs/pdf20/DEN200080.pdf (accessed on 4 November 2021).
14. Echle, A.; Rindtorff, N.T.; Brinker, T.J.; Luedde, T.; Pearson, A.T.; Kather, J.N. Deep learning in cancer pathology: A new generation of clinical biomarkers. *Br. J. Cancer* **2021**, *124*, 686–696. [CrossRef] [PubMed]
15. Oliveira, S.P.; Neto, P.C.; Fraga, J.; Montezuma, D.; Monteiro, A.; Monteiro, J.; Ribeiro, L.; Gonçalves, S.; Pinto, I.M.; Cardoso, J.S. CAD systems for colorectal cancer from WSI are still not ready for clinical acceptance. *Sci. Rep.* **2021**, *11*, 14358. [CrossRef] [PubMed]
16. Royal College of Pathologists. Best Practice Recommendations for Digital Pathology. 2018. Available online: https://www.rcpath.org/resourceLibrary/best-practicerecommendations-for-implementing-digital-pathology-pdf (accessed on 20 December 2021).
17. Williams, B.J.; Treanor, D. Practical guide to training and validation for primary diagnosis with digital pathology. *J. Clin. Pathol.* **2020**, *73*, 418–422. [CrossRef] [PubMed]
18. Baidoshvili, A.; Bucur, A.; van Leeuwen, J.; van der Laak, J.; Kluin, P.; van Diest, P.J. Evaluating the benefits of digital pathology implementation: Time savings in laboratory logistics. *Histopathology* **2018**, *73*, 784–794. [CrossRef] [PubMed]
19. Ho, J.; Ahlers, S.M.; Stratman, C.; Aridor, O.; Pantanowitz, L.; Fine, J.L.; Kuzmishin, J.A.; Montalto, M.C.; Parwani, A.V. Can digital pathology result in cost savings? A financial projection for digital pathology implementation at a large integrated health care organization. *J. Pathol. Inform.* **2014**, *5*, 33. [CrossRef]
20. Eloy, C.; Vale, J.; Curado, M.; Polónia, A.; Campelos, S.; Caramelo, A.; Sousa, R.; Sobrinho-Simões, M. Digital Pathology Workflow Implementation at IPATIMUP. *Diagnostics* **2021**, *11*, 2111. [CrossRef] [PubMed]
21. Hanna, M.G.; Ardon, O.; Reuter, V.E.; Sirintrapun, S.J.; England, C.; Klimstra, D.S.; Hameed, M.R. Integrating digital pathology into clinical practice. *Mod Pathol. Mod. Pathol.* **2021**, *35*, 152–164. [CrossRef]
22. Hanna, M.G.; Reuter, V.E.; Ardon, O.; Kim, D.; Sirintrapun, S.J.; Schüffler, P.J.; Busam, K.J.; Sauter, J.L.; Brogi, E.; Tan, L.K.; et al. Validation of a digital pathology system including remote review during the COVID-19 pandemic. *Mod. Pathol.* **2020**, *33*, 2115–2127. [CrossRef] [PubMed]
23. Retamero, J.A.; Aneiros-Fernandez, J.; Del Moral, R.G. Microscope? No, Thanks: User Experience With Complete Digital Pathology for Routine Diagnosis. *Arch. Pathol. Lab. Med.* **2020**, *144*, 672–673. [CrossRef]
24. Evans, A.J.; Salama, M.E.; Henricks, W.H.; Pantanowitz, L. Implementation of Whole Slide Imaging for Clinical Purposes: Issues to Consider From the Perspective of Early Adopters. *Arch. Pathol. Lab. Med.* **2017**, *141*, 944–959. [CrossRef] [PubMed]
25. Griffin, J.; Treanor, D. Digital pathology in clinical use: Where are we now and what is holding us back? *Histopathology* **2017**, *70*, 134–145. [CrossRef] [PubMed]
26. Fraggetta, F.; L'Imperio, V.; Ameisen, D.; Carvalho, R.; Leh, S.; Kiehl, T.R.; Serbanescu, M.; Racoceanu, D.; Della Mea, V.; Polonia, A.; et al. Best Practice Recommendations for the Implementation of a Digital Pathology Workflow in the Anatomic Pathology Laboratory by the European Society of Digital and Integrative Pathology (ESDIP). *Diagnostics* **2021**, *11*, 2167. [CrossRef] [PubMed]

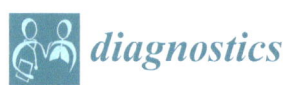 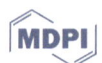

Review

Implementation of Artificial Intelligence in Diagnostic Practice as a Next Step after Going Digital: The UMC Utrecht Perspective

Rachel N. Flach [1], Nina L. Fransen [1], Andreas F. P. Sonnen [1], Tri Q. Nguyen [1], Gerben E. Breimer [1], Mitko Veta [1,2], Nikolas Stathonikos [1], Carmen van Dooijeweert [1] and Paul J. van Diest [1,*]

[1] Department of Pathology, University Medical Center Utrecht, 3508 GA Utrecht, The Netherlands; r.n.flach-2@umcutrecht.nl (R.N.F.); n.l.fransen@umcutrecht.nl (N.L.F.); a.f.p.sonnen-3@umcutrecht.nl (A.F.P.S.); t.q.nguyen@umcutrecht.nl (T.Q.N.); g.e.breimer-2@umcutrecht.nl (G.E.B.); mitko.veta@gmail.com (M.V.); nstatho2@umcutrecht.nl (N.S.); c.vandooijeweert-3@umcutrecht.nl (C.v.D.)

[2] Department of Biomedical Engineering, Eindhoven University of Technology, 5600 MB Eindhoven, The Netherlands

* Correspondence: p.j.vandiest@umcutrecht.nl

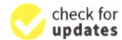

Abstract: Building on a growing number of pathology labs having a full digital infrastructure for pathology diagnostics, there is a growing interest in implementing artificial intelligence (AI) algorithms for diagnostic purposes. This article provides an overview of the current status of the digital pathology infrastructure at the University Medical Center Utrecht and our roadmap for implementing AI algorithms in the next few years.

Keywords: artificial intelligence; machine learning; digital pathology; roadmap; implementation

Citation: Flach, R.N.; Fransen, N.L.; Sonnen, A.F.P.; Nguyen, T.Q.; Breimer, G.E.; Veta, M.; Stathonikos, N.; van Dooijeweert, C.; van Diest, P.J. Implementation of Artificial Intelligence in Diagnostic Practice as a Next Step after Going Digital: The UMC Utrecht Perspective. *Diagnostics* **2022**, *12*, 1042. https://doi.org/10.3390/diagnostics12051042

Academic Editor: Catarina Eloy

Received: 28 March 2022
Accepted: 19 April 2022
Published: 21 April 2022

Publisher's Note: MDPI stays neutral with regard to jurisdictional claims in published maps and institutional affiliations.

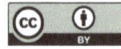

Copyright: © 2022 by the authors. Licensee MDPI, Basel, Switzerland. This article is an open access article distributed under the terms and conditions of the Creative Commons Attribution (CC BY) license (https://creativecommons.org/licenses/by/4.0/).

1. Background

In 2007, we started with the first implementation of a digital pathology system, initially by building up a digital archive for quick revision of cases for and in support of multidisciplinary team meetings, research, and teaching [1]. For scanning roughly 137,000 histological stains and 30,000 immunohistochemical (IHC) stains annually, at that time, we acquired three Aperio ScanScope XT scanners that provided the desired capacity of 700 slides per day. Images acquired at 20× were stored in proprietary pyramid multiresolution.svs file format in a resolution of 0.50 μm/pixel. After the diagnostic process was finished in the traditional microscopic way, slides were scanned. At the time, no quality control of the whole slide images (WSI) was performed. Only scanning failures that were seen by chance were manually corrected. Making use of the vendor's application programming interface (API) and software development kit (SDK), we were able to integrate with our pathology reporting system and laboratory information system.

As to storage, the first iteration was a hierarchical storage management solution (Sun Microsystems, Santa Clara, CA, USA). Initially, all images were stored on fiber channel hard disk drives for rapid access and also copied to a scalable tape library in a buffered way. This storage hardware remained in place until migration to an all object based storage disk system. Because of performance problems of the first iteration of the all disk storage system [1], we migrated to the new hospital-wide disk-based bulk storage system with a superb performance.

The first generation of our digital pathology system started to show signs of aging by the end of 2014. Scanning capacity was no longer sufficient because of our growing practice, so we decided to go for a completely new setup to enable fully digital diagnostics, which was implemented in 2015. It comprised three high throughput Hamamatsu XR scanners and one Hamamatsu RS scanner (Hamamatsu City, Japan) for fluorescence and big slides, and the Sectra Picture Archiving Communication System (PACS) (Sectra AB, Linkoping, Sweden).

The system has performed adequately for 6 years, signing out >95% of our histology cases digitally. Occasionally, we revert back to slides for pediatric pathology, mitoses, microorganisms recognition, birefringence assessments, and hematopathology. We do cytology still with the microscope because of a lack of scanning capacity and storage for Z-stack scanning, since this would result in a lack of confidence in digital diagnostics with current image quality. We have seen several important developments in the PACS, such as the implementation of tools to support mitoses and Ki67 counting, a bidirectional link between our reporting system and the PACS, placeholder thumbnails for stains requested and for lacking images. Also, patient safety increased by magnification-sensitive tracking of our movements through the slides to preclude missing tissue parts and flagging thumbnails of unreviewed slides.

2. Current Setup and Activities

We have recently renewed the contracts with Sectra and Visiopharm (the reseller of Hamamatsu in The Netherlands) and have migrated to a new single pathology reporting system with LIMS (Delphic AP, Sysmex, New Zealand). In 2022, we expect to incorporate two regional pathology laboratories into our digital pathology infrastructure. The recent versions of Sectra PACS and Delphic AP are ready to function as a multicenter digital pathology workflow system, which will allow us to work as one virtual team of fully superspecialized pathologists over three locations. In addition, we will be installing four NanoZoomer S360 Hamamatsu high throughput scanners and one NanoZoomer S60 Hamamatsu scanner for fluorescence and whole mounts.

In 2022, dedicated cytology whole slide scanners are expected to enter the market, which we hope to evaluate and purchase to make the jump to digital cytology, without seriously impacting storage.

3. AI Implementation: Current Status and Road Map

At UMC Utrecht, we aspire to implement AI as much and as soon as possible, thereby unleashing the full potential of digital pathology, with benefits for both patients and pathologists. Various studies on AI-implementation, both prospective and retrospective, are currently ongoing within the UMC Utrecht. Examples are the CONFIDENT trials, which will be discussed below. Several algorithms are available that have been developed through collaborations with the Radboud University in Nijmegen and the Technical University of Eindhoven, The Netherlands, that are ready for further testing and validation in daily practice [2–4]. Besides, we work with several companies bringing AI algorithms to the market on implementation. We expect to make pathology diagnostics more objective, faster and intellectually more satisfying, while more importantly our patients will also benefit from the best tissue diagnostics that forms the basis for personalized treatment.

Pathology has always been a medical specialty that was in the frontline of automation (e.g., electronic reporting, speech recognition, image analysis, structured reporting). Although lagged several decades behind radiology in going digital, this was largely due to lack of affordable and fast scanners and infrastructure to handle big image files. There is at this moment a big wave in pathology to catch up with going digital, and we expect AI to be adopted fairly organically. Likely, in view of our inclination towards automation and use of computers, pathologists will easily learn to use and interpret AI interactively, so probably not much education will be necessary. This does not take away that using AI should be user-friendly and integrated into PACS systems [5].

Our Sectra PACS includes an algorithm for assessing the percentage of Ki67 positive nuclei, which is based on AI. Further, we have integrated an in-house developed AI algorithm for recognizing mitotic figures. In an interactive way, an area of interest can within the PACS be demarcated on the WSI after which the algorithm finds mitoses and mitosis-like objects and displays them in galleries. Objects can easily be moved between these galleries to arrive at a final AI-assisted mitotic count (Figure 1).

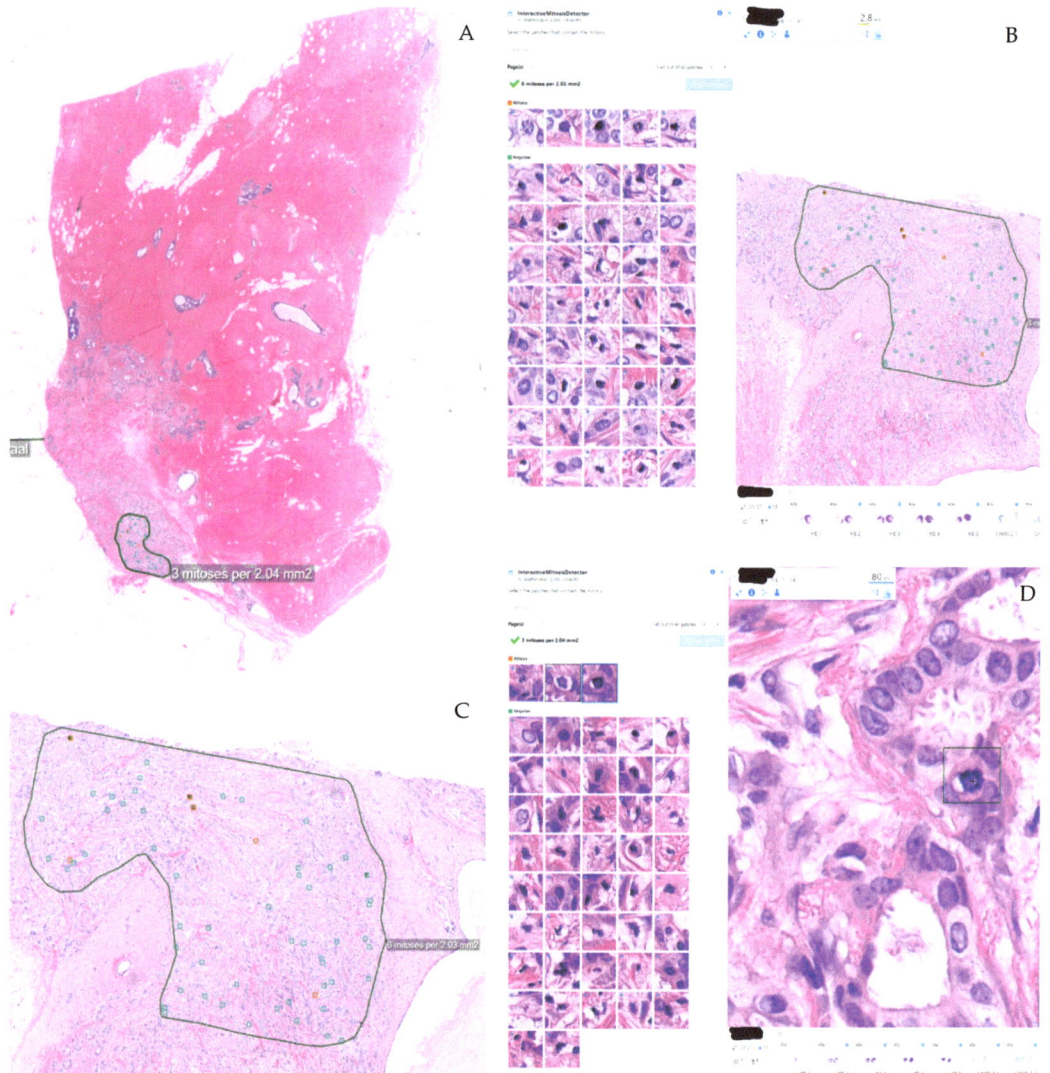

Figure 1. In-house developed AI algorithm for mitotic figures recognition. (**A**) Selecting a region of interest. (**B**,**C**) Interactive Mitosis Detector, with gallery (**B**) and without gallery (**C**). The detector highlights those areas suspicious for mitosis with orange, those negative for mitosis as green. (**D**) Close-up of mitotic figure (mitotic figure selected by the pointer on the right in the gallery), recognized by the algorithm.

At this moment, we are evaluating Qualitopix, a new stain quality control algorithm from Visiopharm, and Derm-AI, a Proscia algorithm for workflow stratification of dermatopathology cases. Within the framework of our new contract with Visiopharm, we will soon implement their breast cancer AI package, consisting of algorithms for ER, PR,

HER2, Ki67, and lymph node metastases. We aim to run these algorithms entirely in the background so results will be ready when the pathologist opens up the case.

4. Developing AI-Implementation Studies

AI algorithms might be implemented in various ways, depending on the algorithm. Some algorithms can be used solely for workflow optimization; for example, for identifying cases that do not need additional diagnostics, or assigning difficult cases to expert pathologists [6]. It might also improve tumor grading consistency [2,7,8]. Whereas currently most AI validating studies are designed retrospectively, useful prospective trials are currently lacking [9].

The design of prospective studies is based on the interests of the many parties involved in AI-implementation in daily clinical practice. First, patients need an accurate diagnosis. For example, no tumor cells may be missed, and tumors must be graded accurately and consistently. While the former is currently achieved in daily clinical practice by using IHC stainings in all negative cases, the latter is not. Significant inter- and intra-laboratory variation in grading of various tumor types (colorectal, breast, prostate) has been observed nationwide [10–14]. As grade can be decisive in treatment choice, the pathologist is pivotal in guiding treatment of cancer patients, and consistency is warranted [15,16]. [Flach, under review] Here, AI algorithms may help pathologists grade more accurately and consistently, and might even serve as a second 'reviewer'.

From a pathologist's point of view, in a field with an ever growing workload, searching, for example, for tumor metastases in (sentinel) lymph nodes is a time-consuming task. It requires meticulous assessment of slides, in general with an overall low yield. Therefore, looking diligently may not be compelling, and pathologists may be prone to use IHC stainings in most, if not all cases, thereby putting pressure on the budget of the pathology department. AI assistance of pathologists on this task may not only save on IHC, but it may lower pathologists' workload, as it has been shown that AI-assisted grading is less time consuming than traditional grading [8].

From the department's financial point of view, costs of the growing number of IHC stainings sometimes even exceed the compensation for assessment of the complete resection specimen. Calculations from our hospital showed, for example, that we spent over €13,000 to detect nine cases of lymph node metastases in 95 sentinel nodes from 68 breast cancer patients. The majority of these (6/9) were not even deemed clinically relevant by medical oncologists, who consider isolated tumor cells in patients without neoadjuvant treatment irrelevant in relation to treatment strategy [17].

In cervical cancer, IHC identified only three patients with micrometastasis and five patients with isolated tumor cells undetected with H&E staining in 630 sentinel nodes from 234 patients. To achieve this, 3791 slides were stained with IHC at an estimated additional cost of €94,775. In 1.4% (95% CI 0.3–4.3%) of patients, routine use of IHC adjusted the adjuvant treatment [18].

For prostate cancer, performing IHC staining as standard of care is not necessarily advised when carcinoma is obviously present or absent [19]. However, it does help pathologists identify small foci, the extent of the tumor and can assist in tumor grading, which is critical in prostate cancer risk stratification and decision-making for performing pelvic lymph node dissection [20]. For this purpose, we spent €22,000 on triple p63/CK5/AMACR IHC staining in a 3-month period in 27 cases.

This financial point of view has to be considered when assessing the viability of business cases for digital pathology and AI implementation. A complex matter, as digital pathology is often seen as an 'add-on', as it does not replace the physical slides, which also need to be kept and stored, at least for now. AI, however, may tip this balance to the side of benefit as it has the potential to improve cancer grading and reproducibility, thereby improving patient treatment and potentially outcome, while lowering costs. This is specifically promising, as the current trend in oncology seems to be that improving patient care may only be realized at higher costs [21].

Lastly, from a legal perspective, algorithms for clinical use must be certified (FDA-approved or IVDR-approved). Currently, the first algorithms are reaching this stage, enabling pathologists to implement and evaluate them in prospective trials (see also below). Nevertheless, it was presumed too big a step to implement them without a safety net (for example, IHC-stainings) in the first implementation phase.

Another imperative ethical point to raise, is that it is currently unimaginable that AI-algorithms will diagnose cases unsupervised or communicate results without human input. Therefore, previous studies evaluating and comparing independent AI-algorithms to pathologists may seem nice, but situations simulated in these studies are highly unlikely to be implemented in current daily clinical practice. Therefore, we strongly feel that the aim is augmented intelligence, rather than AI independently, since pathologists and AI together have been shown to outperform either one alone [5,8,22]. For example, it has been shown that scoring of HER2 IHC staining intensity (which is relevant for treatment decision in breast cancer patients) is done more accurately by a pathologist using an AI assisted digital microscope tool compared to a non-AI assisted pathologist [23]. This is also illustrated by an international survey amongst 718 pathologists in dermatopathology, that showed that only 6% of the pathologists feared that the human pathologist would be replaced by AI in the foreseeable future. The vast majority agreed that AI will improve dermatopathology, while most of these pathologists did not have any experience with AI in their daily practice [24].

Overall, the hope is that AI will improve the quality of diagnosis, reduce the workload of pathologist's performing these diagnostics, and reduce costs of the entire diagnostic process. However, as pointed out by Van der Laak et al., the hope is still to be distinguished from the hype in prospective trials [9].

5. Challenges in Trial Designs

A major challenge in prospective implementation trials is implementing a reference standard in the workflow. Here, it is essential to distinguish assessing biomarkers or other factors, for which currently no reference standard is implemented (like histologic grading or scoring percentages of cells), from tumor detection, for which a reference standard is in place, such as using IHC stainings in all negative cases [17,19].

6. Confident Trials

At the UMC Utrecht, we are currently running two prospective trials on clinical implementation of AI-assisted tumor detection in digital pathology (CONFIDENT). The first is the CONFIDENT B-trial which evaluates the detection of sentinel lymph node metastases in breast cancer. The second is the CONFIDENT-P trial, which evaluates tumor detection in prostate cancer. These studies aim to safely introduce an AI-assisted workflow, and should be easy to use for other algorithms in pathology practice as well. Within these prospective CONFIDENT trials, we investigate the value of AI-assistance in tumor detection in pathology specimens in the current pathology workflow.

7. Interactive vs. Background Processing

There are basically two forms of deployment for AI algorithms in clinical practice: on-demand and background batch analysis. The former approach is interactive, fulfilling the need of the pathologist when encountering a situation during diagnostics (Figure 2). The advantage of this approach is that analysis can be limited to relevant areas in relevant slides selected by the pathologist. The disadvantage is that, depending on the model, runtime might be long, especially if the selected area is too large. Also, the biased nature of interactively selecting certain areas in specific slides (e.g., for mitoses counting) can be considered a disadvantage. Therefore, running algorithms in the background that process full WSI may be the default approach for deploying AI models in practice (Figure 3). It is imperative that results are ready by the time the pathologist opens up the case. However, implementing such automatic processes is not trivial from a technical and functional perspective.

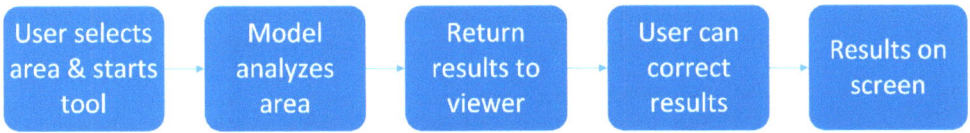

Figure 2. Flowchart showing a workflow for on-demand, interactive processing.

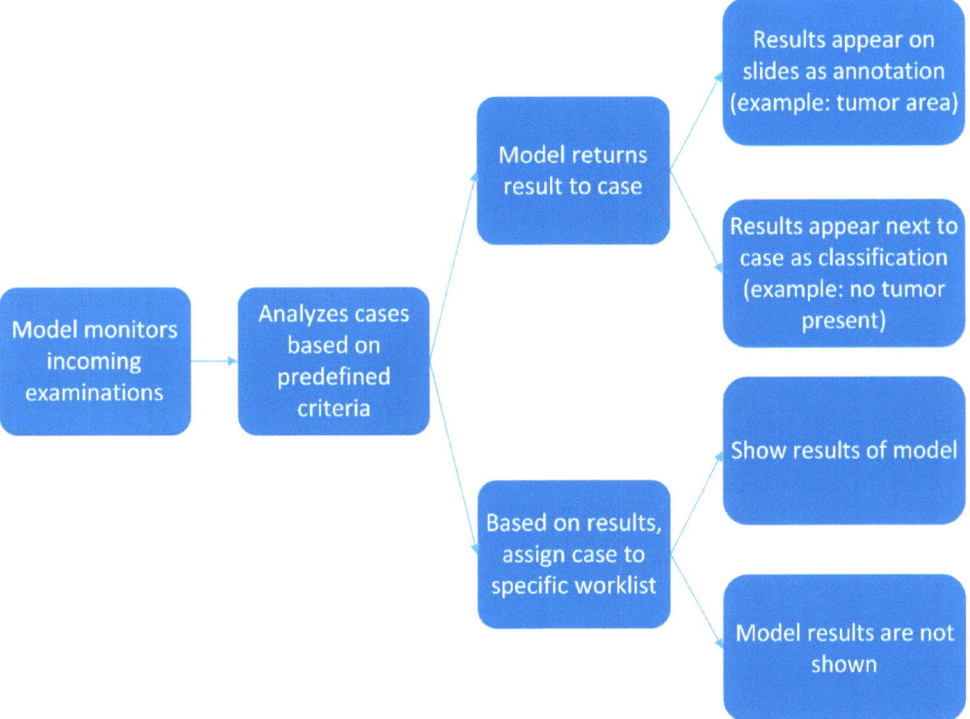

Figure 3. Flowchart showing workflow for background batch analysis, a workflow driven process.

In order to trigger an AI system to start analysis on a WSI, it will have to either have some well-defined criteria to analyze a case, which means that well defined metadata of a case or advanced text mining of grossing description will be used to start the analysis. In absence of such information, the alternative is to perform the analysis on all possible WSI that might fit a broader selection criteria to ensure that the pathologist has access to the results. That would require an extensive hardware infrastructure to ensure that there is no latency between the time the case is ready and the time that the results are ready.

8. Hardware Issues

Running AI algorithms requires significant computing, especially when processing entire WSI, which are easily 10 Gigapixels. Installing and maintaining a local GPU server cluster for AI purposes at a pathology department is costly and, most of the time, an overkill since the GPU capacity will need to accommodate peak loads. This means that using an existing hospital GPU cluster or a cloud solution would be necessary. However, external cloud solutions can be a security and privacy concern. Analyzing WSI entails transferring data outside of the hospital firewall which would either have to be anonymized prior to export or the connection to cloud solution would have to be over a VPN. In addition, the security issues related to anonymizing and exporting images outside the firewall and importing AI algorithm output are not trivial, but can probably be solved.

9. Certification Issues

Historically, healthcare may not be in the frontline of implementing technology tools that have already transformed other areas of commerce and daily life [25]. One factor, among others, that hampers the implementation of new technology tools in health care is the regulation that accompanies medical products. With the promising developments in AI software technology that will assist pathologists in making a more accurate diagnosis, pathologists will in the future increasingly depend on software technology to make their diagnosis. Implementing such AI software tools in clinical practice will improve diagnosis accuracy and therapy response prediction. Therefore, the development and implementation of these tools must not be hampered by unnecessary regulation.

However, these software tools will process sensitive personal medical data, and therefore regulation on the use of this data is necessary to prevent unconsented and secondary use of personal data. In May 2021, the new European regulation on software as a medical device (Medical Device Regulation, MDR) came into effect. This regulation changed the definition of software as a medical device and the risk classification of software. AI software tools that will help pathologists make a more accurate diagnosis now fall in a higher risk score and must be assessed by an officially appointed organization [26]. The MDR aims to improve the regulation and safety of the software used for diagnosing and treating patients. The GDPR (General Data Protection Regulation) from the European Union reduces the obligations regarding administrative formalities before accessing health data. They aim to make data actors more accountable rather than restricting their ability to develop new tools in the first place [27]. The FDA also proposes that the regulation of software development and design for health care needs a different approach than the traditional regulation of hardware-based medical devices [25]. They have therefore proposed a software pre-certification program where they assess organizations that perform high-quality software design, testing, and monitoring. The FDA program aims to develop effective medical device software, drive faster innovation, and enable timely patient access while keeping pragmatic and least burdensome regulatory oversight to verify the continued safety and performance of software tools in the real world [25]. To date, several companies have obtained CE-IVD, IVDR, or FDA approval of their algorithms. For locally developed algorithms, thorough local validation will probably be required in many countries.

10. Deployment of Models in Clinical Practice

The development and training of AI models that can reach decent performance has become increasingly easier in practice thanks to frameworks released by major companies like Google and Facebook (PyTorch and Tensorflow) [28,29] as well as libraries like FastAI, which offer tools to rapidly train new models in a matter of days [30]. However, despite the rapid development tools and resources available, the deployment of such models have proven much more challenging in practice. Apart from the regulatory framework needed to validate a model for clinical practice, the effort required to develop a model into a full-fledged product is a multiple of the effort to train the model. In order to effectively deploy a model in production, there has to be:

- The necessary infrastructure to retrain the model if and when performance drops.
- Records of data versions used with every version of the model released.
- Monitoring infrastructure.
- Serving infrastructure—infrastructure needed to deploy the model.

The AI field is rapidly developing, which means that the technology developed around it is also developing with the same rate. Top-performing models dating from 2 years ago, will be outdated today and will have suffered from model drift. Computer vision models trained on a first generation platform (for example Tensorflow v1), would be almost impossible to port to the latest version without redeveloping/rewriting. That rapid development, which has served as a boom for AI proliferation, has brought along long standing issues found in the rapid software development community namely technical debt [31].

Another issue in deploying AI-models in practice, is trust of the application of AI models. Recently, a lot of discussion and efforts have gone into the topic of explainable AI for medical image analysis. Explainability methods are seen as a tool that can enable or increase the transparency of AI models thus addressing some of the ethical and regulatory concerns of their use [32]. Ghassemi et al. have recently expressed scepticism about state-of-the-art explainability methods and argued that more effort should be put toward proper validation of AI methodology [33]. We generally agree with this sentiment and see explainability methods as just another tool in the toolbox of AI development and validation methods.

11. The Business Case

For patients, implementation of AI algorithms might result in an improved diagnostic process. However, Ho et al. already stated that digital pathology is not likely to be implemented, unless a viable business case is presented, as digital pathology diagnostics workflow comes with significant costs [34]. Next to high acquisition costs, also additional histopathology, IT personnel and costs for integrating with other medical devices and system raise costs, which laboratories cannot easily afford without external help, especially when considering future developments outlined below [34]. Ho et al. found that improving speed and quality of pathology diagnostics, which is necessary for digital pathology, comes with significant savings elsewhere in the healthcare system. The same holds for AI implementation. However, Ho et al. made their financial projections for digital pathology implementation in an integrated health care organization, serving as both a health care provider and the payor [34]. In organizations where this is not the case, it is challenging to turn budget silos into communicating vessels, so it will mostly be the pathology labs themselves that need to build a business case for AI implementation. Bluntly, time savings will likely make pathologists go home earlier, but those will rarely be on such a scale that fewer pathologist FTEs will suffice. Therefore, tangible, straightforward cost savings associated with some key AI algorithms will have to pave the budgetary way for larger-scale AI implementation. For instance, the Visiopharm company claims that their HER2 IHC algorithm reduces the 2+ category, comprising about 20% of breast cancer cases and for which expensive reflex FISH testing is indicated, by some 75%, which would amount to saving €3600 per 100 random breast cancer cases. Second, a prostate cancer algorithm facilitating finding cancer spots may obviate the need for the expensive triple p63/CK5/AMACR IHC staining, besides saving much time with regard to measurements and grading. Third, an AI algorithm that finds micro metastases and isolated tumor cells in sentinel nodes may obviate the need for cytokeratin IHC on step sections, saving up to €100 per sentinel node.

12. AI 2.0

With our experiences in implementing a fully digital pathology workflow, including the first AI algorithms used in daily practice, where do we see AI in pathology going in the future? Considering the current rise of genetic and proteomic methods in pathology diagnostics and the development of spatially-resolved molecular imaging modalities, i.e., spatial transcriptomics and spatial proteomics, it becomes evident that advanced machine learning algorithms will play a key role in making sense of the ever growing amount of data. Especially in the context of precision medicine in a personalized care setting, leveraging on the full potential of all data available is of the utmost importance to select the proper treatment for each patient and prevent unwanted treatments, thus saving overtreatment for the patient, and costs for society. Again, as detailed in the example of the introduction of digital pathology and AI in the UMC Utrecht, careful and stepwise introduction of algorithms will be needed in the future for both quality control and financial reasons.

The following years we will see a rise in research that will try to stratify patient and treatment options based on models that include classical histology, IHC, DNA- and RNA sequencing in bulk, and spatially-resolved molecular imaging methods. Models that will be generated will rely on tabular data (sequencing) and potentially multiscale image data, making an integration and assessment of classifiers without machine learning algorithms unlikely [35,36].

However, as with digital pathology itself, the basis will initially be a well-organized data infrastructure/repository for tabular and image data on which the algorithms can work. In a modest step towards digital pathology 2.0/AI 2.0 at the UMC Utrecht, we are working towards integrating (spatially)-resolved proteomics into our diagnostics routines. We use matrix assisted laser desorption/ionization-based mass spectrometry imaging (MALDI-MSI) in various research projects using patient tissues. MALDI-MSI can provide a molecular profile of thousands of molecules at each image pixel without the loss of tissue architecture. This opens the way, for example, to assess molecular tumor heterogeneity or to look at amyloid composition together with classical histology on the same image, by carefully selecting peaks from the measured mass spectra [37]. Integrating these data into our digital pathology environment/PACS system seems natural, as pathologists are already used to annotating different regions for diagnostics. Eventually, AI algorithms will annotate regions of interest and, from these regions, pick peaks on the mass spectrum to assess molecular composition. As this example shows, there are many hows, buts, and ifs associated with such projects, ranging from file/data framework issues to acceptance by pathologists [36]. However, as our "road-trip" from fully glass-based pathology to "fully-digital" pathology at the UMC Utrecht shows, early investment into the future eventually pays off, and we believe that multiscale integration of molecular and image data—pathomics—is the future of pathology.

Author Contributions: Conceptualization—P.J.v.D.; Visualization—N.S.; Writing—original draft preparation, R.N.F., N.L.F., A.F.P.S., N.S., C.v.D. and P.J.v.D.; Writing—review and editing, R.N.F., N.L.F., A.F.P.S., T.Q.N., G.E.B., M.V., N.S., C.v.D. and P.J.v.D. All authors have read and agreed to the published version of the manuscript.

Funding: This research received no external funding.

Institutional Review Board Statement: Not applicable.

Informed Consent Statement: Not applicable.

Data Availability Statement: Not applicable.

Conflicts of Interest: The authors declare no conflict of interest.

References

1. Stathonikos, N.; Nguyen, T.Q.; Van Diest, P.J. Rocky road to digital diagnostics: Implementation issues and exhilarating experiences. *J. Clin. Pathol.* **2021**, *74*, 415–420. [CrossRef] [PubMed]
2. Bejnordi, B.E.; Veta, M.; Van Diest, P.J.; van Ginneken, B.; Karssemeijer, N.; Litjens, G.; van der Laak, J.A.W.M.; CAMELYON16 Consortium. Diagnostic assessment of deep learning algorithms for detection of lymph node metastases in women with breast cancer. *JAMA* **2017**, *318*, 2199–2210. [CrossRef] [PubMed]
3. Veta, M.; van Diest, P.J.; Willems, S.M.; Wang, H.; Madabhushi, A.; Cruz-Roa, A.; Gonzalez, F.; Larsen, A.B.L.; Vestergaard, J.S.; Dahl, A.B.; et al. Assessment of algorithms for mitosis detection in breast cancer histopathology images. *Med. Image Anal.* **2015**, *20*, 237–248. [CrossRef] [PubMed]
4. Swiderska-Chadaj, Z.; Pinckaers, H.; van Rijthoven, M.; Balkenhol, M.; Melnikova, M.; Geessink, O.; Manson, Q.; Sherman, M.; Polonia, A.; Parry, J.; et al. Learning to detect lymphocytes in immunohistochemistry with deep learning. *Med. Image Anal.* **2019**, *58*, 101547. [CrossRef] [PubMed]
5. Harrison, J.H.; Gilbertson, J.R.; Hanna, M.G.; Olson, N.H.; Seheult, J.N.; Sorace, J.M.; Stram, M.N. Introduction to Artificial Intelligence and Machine Learning for Pathology. *Arch. Pathol. Lab. Med.* **2021**, *145*, 1228–1254. [CrossRef] [PubMed]
6. Litjens, G.; Sánchez, C.I.; Timofeeva, N.; Hermsen, M.; Nagtegaal, I.; Kovacs, I.; van de Kaa, C.H.; Bult, P.; van Ginneken, B.; van der Laak, J. Deep learning as a tool for increased accuracy and efficiency of histopathological diagnosis. *Sci. Rep.* **2016**, *6*, 1–11. [CrossRef] [PubMed]

7. Bulten, W.; Pinckaers, H.; van Boven, H.; Vink, R.; de Bel, T.; van Ginneken, B.; van der Laak, J.; Hulsbergen-van de Kaa, C.; Litjens, G. Automated deep-learning system for Gleason grading of prostate cancer using biopsies: A diagnostic study. *Lancet Oncol.* **2020**, *21*, 233–241. [CrossRef]
8. Raciti, P.; Sue, J.; Ceballos, R.; Godrich, R.; Kunz, J.D.; Kapur, S.; Reuter, V.; Grady, L.; Kanan, C.; Klimstra, D.S. Novel artificial intelligence system increases the detection of prostate cancer in whole slide images of core needle biopsies. *Mod. Pathol.* **2020**, *33*, 2058–2066. [CrossRef]
9. Van der Laak, J.; Litjens, G.; Ciompi, F. Deep learning in histopathology: The path to the clinic. *Nat. Med.* **2021**, *27*, 775–784. [CrossRef]
10. Flach, R.; Willemse, P.P.; Suelmann, B.; Deckers, I.A.G.; Jonges, T.; van Dooijeweert, C.; van Diest, P.J.; Meijer, R.P. Significant Inter- and Intra-Laboratory Variation in Gleason Grading of Prostate Cancer: A Nationwide Study of 35,258 Patients in the Netherlands. *Cancers* **2021**, *13*, 5378. [CrossRef]
11. Van Dooijeweert, C.; van Diest, P.J.; Willems, S.M.; Kuijpers, C.C.H.J.; van der Wall, E.; Overbeek, L.I.H.; Deckers, I.A.G. Significant inter- and intra-laboratory variation in grading of invasive breast cancer: A nationwide study of 33,043 patients in the Netherlands. *Int. J. Cancer* **2020**, *146*, 769–780. [CrossRef] [PubMed]
12. Van Dooijeweert, C.; van Diest, P.J.; Willems, S.M.; Kuijpers, C.C.H.J.; Overbeek, L.I.H.; Deckers, I.A.G. Significant inter- and intra-laboratory variation in grading of ductal carcinoma in situ of the breast: A nationwide study of 4901 patients in the Netherlands. *Breast Cancer Res. Treat.* **2019**, *174*, 479–488. [CrossRef] [PubMed]
13. Kuijpers, C.C.H.J.; Sluijter, C.E.; von der Thüsen, J.H.; Grünberg, K.; van Oijen, M.G.H.; van Diest, P.J.; Jiwa, M.; Nagtegaal, I.D.; Overbeek, L.I.H.; Willems, S.M. Interlaboratory variability in the grading of dysplasia in a nationwide cohort of colorectal adenomas. *Histopathology* **2016**, *69*, 187–197. [CrossRef] [PubMed]
14. Kuijpers, C.C.H.J.; Sluijter, C.E.; von der Thüsen, J.H.; Grünberg, K.; van Oijen, M.G.H.; van Diest, P.J.; Jiwa, M.; Nagtegaal, I.D.; Overbeek, L.I.H.; Willems, S.M. Interlaboratory variability in the histologic grading of colorectal adenocarcinomas in a nationwide cohort. *Am. J. Surg. Pathol.* **2016**, *40*, 1100–1108. [CrossRef] [PubMed]
15. The AACR Pathology Task Force. Pathology: Hub and Integrator of Modern, Multidisciplinary [Precision] Oncology. *Clin. Cancer Res.* **2022**, *28*, 265–270. [CrossRef]
16. Van Dooijeweert, C.; Baas, I.O.; Deckers, I.A.G.; Siesling, S.; van Diest, P.J.; van der Wall, E. The increasing importance of histologic grading in tailoring adjuvant systemic therapy in 30,843 breast cancer patients. *Breast Cancer Res. Treat.* **2021**, *187*, 577–586. [CrossRef]
17. NABON; NVI. *Breast Cancer Guideline*. Available online: https://richtlijnendatabase.nl/richtlijn/borstkanker/tnm_8.html (accessed on 20 April 2022).
18. Baeten, I.G.T.; Hoogendam, J.P.; Jonges, G.N.; Jürgenliemk-Schulz, I.M.; Braat, A.J.A.T.; van Diest, P.J.; Gerestein, G.; Zweemer, R.P. Value of routine cytokeratin immunohistochemistry in detecting low volume disease in cervical cancer. *Gynecol. Oncol.* **2022**. [CrossRef]
19. Epstein, J.I.; Egevad, L.; Humphrey, P.A.; Montironi, R. Best Practices Recommendations in the Application of Immunohistochemistry in the Prostate. *Am. J. Surg. Pathol.* **2014**, *38*, e6–e19. [CrossRef]
20. Mottet, N.; van den Bergh, R.C.N.; Briers, E.; van den Broeck, T.; Cumberbatch, M.G.; de Santis, M.; Fanti, S.; Fossati, N.; Gandaglia, G.; Gillessen, S.; et al. EAU-EANM-ESTRO-ESUR-SIOG Guidelines on Prostate Cancer—2020 Update. Part 1: Screening, Diagnosis, and Local Treatment with Curative Intent. *Eur. Urol.* **2021**, *79*, 243–262. [CrossRef]
21. Schnog, J.J.B.; Samson, M.J.; Gans, R.O.B.; Duits, A.J. An urgent call to raise the bar in oncology. *Br. J. Cancer* **2021**, *125*, 1477–1485. [CrossRef]
22. Wang, D.; Khosla, A.; Gargeya, R.; Irshad, H.; Beck, A.H. Deep Learning for Identifying Metastatic Breast Cancer. *arXiv* **2016**, arXiv:1606.05718.
23. Yue, M.; Zhang, J.; Wang, X.; Yan, K.; Cai, L.; Tian, K.; Niu, S.; Han, X.; Yu, Y.; Huang, J.; et al. Can AI-assisted microscope facilitate breast HER2 interpretation? A multi-institutional ring study. *Virchows Arch.* **2021**, *479*, 443–449. [CrossRef] [PubMed]
24. Polesie, S.; McKee, P.H.; Gardner, J.M.; Gillstedt, M.; Siarov, J.; Neittaanmäki, N.; Paoli, J. Attitudes Toward Artificial Intelligence Within Dermatopathology: An International Online Survey. *Front. Med.* **2020**, *7*, 1–9. [CrossRef] [PubMed]
25. US FDA. *Developing a Software Precertification Program: A Working Model*; US Food and Drug Administration: White Oak, MD, USA, 2019. Available online: https://www.fda.gov/downloads/MedicalDevices/DigitalHealth/DigitalHealthPreCertProgram/UCM629276.pdf (accessed on 18 March 2022).
26. Regulation (EU) 2017/745 of the European Parliament and of the Council of 5 April 2017 on Medical Devices, Amending Directive 2001/83/EC, Regulation (EC) No 178/2002 and Regulation (EC) No 1223/2009 and Repealing Council Directives 90/385/EEC and 93/42/EE. 05-04-2017. 2020. Available online: https://eur-lex.europa.eu/eli/reg/2017/745/oj (accessed on 17 March 2022).
27. Forcier, M.B.; Gallois, H.; Mullan, S.; Joly, Y. Integrating artificial intelligence into health care through data access: Can the GDPR act as a beacon for policymakers? *J. Law Biosci.* **2019**, *6*, 317–335. [CrossRef]
28. PyTorch. From Research to Production. Available online: https://pytorch.org/ (accessed on 18 March 2022).
29. Tensorflow. An End-to-End Open Source Machine Learning Platform. Available online: https://www.tensorflow.org/ (accessed on 18 March 2022).
30. FastAI. Available online: https://www.fast.ai/ (accessed on 18 March 2022).

31. Sculley, D.; Holt, G.; Golovin, D.; Davydov, E.; Phillips, T.; Ebner, D.; Chaudhary, V.; Young, M.; Crespo, J.; Dennison, D. Hidden technical debt in machine learning systems. *Adv. Neural Inf. Process. Syst.* **2015**, *28*, 2503–2511.
32. McKay, F.; Williams, B.J.; Prestwich, G.; Bansal, D.; Hallowell, N.; Treanor, D. The ethical challenges of artificial intelligence-driven digital pathology. *J. Pathol. Clin. Res.* **2022**, *8*, 209–216. [CrossRef]
33. Ghassemi, M.; Oakden-Rayner, L.; Beam, A.L. The false hope of current approaches to explainable artificial intelligence in health care. *Lancet Digit. Health* **2021**, *3*, e745–e750. [CrossRef]
34. Ho, J.; Kuzmishin, J.; Montalto, M.; Ahlers, S.M.; Stratman, C.; Aridor, O.; Pantanowitz, L.; Fine, J.L.; Parwani, A.V. Can digital pathology result in cost savings? A financial projection for digital pathology implementation at a large integrated health care organization. *J. Pathol. Inform.* **2014**, *5*, 33. [CrossRef]
35. Rakha, E.A.; Toss, M.; Shiino, S.; Gamble, P.; Jaroensri, R.; Mermel, C.H.; Po-Hsuan, C.C. Current and future applications of artificial intelligence in pathology: A clinical perspective. *J. Clin. Pathol.* **2021**, *74*, 409–414. [CrossRef]
36. Ahmad, Z.; Rahim, S.; Zubair, M.; Abdul-Ghafar, J. Artificial intelligence (AI) in medicine, current applications and future role with special emphasis on its potential and promise in pathology: Present and future impact, obstacles including costs and acceptance among pathologists, practical and philosoph. *Diagn. Pathol.* **2021**, *16*, 24. [CrossRef]
37. Ucal, Y.; Durer, Z.A.; Atak, H.; Kadioglu, E.; Sahin, B.; Coskun, A.; Baykal, A.T.; Ozpinar, A. Clinical applications of MALDI imaging technologies in cancer and neurodegenerative diseases. *Biochim. Biophys. Acta Proteins Proteomics* **2017**, *1865*, 795–816. [CrossRef] [PubMed]

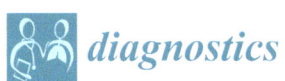

Review

Cultivating Clinical Clarity through Computer Vision: A Current Perspective on Whole Slide Imaging and Artificial Intelligence

Ankush U. Patel [1,*], Nada Shaker [2], Sambit Mohanty [3,4], Shivani Sharma [3], Shivam Gangal [2,5], Catarina Eloy [6,7] and Anil V. Parwani [2,8]

1. Mayo Clinic Department of Laboratory Medicine and Pathology, Rochester, MN 55905, USA
2. Department of Pathology, Wexner Medical Center, The Ohio State University, Columbus, OH 43210, USA; nada.shaker@osumc.edu (N.S.); gangal.6@osu.edu (S.G.); anil.parwani@osumc.edu (A.V.P.)
3. CORE Diagnostics, Gurugram 122016, India; sambit04@gmail.com (S.M.); shivani.sharma@corediagnostics.in (S.S.)
4. Advanced Medical Research Institute, Bareilly 243001, India
5. College of Engineering, Biomedical Engineering, The Ohio State University, Columbus, OH 43210, USA
6. Institute of Molecular Pathology and Immunology of the University of Porto (IPATIMUP), Rua Júlio Amaral de Carvalho, 45, 4200-135 Porto, Portugal; catarinaeloy@hotmail.com
7. Institute for Research and Innovation in Health (I3S Consortium), Rua Alfredo Allen, 208, 4200-135 Porto, Portugal
8. Cooperative Human Tissue Network (CHTN) Midwestern Division, Columbus, OH 43240, USA
* Correspondence: ankushpatel@rcsi.ie; Tel.: +1-206-451-3519

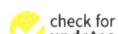

Citation: Patel, A.U.; Shaker, N.; Mohanty, S.; Sharma, S.; Gangal, S.; Eloy, C.; Parwani, A.V. Cultivating Clinical Clarity through Computer Vision: A Current Perspective on Whole Slide Imaging and Artificial Intelligence. *Diagnostics* **2022**, *12*, 1778. https://doi.org/10.3390/diagnostics12081778

Academic Editor: Andreas Kjaer

Received: 19 June 2022
Accepted: 11 July 2022
Published: 22 July 2022

Publisher's Note: MDPI stays neutral with regard to jurisdictional claims in published maps and institutional affiliations.

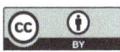

Copyright: © 2022 by the authors. Licensee MDPI, Basel, Switzerland. This article is an open access article distributed under the terms and conditions of the Creative Commons Attribution (CC BY) license (https://creativecommons.org/licenses/by/4.0/).

Abstract: Diagnostic devices, methodological approaches, and traditional constructs of clinical pathology practice, cultivated throughout centuries, have transformed radically in the wake of explosive technological growth and other, e.g., environmental, catalysts of change. Ushered into the fray of modern laboratory medicine are digital imaging devices and machine-learning (ML) software fashioned to mitigate challenges, e.g., practitioner shortage while preparing clinicians for emerging interconnectivity of environments and diagnostic information in the era of big data. As computer vision shapes new constructs for the modern world and intertwines with clinical medicine, cultivating clarity of our new terrain through examining the trajectory and current scope of computational pathology and its pertinence to clinical practice is vital. Through review of numerous studies, we find developmental efforts for ML migrating from research to standardized clinical frameworks while overcoming obstacles that have formerly curtailed adoption of these tools, e.g., generalizability, data availability, and user-friendly accessibility. Groundbreaking validatory efforts have facilitated the clinical deployment of ML tools demonstrating the capacity to effectively aid in distinguishing tumor subtype and grade, classify early vs. advanced cancer stages, and assist in quality control and primary diagnosis applications. Case studies have demonstrated the benefits of streamlined, digitized workflows for practitioners alleviated by decreased burdens.

Keywords: computer vision; digital pathology; whole slide imaging (WSI); artificial intelligence (AI); machine learning; deep learning; diagnostics; laboratory medicine; digital workflow; informatics

1. Introduction

Nearly 2000 years have passed since Emperor Marcus Aurelius sought reinforcement for a society decimated by the first wave of the deadliest pandemic to impact ancient Rome. The same factors lauded as strengths for the seemingly impenetrable empire, e.g., expansive trade networks and large, crowded populations, were those which ultimately led to its demise. These precarious elements had long lingered as a silent plague within a territorial superpower fully primed to combat the fiercest of invaders, yet one which succumbed to those overlooked behind its volcanic rock fortifications. A hidden tinderbox of similar proportion was ignited to plume within many pathology departments upon inception of the 2019 coronavirus (COVID-19) pandemic [1]. New safety and practice restrictions following the wake of the pathogen's propagation increased the demand for digital pathology (DP) solutions and remote services. Issues that had lingered throughout many departments were fervently exacerbated, e.g., specialist deficits and demands of shorter turnaround times (TAT) amidst increasing caseloads and complexity of pathology reports for aging patient demographics harboring higher disease incidence. New solutions were necessitated upon the exhumation of long withstanding problems [2,3]. Diagnostic surgical pathology remains the 'gold standard' for cancer diagnosis despite substantial inter-observer variability from human error, e.g., bias and fatigue, leading to misdiagnosis of challenging histological patterns and missed identification of small quantities of cancer within biopsy material. Digital (whole slide) imaging, now synonymous with DP, has achieved significant milestones within the last 20 years, with whole slide image (WSI) scanning devices evolving in tandem with challenges pervasive throughout the modern pathology landscape. Batch-scanning and continuous or random-access processing capabilities enabling the concurrent uploading of glass slides during the image capture and digitization processes of others have improved laboratory efficiency [4,5]. Many WSI devices can now handle an array of mediums cast on slides of varying dimensions, with single slide load capacity of some devices reaching up to 1000 [2]. WSI scanning cameras and image sensors deliver superior sensitivity, resolution, field-of-view (FOV), and frame rates for optimal capture and digitization of glass slide specimens [2]. Newer scientific CMOS (sCMOS) sensors are featured in many current WSI scanning devices, often as adjunctive to multiple CCD and CMOS sensors for optimization of image quality.

The Ohio State University (Columbus, OH, USA) was among the first academic institutions to invest in DP devices initially purposed for research and archival, i.e., retrospective scanning of oncology cases [6]. Complete transition to a fully integrated digitized workflow for primary diagnosis followed one year after initial steps toward DP adoption in 2016 (Figure 1).

Beneficial returns from the preemptive digital transformation were evidenced throughout the first wave of the coronavirus pandemic in 2020, during which the department was well positioned to continue educational and research activities with minimal disruption [6]. Clinical services persisted with relative fluidity with digital workflow emerging as a pillar of stability during an otherwise catastrophic downtime event for many. Temporary remote sign-out authority issued by the Centers for Medicare and Medicaid Services (CMS) emphasized a growing acknowledgment of the utility that digital practice may afford during such times. The substantial percentage of pathologists (71.4%) who were already trained and approved for on-site WSI for primary diagnosis at the department increased to 90.6% during the pandemic (reflecting a conglomerate percentage of pathologists using WSI exclusively for primary diagnosis and those using WSI in conjunction with glass slides). Diagnostic quality assurance (QA) evaluation noted little discrepancy pertaining to the percentage of major and minor diagnostic errors accrued prior to and following the viral catalyzation of digital workflow. Intraoperative consultation services also remained considerably unaffected from digital deployment. Real-time rerouting of slides to available pathologists in different locations increased staffing flexibility. Loosening of work-from-home restrictions including sign-out fostered greater pathologist latitude. Reduction in in-person interactions and the number of individuals handling case materials served to reduce viral transmission while also reducing glass slide contamination potential. An aging population of pathologists at the department, reflective of US specialist demographics, reported greater satisfaction from improved office ergonomics following DP implementation, e.g., forward screen-viewing fostered a more natural reading position in comparison to microscopy techniques requiring bending movements [3]. Lastly, WSI viewing software equipped with tools for WSI annotation, precision measurements, and side-to-side WSI viewing programs with virtual magnification and annotation tools enabled pathologists to effectively collaborate via image sharing and real-time slide examination mimicking laboratory conditions despite working from remote locations. WSI viewing software also facilitated comparison of H&E images to corresponding immunohistochemistry (IHC) or special stained slides, further aiding the ease and efficiency of intradepartmental consultations.

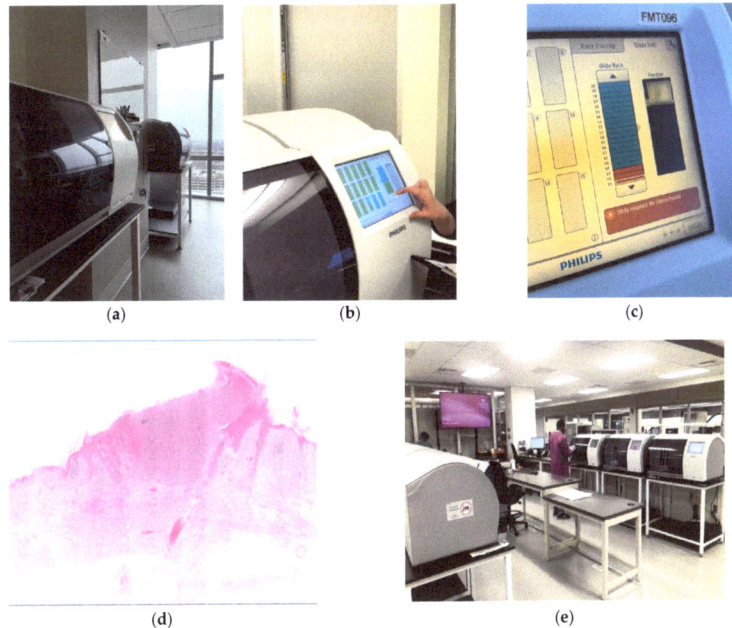

Figure 1. Digital pathology integration at the Ohio State University James Cancer Hospital and Solove Research Institute (captured by David Kellough of The Ohio State University Comprehensive Cancer Center—Arthur G. James Cancer Hospital and Richard J. Solove Research Institute): (**a**) Philips UFS scanners; (**b**) Integrated LCD touchscreen for WSI review; (**c**) Scan failure indicator; (**d**) example of scanning error ("Venetian blinding"); (**e**) Histology laboratory.

Diagnostic merits of WSI are evidenced in scores of investigations reporting significantly high concordance rates with conventional microscopy throughout numerous disciplines and increasingly for arenas formerly posing hurdles curtailing digital adoption, e.g., cytopathology [7–10]. Obstacles in modeling business viability for laboratory digitization are surmounted as advanced technology enables a similar roadmap to ubiquitous DP diagnostics already traversed by radiology [10]. The interconnectivity of pathologists, staff, and resources observed following WSI implementation at The Ohio State University reflect a primary endpoint of laboratory digitization. Augmentation of DP tools with artificial intelligence (AI)-based algorithms reflect another. As the university's primary diagnostic novelty recedes amongst a growing global normalcy of automated workflows, increased efforts for diagnostic quality, and the creation of integrated ecosystems supportive of computational pathology [2,11–13], further capitalization from digital integration is now within reach for digitized departments primed to actuate the clinical potential of predictive diagnostic AI-technology for WSI.

2. Development of Computer Vision for Pathology

Computer-aided image processing and pattern recognition, e.g., classification, of histological and cytological structures for pathology has developed from the early 1970s [14,15].

Primordial AI tools for pathology classification tasks typically find genesis at the same vantage point from which modern machine learning (ML) tools began their evolution. Pixel-based analysis, e.g., computer-recognition of a unique series of numerical values that form a shape of interest, is used for classification, e.g., segmentation, tasks that are now among the most essential applications included within integrative workflow image analysis (IA) tools. Traditional morphometric feature evaluation entailed calculation of object size via computational counting of pixels occupied by an object followed by calibration for magnification [16]. Description of object shape resulted from computer determination of a specific shape from a rigid set of preprogrammed rules. Traditional programming directives utilized shape descriptors, e.g., elongation factor and nuclear roundness factor, to identify structures such as peripheral blood erythrocytes. Substantial focus has been directed toward development of computational IA for genitourinary (GU) pathology. Prototypal quantitative light microscopy applications for urological oncology were initially applied to histological sections for rudimentary tumor recurrence and grading predictions [16].

As evidenced from early explorations in computer vision for pathology, traditional programming methods were inherently prone to rapid devolution when image shapes did not adhere to specific pre-programmed rules/definitions, thereby confounding the narrow window of computational interpretability allotted through the ridged training modus. For example, nuclear roundness factor (NRF), defined as the ratio of an area to a perimeter, was observed to decrease when an object shape, e.g., ellipse, deviated from congruence with a perfect circle. The restrictive nature of the programmed code for NRF had predisposed it to conflating "roundness" with "circularity".

ML techniques have widened the window of interpretability through algorithmic modeling via the use of images rather than preprogrammed rules as input data for algorithm training, allowing computers to correctly visualize shapes regardless of their size, symmetry, or rotation. ML for computational pathology has enabled the interpretive ability of algorithmic tools to extend beyond the limited output yielded from cast-iron programming codes to a system that is able to deduce patterns with increasing accuracy through training. Most current ML approaches utilize methods such as "Random Forest classification", an algorithmic approach developed in 2001 (the same year as the Leica Aperio T1 gained distinction as the first WSI device released for commercial use) by which a series of decision trees are employed to make an aggregated prediction (Figure 2) [17].

Machine learning allows computers to recognize patterns and make predictive decisions without explicit, step-by-step programming. Trial, error, and extensive "practice" are the core elements of model building for ML, the essence of which follows an iterative approach akin to flashcard memorization. Algorithms are fashioned from a point of zero training data through learning from an output set. A preselected group of image/shape descriptors are chosen by a computer, initially at absolute random, to describe input data fed into the system by a developer. An incorrect label ascribed to an input image by a computer will be amended to display the correct image description from which a machine may demonstrate its learning capacity via correct attribution of the label to a future input image. The ML system takes account of every image pixel and its surrounding pixels with each estimation to ultimately build its own set of rules/algorithms, progressively fashioning an adroit apparatus for predictive accuracy and precision as the cycle continues. Predictive classification models may be tuned and optimized via additional data input providing more opportunities for improvement through trial-and-error for increased accuracy of pattern recognition within new images.

Deep learning (DL) has further expounded upon the cognitive model of ML algorithms, achieving remarkable mimicry to the neural network of the human brain. Artificial neural networks (ANNs) consisting of weighted, interconnected nodes comprise the scaffolding of DL modeling for pathology (Figure 3).

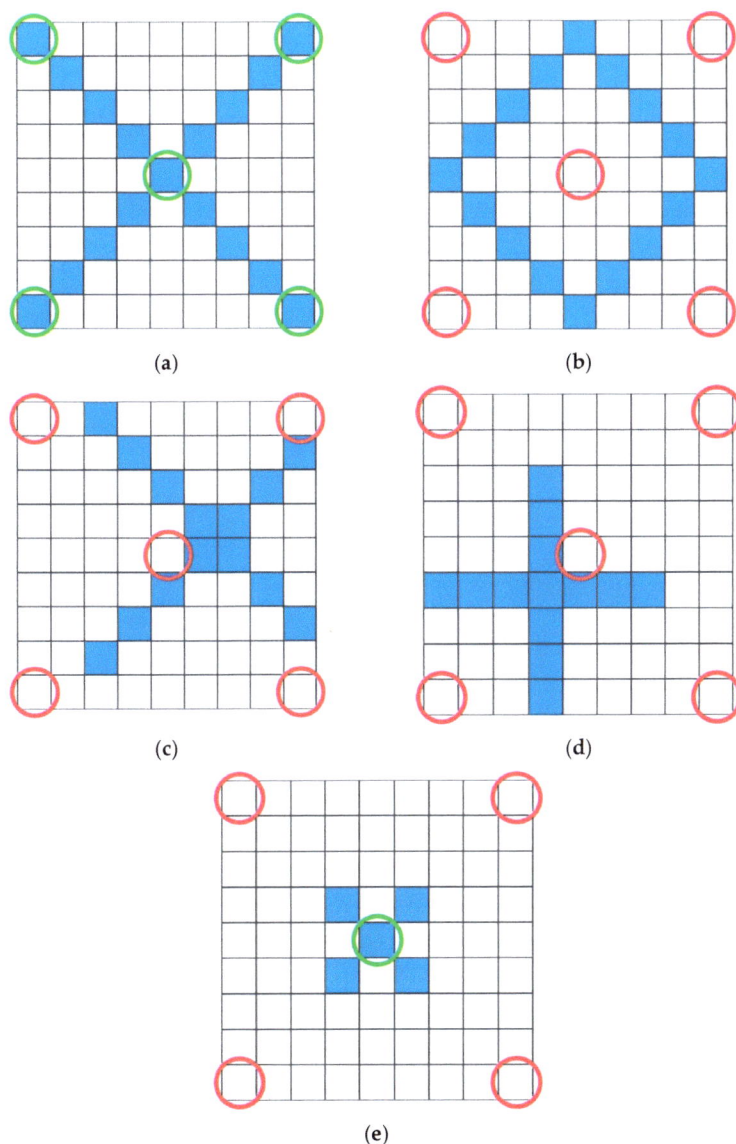

Figure 2. Traditional Programming vs. Machine Learning for Computer Vision (original figures). Squares are representative of pixels comprised of binary graphical indicators for computer recognition, with blue squares comprising a pixelated "input" shape to be recognized by a preset formula that may direct the computer to correctly identifying the shape in its output determination. Green circles are indicative of computer-recognized elements of the pixelated input shape per input programming rules. Red circles represent areas in which programming rules neglected to recognize blue input image elements. Computer programmed rules for defining shapes in figures (**a**) through (**e**) are (1) shape is "X" if the center and corner pixels are full and "O" if the center and corner pixels are empty:

(**a**) Pathologist/human interpretation of image: shape is "X". Computer interpretation of image: shape is "X", as dictated by rule. Outcome: concordant with pathologist visual interpretation; (**b**) Pathologist interpretation of image: shape is "O". Computer interpretation of image: Shape is "O", as dictated by rule. Outcome: concordant with pathologist visual interpretation; (**c,d**) Pathologist interpretation of image: shape is "X". Computer interpretation of images: shape is "O", as dictated by rules. Outcome: discordant with pathologist visual interpretation; (**e**) Pathologist interpretation of image: shape is "X". Computer interpretation of image: image is not recognized, as complete criteria are not fulfilled for either rule. Outcome: discordant with pathologist visual interpretation, i.e., unidentifiable image.

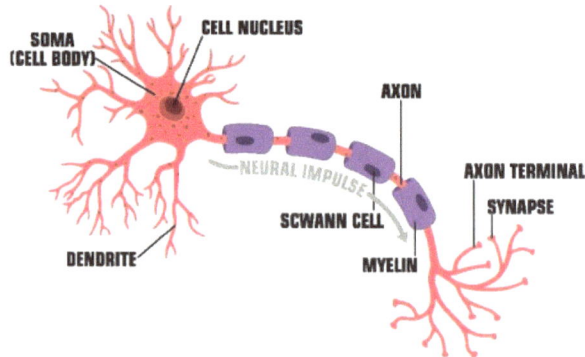

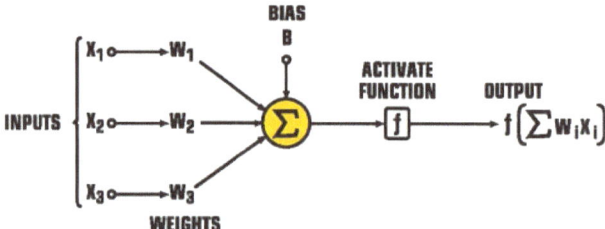

Figure 3. Artificial Neuron Model (ShadeDesign/Shutterstock.com, accessed on 27 April 2022).

Powerful neural networks contain up to millions of nodes arranged in layers including input layers, hidden layers, and output layers (Figure 4).

Outputs from one layer of a neural network act as inputs which feed into the nodes of another layer. Convolutional neural networks (CNNs) are a complex derivative from the ANN model fashioned for outcome prediction from WSI data inputs without the assistance of a predefined output set. CNNs for WSI analysis have demonstrated substantial capacity to effectively aid in primary diagnostic and quality control (QC) applications. Other DL models such as the recurrent neural network (RNN) may be used to enhance CNN analysis through provision of spatial and contextual modeling enabled from a bi-directional framework equipped to process high-resolution gigapixel WSIs without image-patch modeling techniques suggested to compromise overall tumor size and sub-structures present within a WSI (Figure 5).

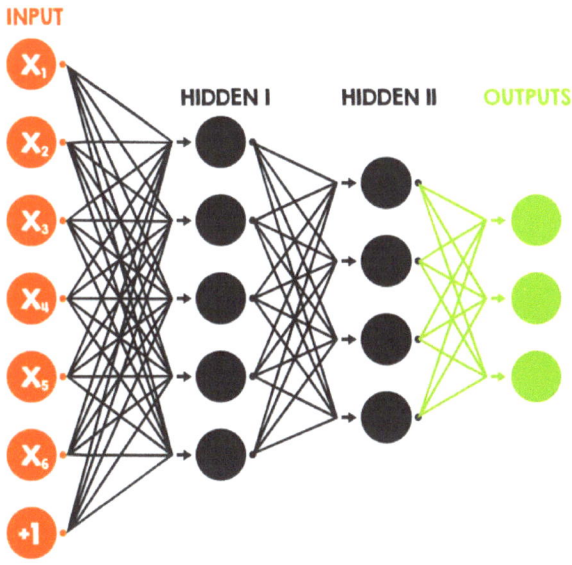

Figure 4. Artificial Neural Network (ShadeDesign/Shutterstock.com, accessed on 27 April 2022).

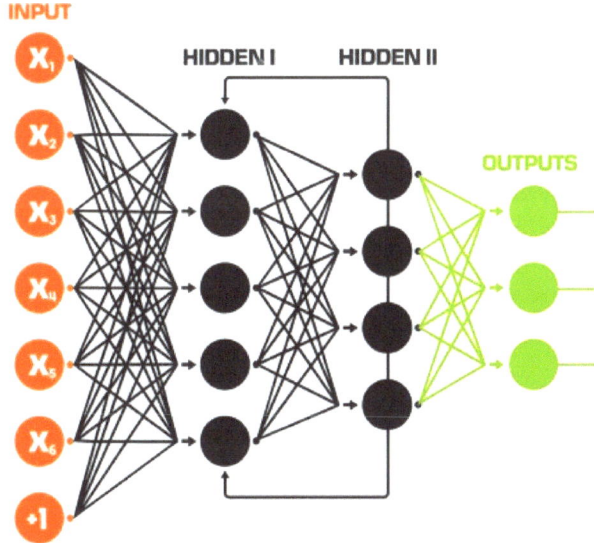

Figure 5. Recurrent Neural Network (ShadeDesign/Shutterstock.com, accessed on 27 April 2022).

CNN models may use WSIs ascribed individual diagnostic target-labels per associated pattern, e.g., Gleason grade, or up to millions of unlabeled WSI image-patches for autodidactic training during which the AI-model will learn to identify and extract important features without developer assistance (Figure 6).

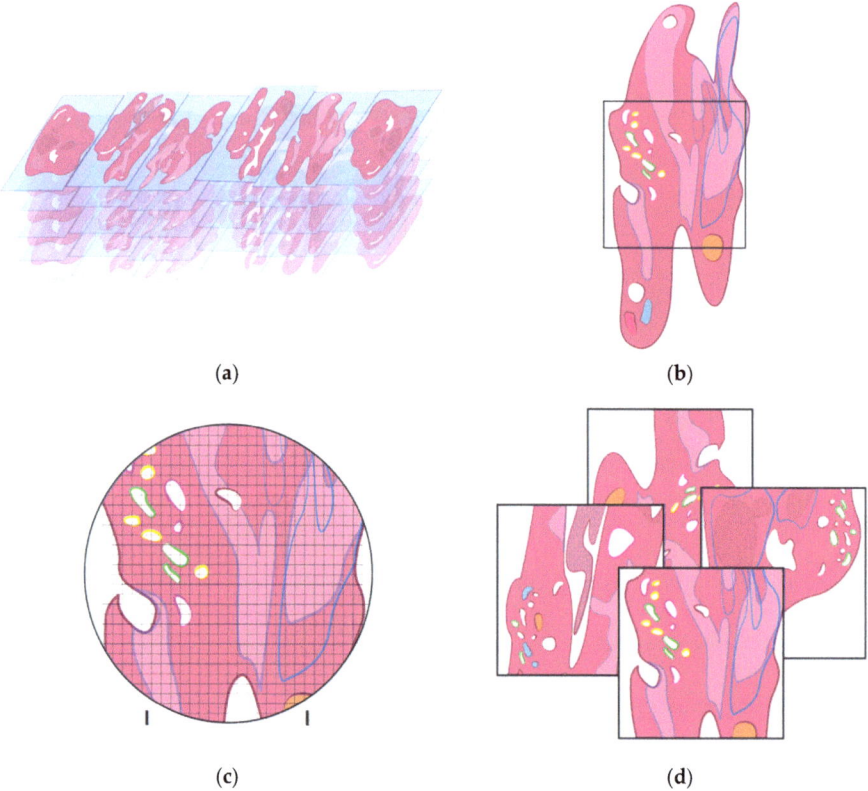

Figure 6. WSI patch extraction for algorithm training (original figures). (**a**) WSI dataset; (**b**) WSI region of interest for patch selection; (**c**) patch selection; (**d**) extracted patches used for algorithm training. Demarcated and colored areas on pink WSI specimen represent computer-assisted pathologist annotations.

"End-to-end" methods for training DL models for WSI have greatly mitigated and outperformed highly supervised, effort-intensive methods of algorithmic training dependent upon manually annotated, pixel-based feature extraction techniques (Figure 7).

Algorithm development is typically divided into a series of steps beginning with procurement of clinically annotated samples followed by WSI annotation. An algorithm is developed via a training set and tested via an independent validation set (Figure 8).

A clinical cause pertaining to a relevant population of interest formulates the origin and endpoint for algorithm development driven by a computational pathology team. Pathologists act to direct the genesis and culmination of clinical algorithms while data scientists, e.g., statisticians and bio-informaticians, assist in algorithm design and training. Engineers maintain hardware and software for the operating environment. Pathologists invoke downstream development though providing context through clinically relevant questions that spearhead algorithmic solutions. They are essential for the verification and validation processes for application and monitoring of the algorithm prior to and following clinical deployment, such that feedback is relayed to developers for optimization (Figure 9).

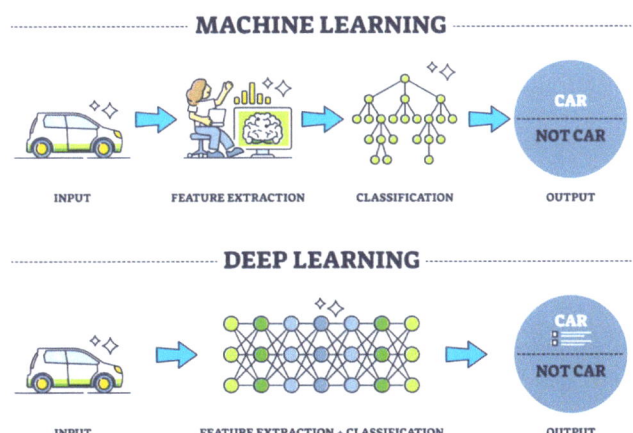

Figure 7. Machine learning vs. Deep learning (VectorMine/Shutterstock.com, accessed on 27 April 2022).

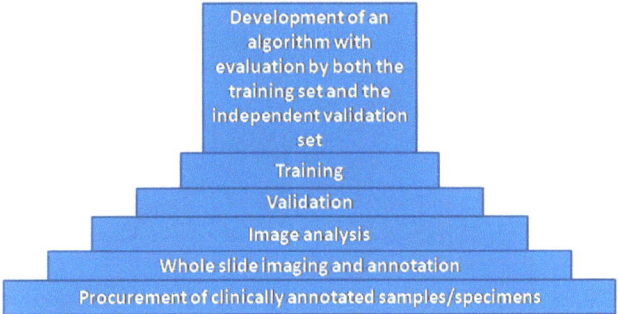

Figure 8. Algorithm Development (original diagram).

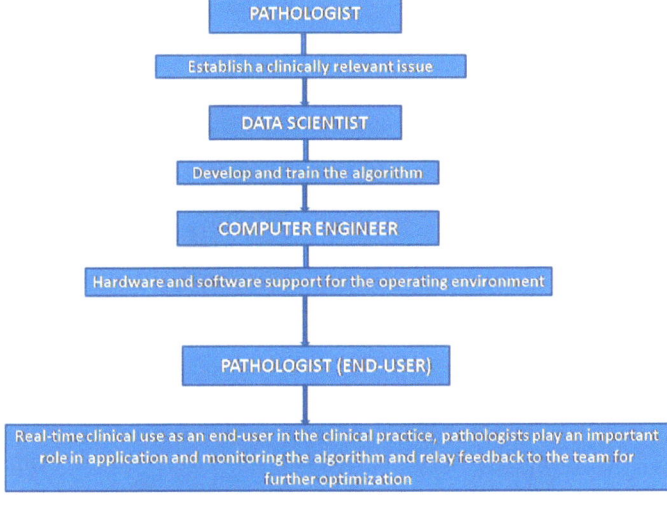

Figure 9. Computational pathology team (original diagram).

3. Realizing the Clinical Potential of AI

The potential for AI to catalyze clinical transformation has been exemplified through recent research, academic, and translational investigations in algorithm development for predictive diagnostic and prognostic analysis made directly from H&E-stained WSIs [18]. Such studies, indicative of the potential for AI to enhance pathologist understanding of disease and improve patient quality of care, encourage further investigations where algorithms may be deployed and evaluated within standardized settings. AI for primary diagnostic and quality control applications may be optimized through clinical trials. Algorithmic development for prostate cancer needle biopsies [19–28], radical prostatectomies [29,30], and tissue microarrays [21,31–33], has held the brunt of focus for the transition of such tools into utilization within clinical forums thus far. Though such investigations have shown promise for AI-assisted grading for prostate cancer and pathologist-review, many have been susceptible to biases and limitations during both development and validation processes, many of which affect the clinical translatability of algorithms developed within non-clinical, e.g., research, settings. The most prominent hurdles affecting clinical implementation of ML and DL tools stem from data availability, generalizability, and transparency ("black box") concerns (Figure 10).

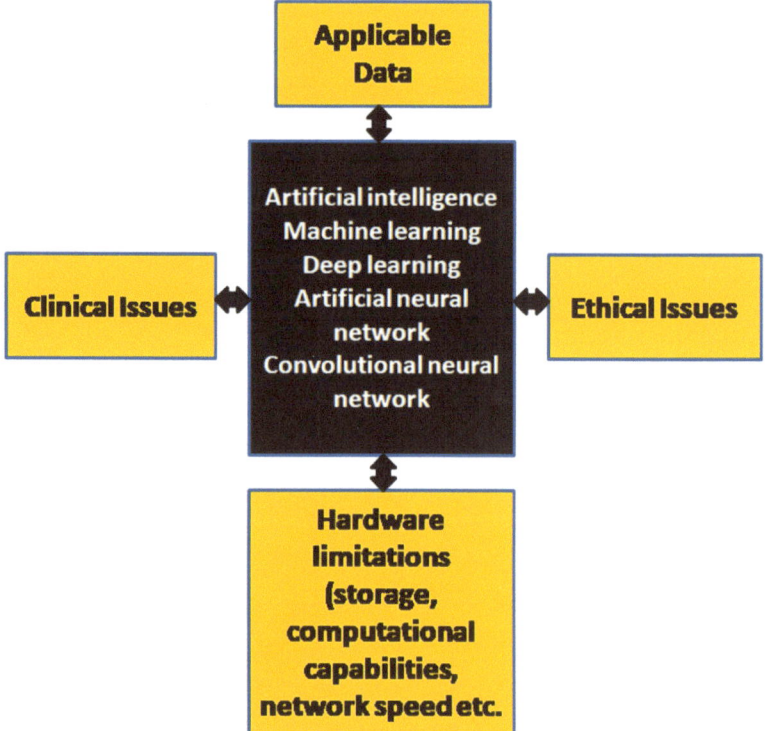

Figure 10. Limitations affecting AI development and deployment (original diagram).

3.1. Overcoming Inter-Observer Variability for Challenging Diagnosis with AI

Challenging histology and morphology is often met with enduringly high rates of inter- and intra-observer variability and increased time-to-diagnosis from pathologists using light microscopy [34]. Discordance is further emphasized within the focuses of genitourinary and renal pathology, where interpretation of complex grading systems, e.g., Fuhrman and Gleason, and prognostic patterns, e.g., cribriform and glomerulosclerotic, is concerningly incongruent even amongst specialists [35–48]. Inter-pathologist grading assessments for prostate cancer grading have elicited concerning results, with kappa values reported as low as 0.3 [38,49]. The last 7 years of ML development for prostatic adenocarcinoma has yielded results demonstrating potential for greater diagnostic objectivity.

2016 marked the first account of DL network development for the detection of prostate adenocarcinoma in core needle biopsy (CNB) tissue. Slide patches extracted from H&E-stained prostate biopsy tissue slides from 254 patients were separated into training, testing, and validation sets. Mean ROC for the median analysis was 0.98–0.99 for the 90th percentile analysis [19].

An advanced CNN derivative was trained for prostate cancer grading using 0.6 mm diameter cores from primary prostate carcinomas in TMAs from 641 patients and tested using TMA cores from 245 prostatectomy cases from another cohort graded independently by two pathologists. Agreement between the DL model and each pathologist was 0.75 and 0.71, respectively, per Cohen's quadratic kappa statistic, with an inter-pathologist agreement of 0.71. Furthermore, the model demonstrated significantly greater accuracy in distinguishing low-risk from intermediate-risk ($p = 0.098$) cancer than either pathologist ($p = 0.79$ and $p = 0.29$, respectively) [32].

A total of 752 tissue biopsies from multiple sites were used to train a DL system for Gleason grade (GG) identification. Model agreement with pathologists was 72% (68–75%) for specialists and 58% (54–61%) for general pathologists. The model was less likely to over-grade WHO grade group 1 than grade group 2 and more likely to undergrade higher grades in comparison to general pathologists. ROC curves distinguished model-based grade groups 1 and 2 from grade groups 3 through 5 (AUC = 0.97) [50].

Another study in which a CNN was trained for GG classification using 5759 biopsies from 1243 patients yielded a kappa value of 0.85 when compared to three genitourinary pathologists, superior to the kappa of 0.82 obtained from a pathologist panel [51].

Corroborating the potential for AI to improve pathologist grading of prostate biopsies, Bulten et al. recruited fourteen genitourinary specialists to evaluate 160 biopsies with and without assistance of AI algorithms. Using AI, the panel of pathologists demonstrated significantly greater agreeability, yielding kappa values of 0.87 vs. 0.799 when graded independently [52].

ML tools have recently seen development for the automated detection of cribriform pattern in prostate WSIs [41,46,47]. The first instance of ML applications applied to investigate the prognostic utility of invasive cribriform adenocarcinoma (ICC) within specific Gleason grade groups provided insight on the strong prognostic role of ICC morphology fraction of tumor area (cribriform area index(CAI)) in patients with Gleason grade 2 cancer due to the morphology conferring a higher concordance index for biochemical recurrence than patients without evidence of ICC. A CAI increase by a factor of two was determined to be prognostic in patients with ICC morphology after controlling for Gleason grade, surgical margin positivity, preoperative prostate-specific antigen level, pathological T stage, and age (hazard ratio: 1.19) [47].

AI-approaches have demonstrated the capacity identify subtle morphological differences, e.g., sarcomatoid vs. spindle cell pattern, in clinical groups of patients with clear cell renal cell carcinoma (ccRCC) [34]. ML-models have demonstrated the ability to classify early vs. advanced stages of ccRCC, with recent algorithms using gene expression profiling to classify ccRCC stages. One study analyzed gene expression of 523 samples to identify genes differentially expressed in early and late stages of ccRCC, achieving a maximum accuracy of 72.64% and 0.81 ROC using 64 genes on validation dataset [53].

Fenstermaker et al. [54] developed a CNN model to detect, grade (Fuhrman 1–4), and distinguish RCC subtypes (clear cell, chromophobe, papillary). The model was trained on 3000 normal and 12,168 RCC H&E-stained tissue samples of RCC from 42 patients (acquired from the Cancer Genome Atlas). The model classified normal parenchyma vs. RCC tissue with 99.1% accuracy, demonstrating an additional 97.5% accuracy in distinguishing RCC subtypes. Model accuracy in predicting Fuhrman grade was 98.4%.

Two studies using ML models developed from features extracted from single and multi-omics data for classification of early and late stages of papillary RCC emphasized the utility of model-training from multiple data sources. Gene expression and DNA methylation data were used in the later (2020) study, demonstrating slightly better predictive performance than the former (2018) study (MCC 0.77, PR-AUC 0.79, accuracy 90.4) [55–57]. A total of 104 genes from Cancer Genome Project expression profiles of 161 patients were used as data in both studies.

Misdiagnoses may lead to delays in appropriate treatment regimens for patients presenting with challenging morphology that is often misidentified. The subtle morphologic characteristics which differentiate the TFE2 Xp11.2 translocation variant of RCC (TFE3-RCC) from other RCC subtypes often leads to the misdiagnosis of this aggressively progressive form of RCC and was the basis for a recent ML development for its identification. An automated ML pipeline was developed to extract TFE3-RCC features and used to differentiate subtle morphological differences between TFE3-RCC and ccRCC with high accuracy. AUCs ranged from 0.84 to 0.89 when evaluating classification models against an external validation set [58].

3.2. Exploring AI Development for Nephropathology Applications

Glomerulosclerosis and IFTA are histologic indicators of irreversible kidney injury, with cortical fibrosis holding distinction as the single greatest morphologic predictor of chronic kidney disease, regardless of disease etiology [59]. Quantification of glomeruli and glomerulosclerosis on kidney biopsy are among the constituents of a standard renal pathology report, yet the prevailing methods for glomerular assessment remain manual, labor intensive, and non-standardized [60]. Although manual evaluation of glomerulosclerotic percentage has consistently demonstrated high inter-observer concordance, traditional visual quantitation of renal cortical involvement incurred by IFTA results in higher variability among pathologists due to the innately complex histology and diverse morphology of the region [59].

The first CNN fashioned for multiclass segmentation of digitized periodic acid-Schiff (PAS) stained nephrectomy samples and transplant biopsies indicated the necessity for more studies interrogating quantitative diagnostic tools for routine kidney histopathology [61]. Significant correlation between pathologist-scored histology vs. the CNN was noted for glomerular counting in whole transplant biopsies (0.94 mean intraclass correlation coefficient). The CNN yielded the best segmentation results for glomeruli in both internal and external validation sets (Dice coefficient of 0.95 and 0.94, respectively), with the model detecting 92.7% of all glomeruli in nephrectomy samples.

The nephropathology landscape has provided fertile grounds for the development of ML tools fashioned to parse and delineate various complex morphological structures, as demonstrated in a slew of recent investigations suggesting the clinical merit of AI within the medical kidney arena [62]. CNN-directed segmentation of morphologically complex image structures, e.g., interstitial fibrosis and tubular atrophy (IFTA), has improved throughout recent years as advances in annotation speed, predictive capacity, and breadth of utility have provided strong arguments for clinical applicability [59].

Recent studies have studied predictive AI-modeling for morphologically complex structures of the kidney using WSIs of human renal biopsy samples [62]. One such study explored the use of CNNs in semantic segmentation of glomerulosclerosis and IFTA from renal biopsies, in which assessment of CNN performance spanned three morphologic areas: IFTA, non-sclerotic glomeruli, and sclerotic glomeruli [59]. Per these respective areas, CNN demonstrated a balanced accuracy of 0.82/0.94/0.86 and MCC of 0.6/0.87/0.68 for intra-institutional holdout cases. For inter-institutional holdout cases, balanced accuracy was 0.70/0.93/0.84 with MCC of 0.49/0.79/0.64 per respective area. Investigators noted the CNN model demonstrating the best performance used a smaller network and low resolution for image analysis. In multiple cases, the CNN demonstrated the capacity to learn to predict IFTA boundaries with greater precision than the ground-truth annotations used for its training. Significant correlation was noted when comparing IFTA and glomerulosclerosis estimations via CNN with ground truth annotations, with IFTA yielding a correlation coefficient of 0.73 (95% CI [0.31, 0.91]) and glomerulosclerosis that of 0.97 (95% CI [0.9, 0.99]). No substantial difference was noted in score agreement concerning comparisons of IFTA grades as per visual assessment conducted by pathologists vs. CNN predictions against ground truth annotations, with inter-rater reliability for pathologists measured to have a kappa value of 0.69 with 95% CI [0.39, 0.99] and that of the CNN to have a kappa value of 0.66 with 95% CI [0.37, 0.96]. The CNN also demonstrated learning capacity in identifying segmental sclerosis, despite having not been trained to identify findings of this nature. Results strongly indicate the feasibility of DL-tools for high-performance segmentation of morphologically complex image structures, e.g., IFTA, by CNN.

Another CNN developed for the identification and segmentation of glomeruli on WSI of human kidney biopsies demonstrated accurate discrimination of non-glomerular images from glomerular images that were either normal or partially sclerosed (NPS) or globally sclerosed (GS) (Accuracy: 92.67% ± 2.02%, Kappa: 0.8681 ± 0.0392) [60]. The segmentation model derived from the CNN classifier demonstrated accuracy in marking GS glomeruli on test data (Matthews correlation coefficient = 0.628).

As tissue volume requirements and annotation quality often mar adoption of CNN training for quantitative analysis, investigators seeking to reduce annotation burden experimented with development of a Human AI Loop (H-AI-L), e.g., "human-in-the-loop" pipeline for WSI segmentation. Annotation speed and accuracy were noted to perform faster than traditional methods limited by data annotation speed [63].

Another ML pipeline was developed for glomerular localization in whole kidney sections for automated assessment of glomerular injury [64]. Average precision for glomerular localization was reported as 96.94%, with an average recall of 96.79%. The localizer did not demonstrate bias in identifying healthy or damaged glomeruli nor did it necessitate manual preprocessing.

Reduced variability from AI-assisted analysis of fine pathologic structures at high resolution may provide accurate quantitative assessment of WSIs for IFTA grade prediction, as demonstrated by a DL framework developed at the Ohio State University Wexner Medical Center using trichrome-stained WSIs. Strong inter-rater reliability was noted regarding IFTA grading between the pathologists and the reference estimate ($\kappa = 0.622 \pm 0.071$). The accuracy of the DL model was 71.8% ± 5.3% on The Ohio State University Wexner Medical Center and 65.0% ± 4.2% on Kidney Precision Medicine Project WSI data sets (from which model performance was evaluated) [65].

The first CNN-based model relevant to kidney transplantation within the literature was developed to address significant intra- and inter-observer variability reported during donor biopsy evaluation [66]. The DL model is the first to have been developed for the identification and classification of non-sclerosed and sclerosed glomeruli in WSI of donor kidney frozen section biopsies. When trained on only 48 WSIs, the model demonstrated slide-level performance in evaluation that was noted to be on par with expert renal pathologists. The model also significantly outperformed, in both accuracy and speed, another CNN model trained using only image patches of isolated glomeruli. Investigators noted that while model training with WSI patches has demonstrated efficacy in WSI classification tasks, this is only when applied to the classification of WSI patches and did not work as effectively for WSI segmentation in the setting of their study. Authors postulated, per results achieved from this CNN model, a future in which its utilization is deemed essential for clinical evaluations of donor kidney biopsies.

A recent publication explored the development of a pipeline for the classification and segmentation of renal biopsies from patients with diabetic nephropathy [67]. The pipeline consisted of a CNN used to detect glomerular features reflective of glomerulopathic structural alteration and a Recurrent Neural Network (RNN) used for analysis of glomerular features for final diagnosis of the biopsy. The pipeline was designed to be extendable to any histologically interpreted glomerular disease, e.g., IgA nephropathy, lupus nephritis, and is trainable for the prediction of any label with a numerically associated indicator of severity such as proteinuria. Strong comparison to traditional, e.g., visual classification methods was noted. The pipeline detected glomerular boundaries from whole slide images with 0.93 ± 0.04 balanced accuracy, glomerular nuclei with 0.94 sensitivity and 0.93 specificity, and glomerular structural components with 0.95 sensitivity and 0.99 specificity. Results were congruent with ground truth classifications annotated by a senior pathologist ($\kappa = 0.55$ with a 95% confidence interval (0.50, 0.60) and two additional renal pathologists $\kappa_1 = 0.68$, 95% interval (0.50, 0.86) and $\kappa_2 = 0.48$, 95% interval (0.32, 0.64).

Percentage assessment for normal and sclerotic glomeruli is vital in determining renal transplant eligibility, with percentage of normal and sclerotic regions serving as, respectively, good or poor indicators for transplant outcome [68]. DL has been leveraged to improve stratification of kidney disease severity via combining patient-specific histologic images with clinical phenotypes of chronic kidney disease (CKD) stage, serum creatinine, and nephrotic-range proteinuria at time of biopsy and afterward [69]. CNN models were demonstrated to outperform score assessments for pathological fibrosis undertaken by pathologists for all clinical CKD phenotypes. In comparison to pathologist estimation, CNN prediction for CKD stage yielded greater accuracy ($\kappa = 0.519$ vs. 0.051). CNN demonstrated an AUC of 0.912 vs. an AUC of 0.840 measured for pathologist estimations for creatinine. For proteinuria estimation, CNN AUC was 0.867 vs. 0.702. CNN estimations for 1-, 3-, and 5-year renal survival yielded respective AUC values of 0.878, 0.875, and 0.904 vs. 0.811, 0.800, and 0.786 via pathologist assessment.

Histopathological images are ripe with information exploitable for clinical survival and therapy response prediction. Such information may be buttressed with supplementation of categorical pathology-report data, as indicated in the previous examples. Histopathological data typically analyzed from WSIs for the prediction of survival and therapy response may also be effectively supplemented with pathology images from multiple sources, as demonstrated in a recent study evaluating an AI-pipeline developed for the prediction of neoadjuvant chemotherapy (NAC) response for patients with breast cancer.

3.3. Optimizing Machine Learning for Neoadjuvant Chemotherapy Response

Immunohistochemistry (IHC) WSIs are replete with data that may be utilized as a powerful adjunctive to histopathology WSIs. IHC images may be quantified for biomarker results, e.g., PD-L1, ER, PR, HER2, Ki67, and distribution of biomarker expression, e.g., PD-L1 (tumor and inflammatory cells), CD8 (cytotoxic tumor-infiltrating lymphocytes/TILs), and CD163 (type 2 macrophages), both metrics of which are important in predicting tumor response to chemotherapy.

3.3.1. Modeling Predictive Response for Neoadjuvant Chemotherapy in Breast Cancer

Up to 50% of HER2-positive breast cancers and a subset of triple-negative breast cancers (TNBCs) achieve pathologic complete response (pCR) following neoadjuvant chemotherapy (NAC), thereby allowing NAC response to act as corollary for disease-free survival in TNBC and HER2+ breast cancer patients [70–72]. Many factors are associated with pCR in breast cancer, e.g., higher mitotic activity and tumor (Nottingham) grade are associated with higher frequency of pCR [73]. Tumor-associated lymphocytes (TIL) occur with greater frequency in TNBC and HER2+ breast cancer subtypes [74]. PD-L1 expression, particularly in HER2+ patients, has demonstrated association with pCR in breast cancer [75,76]. Hormone receptor level is also associated with pCR, with ER-/PR-/HER2+ breast cancers demonstrating the greatest likelihood for pCR amongst all HER2+ tumors [77]. Higher intensity of HER2 IHC expression is associated with significantly higher likelihood for pCR in HER2+ breast cancer than for cases with incomplete pathological response [78]. Intratumoral heterogeneity is independently associated with incomplete response to anti-HER2 NAC in HER2+ breast cancer.

A recent groundbreaking effort compiled multiple image-based features extracted from multiple sources, i.e., H&E-stained WSIs and IHCs (PD-L1, CD8, CD163), quantitative and qualitative breast cancer biomarker results (ER, PR, HER2), and patient demographic and clinical features, e.g., age, to develop a predictive ML model for NAC response in TNBCs and HER2+ breast cancers. An automatic WSI feature extraction pipeline in which H&E-stained WSI tissue segmentation utilized a well-trained neural network model (DeepLabV2) to generate stromal, tumor, and aggregated lymphocyte areas (distinguished by computerized colorization). Multiplexed IHC WSI (CD8, CD163, PD-L1) segmentation was performed using color-based K-means segmentation, in which entire WSIs were segmented into three different IHC areas, then followed by an automatic, multi-step, and non-rigid (changing image size, but not shape) histological image alignment ("registration") of H&E and IHC, upon which an algorithm selected the best non-rigid transformations. Three categories of quantitative IHC image features (CD8, CD163, PD-L1) were extracted from the registered WSIs for subsequent evaluation of expression and distribution within different cellular components/regions (stroma, tumor, lymph) including an overall evaluation of all tissue components. Area ratio, proportion, and purity of IHC image features within cellular regions was evaluated. Breast biomarker results, e.g., positivity/negativity, percentage, were evaluated within inclusion of additional demographic characteristics in relation to different IHC markers, with data pooled from individual and combined H&E/IHC sources.

The ML model predicted NAC outcomes using the various extracted image features using a form of logistic regression. Four groups of image features were compared using AUC, F-1 score, precision, and recall measurements for HER2+ and TNBC patient cohorts:

1. All pipeline-extracted features (36 total) and clinical data patient features, e.g., including biomarker results, age, and additional demographic factors)
2. Automated/pipeline-extracted H&E-stained WSI and clinical patient data features
3. Automated/pipeline-extracted IHC WSI and clinical patient data features
4. Pathologist-extracted WSI features and clinical patient data features

Algorithmic models were developed per each group of pipeline-extracted WSI features/clinical features (with the ML model from the fourth group trained using manually extracted features by pathologists). For both the HER2+ and TNBC cohort, the first group performed best in each measurement, especially for the HER2+ cohort. A feature importance analysis was conducted in which favorable and unfavorable features predictive of pCR or residual tumor, respectively, were determined for both patient cohorts. Favorable features for the HER2+ cohort were determined by the ML model as the independent ratios of CD8, CD163, and PD-L1 in the lymphocytic region, CD163 ration in the tumor area, and the HER2/CEP17 ratio. Unfavorable features for the HER2+ cohort included age, ER and PR ratios, PR positivity, and the stromal CD8 proportion. Overall results demonstrated the effective capacity of the AI-pipeline to automatically extract H&E and IHC image features with accuracy. ML models developed based upon the pipeline-extracted WSI features and clinical features demonstrated the potential for NAC response prediction in breast cancer patients while outperforming the algorithm trained by pathologist-extracted features. The AI-pipeline also generated image features that could be used to predict residual cancer burden in breast cancer cases with residual tumor.

3.3.2. ML for Subspecialty Practice Survival Modeling

Tabibu et al. [34] provided encouraging data following the development of a CNN for the automated subtype classification of renal cell carcinoma (RCC) and identification of features predictive of patient survival outcome. A total of 1027 ccRCC, 303 Papillary RCC, and 254 Chromophobe WSIs with corresponding clinical information were selected for model training from the Cancer Genome Atlas, with 379, 47, and 83 normal tissue images per each respective RCC subtype. An accuracy of 99.39% and 87.34% was recorded for classification of ccRCC from normal tissue and chromophobe RCC from normal tissue, respectively. The AI-model classified ccRCC, chromophobe, and papillary RCC with 94.07% accuracy. High-probability tumor regions identified by the CNN were targeted for morphological feature extraction used for prediction of ccRCC patient survival outcome.

Significant association with patient survival was found after generated risk index was derived based upon tumor shape and nuclei from the extracted regions.

Prediction of RCC recurrence following nephrectomy has also seen focus for ML development, as outlined in a recent study assessing recurrence probability 5- and 10-years post-nephrectomy. Analytical data from 2814 RCC patients were used for model testing, which yielded AUC values of 0.836 and 0.784 5- and 10-years following nephrectomy [79].

4. Actuating Clinical Implementation through Achieving Generalizability

The essence of generalizable AI for clinical pathology lies within the capacity for an AI-tool to remain robust in its precision, accuracy, and efficiency in executing a diagnostic function when confronted with a broad range of tissue variations potentially encountered within a daily clinical workload.

Small, localized cohorts, insufficient ground-truth determination from expert pathologists, non-standardization of training methods and materials and lack of external validation are only some of many risks which have hampered the clinical generalizability of studies that have otherwise presented highly encouraging data. Circumvention of this key barrier to achieving deployment of AI within clinical practice requires equal applicability of an ML tool to different patient populations, pathology labs, WSI scanning device models, and reference standards derived from intercontinental specialist pathologist panels [80].

The largest collective effort for generalizable AI for prostate cancer diagnostics was reached during the Prostate Cancer Grade Assessment (PANDA) challenge, in which 12,625 prostate biopsy WSIs sourced from six international sites were used for model-development, performance evaluation, internal, and external validation [80]. Histological preparation and scanning of WSI data used for external validation was performed by multiple independent laboratories and was compared to pathologist reviews. On United States and European external validation sets, the algorithms achieved agreements of 0.862 (quadratically weighted κ, 95% confidence interval (CI), 0.840–0.884) and 0.868 (95% CI, 0.835–0.900) with expert uropathologists [80].

Well documented accounts of AI-model development for pathology during the last two years have involved large numbers of patient cases for training, testing, and validation data sets, interpretations by multiple expert pathologists to establish 'ground truth' for diagnosis, use of slides from multiple institutions, and use of differing scanners including scanners from external institutions [23,26,28,30,81].

WSIs of 12,132 prostate needle core biopsies digitized by two different WSI device models at Memorial Sloan Kettering (MSK) were used to train a DL system that was tested on 12,727 prostate needle core biopsies from institutions around the world [23]. Investigators found that approximately 10,000 slides were necessary for effective training of their system [82]. Authors noted a 3% difference in AUC recorded between WSI devices used for image capture and digitization attributed to variations in brightness, contrast, and sharpness between the devices. Investigators postulated that the AI-model could remove >75% of slides from a standard pathologist workload without compromising sensitivity and facilitate an increased user-base of non-subspecialized (non-GU pathologists) who may diagnose prostate cancer with greater confidence and efficacy when aided by the algorithmic tool. Weakly supervised AI-model training linking every WSI to synoptic data elements, e.g., benign vs. adenocarcinoma, provided a scalable mechanism of dataset creation circumventing data limitations which often mar the capacity and clinical implementation of highly supervised DL algorithms. Through using only label-based diagnoses for training WSIs, investigators were able to eschew any form of labor-intensive and time-consuming data curation including pixel-wise manual annotations used in highly supervised model training.

High-volume model training using 36,644 WSIs, 7514 of which had cancerous foci, was used in early development of diagnostic software for prostate adenocarcinoma recently granted de novo marketing authorization for in vitro diagnostic (IVD) use, signifying the first ever FDA-approved AI product for clinical pathology [83]. A total of 304 expertly-annotated prostate CNB WSIs were used to establish ground truth for evaluation of the DL system (Paige Prostate Alpha®, Paige AI, New York, NY, USA) [27]. An average diagnostic sensitivity of 74% and specificity of 97% was recorded for general pathologists prior to use of the DL system. When aided by the AI-tool, sensitivity increased to 90% while specificity remained the same. Results suggested the utility of the tool for second-read applications, e.g., quality assurance. Such a device could be deployed in settings where GU pathology subspecialists are not commonly, if at all, present, e.g., underserved climates with substantial healthcare disparity.

The Paige Prostate® system, successor to prototypal version Paige Prostate Alpha®, was subject to extensive multinational validation spanning $\geq$150 different institutions and a diversity of clinical and demographic characteristics from $\geq$7000 patients including differing tumor sizes, grades, and patient ethnicities [23,83–87]. The system achieved a sensitivity of 97.7% and a specificity of 99.3% in detecting cancer in 1876 prostate CNB WSIs, also demonstrating 99% sensitivity and 93% specificity at part-specimen level while upgrading pathologist-ascribed benign/suspicious patient diagnosis to malignant after identification [84,85].

The strengths of many high-volume studies for the validation of Paige Prostate® and other software systems which have since seen clinical deployment throughout the globe now may serve as guidelines for appropriate model evaluation for clinical generalizability. Large cohort sizes, testing sections containing substantial pre-analytic artifacts, e.g., thick cuts, fragmentation, and poor staining, abundance of challenging histological patterns including those seen in benign-mimicking malignant prostatic adenocarcinoma, e.g., pseudo hyperplastic and atrophic pattern variants, along with benign histology that may be mistaken for prostatic adenocarcinoma, all are variables which may confound the appropriate detection and grading of prostatic adenocarcinoma for an insufficiently trained AI-model, yet did not pose hurdles for the DL-models that would later see clinical implementation [88–90].

Clinical Integation of AI

AI tools have demonstrated real-world merit for quality control (QC) support and first read applications for primary diagnostic use within clinical settings. The Paige Prostate® solution notably reduced time-to-diagnosis by 65% when applied to diagnostic histopathologic data from 682 TRUS prostate needle biopsy WSIs acquired from 100 consecutive patients at a laboratory unassociated with its original development and validation [87]. The AI-system notably demonstrated 100% sensitivity and negative predictive values for patient-level diagnostics.

CorePlus (CorePlus Servicios Clínicos y Patológicos LLC, a high complexity CLIA-certified clinical and anatomic pathology laboratory is the first U.S. laboratory to integrate an AI-platform for diagnostics, lab efficiency, and quality control [91]. The Galen™Prostate solution (CE-marked; Ibex Medical Analytics) was integrated into the fully digitized laboratory for routine clinical second-read diagnostic applications. The AI-solution was previously clinically validated for routine clinical diagnostics involving detection, grading, and evaluation of clinically relevant findings within WSIs of prostate CNBs in an extensive study demonstrating the utility of the AI-solution for routine clinical practice [28].

The study was the first to evaluate the performance of a prostate histopathology algorithm deployed within routine clinical practice for assessment of cancer detection, Gleason grading (GG), and proportion of tumor extent in addition to detection of perineural invasion, demonstrating the multifaceted merits of the AI-solution which may fulfil a gamut of clinical reporting needs. Algorithmic interpretation of perineural invasion (PNI) within CNB WSIs, a typically small and relatively uncommon finding bearing large clinical and prognostic significance, presented unique focus for investigators as previous studies had not reported AI-based detection for the feature. The algorithm's capacity to simultaneously evaluate CNBs for PNI (AUC: 0.96 external validation dataset) while interpreting a battery of standard metrics for prostate CNB, e.g., cancer detection, grading, and tumor extent, highlighted the ability of the AI-platform to execute a multitude of functions with high performance.

The second-read application of the AI-platform was again clinically validated for a unique patient population bearing high rates of prostate cancer-specific mortality at the CorePlus laboratory and assessed via comparison to pathologists diagnoses for ground truth, yielding encouraging results including accurate identification of benign vs. cancerous tissue (AUC: 0.994; Specificity: 96.9%; Sensitivity; 96.5%) and GG 1 vs. GG 2+ (AUC: 0.901; Specificity: 81.1%; Sensitivity: 82.0%).

Following clinical implementation of the Galen™Prostate solution at the CorePlus laboratory for primary application in QC, the AI-tool has discovered and corrected 1.97% of over 4000 cases (encompassing over 54,000 WSIs since deployment of the AI platform in June 2020) incorrectly identified as false-negatives. During this period, the second-read application identified 51.4% of cases as benign, 18.16% as GG1, 29.83% as GG2+, while providing technical alert notifications for 1.79% of WSIs. In total, 100% of PCNBs at the laboratory are analyzed with the assistance of AI prior to sign-out.

The Galen™ platform (including Galen™Prostate and Galen™Breast, CE-marked for clinical breast cancer diagnostics) was also integrated into the clinical workflow for second-read applications at Maccabi Healthcare Services (Israel), a large, centralized pathology institute that receives samples from 350 surrounding clinics and hospitals. A significant proportion of yearly histopathology workload at the institution consists of PCNBs (700 cases per year; >8000 slides). Alerts from the second-read application, viewable from the case list and outlined by heatmaps displayed in a slide-viewing module, were raised in 10.1% of PCNB WSIs (583) taken from 232 cases initially given benign diagnoses by pathologists. Gleason 7+ alerts were raised in 5.3% of slides (93) taken from 137 cases initially given diagnoses of Gleason grade 3 + 3. Alerts from the AI-system significantly streamlined the review process and required minimal review time from pathologists (approximately 1% of FTE).

The value of AI-assisted QC was again demonstrated in an earlier study assessing the performance of the Galen™ Prostate algorithm after its validation at Maccabi [92]. Results: Following deployment in four laboratories within the Medipath network, the largest system of pathology institutes in France (averaging an annual workload of 5000 PCNB cases), the AI-solution was noted to have identified 12 cases misdiagnosed as benign, some of which the system identified as having high-grade cancer.

AI-assistance for first read applications offered by the Galen™Prostate solution underwent clinical validation in which superior outcomes were yielded from pathologists using the AI-tool in comparison to those using only light microscopy during interpretation of 100 PCNBs. Results demonstrate a 32% reduction in major discrepancy rate with use of the first read application [93].

Improvements in productivity, clinical-grade accuracy, TAT, and case-level discrepancy resolution were observed after clinical integration of the Galen™first read AI-system at Maccabi Healthcare Services. A 27% overall reduction in time-to-diagnosis and 37% overall gain in productivity compared to manual microscopy followed deployment of the AI-tool, which yielded a 32% reduction in time-to-diagnosis for benign cases and a 25%-time reduction for those with prostate cancer [94]. Diagnostic accuracy did not suffer from increased efficiency, as results for case-level diagnostic accuracy were congruent between AI and manual microscopy. A similar trend was also observed for resolution of case-level discrepancies, of which the Galen algorithm was able to deliver a 97.8% agreement with ground truth following discrepancy resolution in comparison to the almost equivalent 97.5% for diagnosis via microscopy [94]. In total, 160 cases (1224 slides) were used to evaluate case-level agreement for primary diagnosis. A 95.3% agreement was noted between the AI-solution and microscopy diagnosis for 378 cancerous and 789 benign WSIs in a study evaluating the performance of the AI-solution against 310 PCNB cases (totaling 2411 H&E slides) [94]. A total of 99.7% of pathologists using AI-assistance in the study agreed with classifications provided by the adjunctive tool, including reclassifications of three false-negative slides initially classified as benign. It was observed that the use of AI did not yield any false negative diagnosis throughout the duration of the study. Examples of cases misdiagnosed via manual microscopy and detected with AI included high-grade prostate adenocarcinoma (GG4 + GG3) and a case in which only one slide demonstrated findings of prostate cancer [94].

Turnaround time, e.g., total time from first to last review and sign out of one patient case, was also demonstrably reduced with AI-assistance, markedly reducing TAT by 1–2 days while enabling a single review for almost all cases. A total of 80% of cases analyzed via standard microscopy included additional ordering of IHC. Only 0.6% of cases interpreted via AI involved additional IHC ordering to those already automatically pre-ordered based upon AI-classification. In evaluation of 238 cases interpreted via microscopy vs. AI-assistance, the mean sign out time for pathologists using standard microscopy was reported as 1.8 days in comparison to 9.4 min via AI.

5. Discussion

DP technology has revolutionized laboratory practices through enabling the digitization and viewing of entire laboratory histopathological glass slide workloads at microscope resolution. Four generations of WSI scanning instruments have passed since the 2001 release of the Leica Aperio T1, with each generation marking successive improvements in scanning speed, image quality, and batch scanning capacity. Yet, although mature technology to support WSI and laboratory digitization is now readily available, supportive of high-volume laboratory integration, and more cost-effective for implementation than ever before, few laboratories to date have undergone complete digital transformation for routine clinical practice [11,95]. Commercial AI-tools for diagnostic pathology are primed for adoption, offering "plug-and-play", user-friendly systems which now include applications for case triaging, worklists, slide viewing, IHC pre-ordering, tumor grading, sample measurements, reporting, and identification of non-cancerous findings. An increasing number of vendors offer dedicated software with algorithms for WSI image analysis, e.g., estrogen receptor, progesterone receptor, and human epidermal growth factor receptor 2 scoring, including automated multi-class segmentation of H&E stained WSIs demonstrated via 'heatmapping,' i.e., colorized pixel wise classification of tissue (Figure 11) [96].

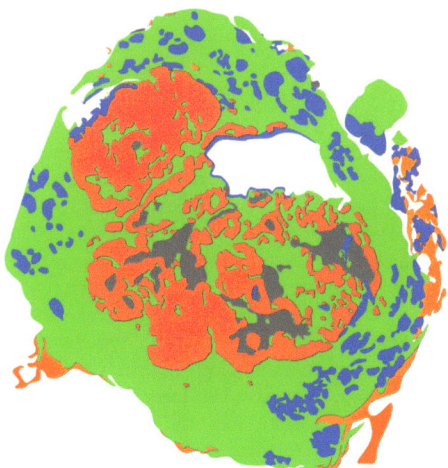

Figure 11. Heatmapping (original figure). Example of heatmapping in which spatial information is delineated by colors indicating carcinomatous region (red), benign epithelium (blue), stroma (green), adipose (orange), and areas of necrosis (gray) on a WSI specimen.

Commercial vendors are now utilizing modern DL techniques including multiple instance learning (MIL) to generate cell-by-cell data, quantify within subregions, and perform feature-based analysis for multiple applications in brightfield and fluorescent WSIs, with recent solutions facilitating the accurate prediction of genomic status from H&E-stained slides [97]. An increasing number of commercially available AI solutions support the construction of bespoke AI models, e.g., custom assay development, whereby pathologists are enabled to train models via annotations rather than complex coding, with some vendors offering built-in learning tools to further assist the annotation process for faster training and increased accuracy. Commercial solutions are capable of high throughput with fast turnaround from rapid generation, visualization, and export of spatial, morphological, and increasingly precise histology data from WSI, e.g., tumor area, cell counts, cell size, staining intensity, collagen area, and blood vessel density [98]. Yet, only 22% of laboratories enrolled in a 2016 College of American Pathologists (CAP) quality improvement survey for histology reported using quantitative tools for image analysis tasks [99].

Following the introduction of IHC and next generation sequencing for clinical practice, AI has been deemed the third revolution of pathology [99]. Such a revolution and the magnificent potential it holds for clinical pathology, as evidenced in our review, may only be unleashed through WSI adoption. Improvements in clinical-grade accuracy, increased productivity, robust QC, and shorter TAT realized through AI-augmented DP laboratories have driven a case for full laboratory digitization as seen in Maccabi Healthcare Services. Integration of AI into clinical workflow at the healthcare network yielded low risks while producing high returns. These findings, in conjunction with increased efficiency, decreased IHC ordering, and increased practitioner satisfaction supported the decision for complete digitization from both practical and financial vantage points.

Van Der Poel et al. had noted in their 1992 review of computational applications in "quantitative light microscopy" for the diagnosis of prostatic adenocarcinoma, transitional cell carcinoma, and renal cell carcinoma, that the purpose for investigating the application of such techniques stemmed from the highly inconsistent nature of visual tumor grading lending to high interobserver variability reported at the time [16]. Authors also noted changes in grading systems that were often descriptively subjective therefore resulting in "disturbingly low reproducibility", further compounding the highly subjective nature of pathologist-directed quantification of histological, cellular, and nuclear features pertaining to malignant potential. The comprehensive review of primordial computational applications for GU pathology concluded with noting that such techniques were valuable in aiding diagnosis only when confined to research settings. The need for standardized automated fixation, embedding, staining, selection, and measuring techniques was emphasized, as the extensive data analyzed within the review had been obtained with varying preparation methods and therefore differed too greatly to support any consistent conclusions.

Twenty years later, Egevad et al. reported on their investigation concerning the shifting approach to Gleason grading following the 2005 change in guidelines by the International Society of Urological Pathologists [36]. New encouragement to incorporate poorly formed glands and cribriform patterns into Gleason pattern (GP) 4 had led to high inter-observer variability amongst even specialist urologic pathologists ($\kappa = 0.34$), who expressed concern regarding the compromised significance of GS 7 in the wake of the amended guidelines [35].

Modern computational pathology tools have facilitated the standardization of workflow components highlighted by Van Der Poel et al., yet most current studies involving the interrogation of AI-development for pathology are still relegated to academia while lacking any consistent methical standardization that may be utilized for clinical relevancy. Though the performance of AI algorithms for GU pathology has, within the cohort of research studies included in our review, demonstrated equivalency to the diagnostic interpretations of GU specialists while surpassing those of general pathologists, training materials and methods for individual AI-models varied when evaluated as a conglomerate. Variations in tissue samples and WSI patch sizes used for model training are two such examples. Firm conclusions pertaining to the clinical relevancy of these investigations were also unreachable, in some instances, due to lack of model-development for correlating cancer grade with clinical outcome.

In his wake, Aurelius left scores of stoic prose directing those seeking understanding almost two millennia later to "look back over the past, with its changing empires that rose and fell ... " to foresee the future. Those pursuing additional directives towards fomenting solutions for change may turn to Socratic texts encouraging avoidance of conflict with the old to build upon the new, words which predated Aurelius' reign by centuries.

Realization of objective diagnostic reproducibility has been a coveted goal for clinical pathology long before the concept of computer vision, or computers in any respect. Newer studies featured in our review have highlighted instances of clinical implementation, groundbreaking generalizability, and MIL methods for algorithm development incorporating data from entire clinical pathology reports into training for enhanced clinical relevancy. Newer CNN derivatives and methods for model training have emerged to combat data concerns which have been a primary limitation to algorithmic clinical implementation.

Integration of a fully digitized, LIS-centric laboratory was a response to overwhelming workload burdens at the Gravina Hospital in Caltagirone (Sicily, Italy) [95]. Such problems had been compounded by the Coronavirus pandemic, though were omnipresent in similar departments throughout the globe struggling to combat long withstanding problems that had fervently resurged after lying dormant for years. Digital transformation of all workflow steps through departmental LIS allowed practitioners and staff at the Gravina Hospital to alleviate burdens through a completely interconnected, easily streamlined workflow. DP transformation of the laboratory would later be followed by augmentation of the digitized workflow processes with AI-tools. Superior diagnostic concordance amongst pathologists and increased WSI quality was observed shortly following implementation of AI, as algorithmic adjuncts to digital workflow processes created a cause for upholding a high standard of workflow quality. Through shining a light upon areas for improvement within the existing workflow it was embedded within, AI had uncovered problem areas otherwise overlooked existing prior to its arrival, which would then be amended to optimize the conjunctive potential of both diagnostic utilities.

Unearthed depths of clinical potential embedded within millions of WSI pixels has driven the development of effective, accurate, and precise AI algorithms purposed for transforming such potential into meaning. The same prospects have inspired the evolution of four generations of WSI devices to extract and present data from glass slides with greater efficacy, accuracy, and precision with each successive iteration. Driving forward and fueled through shared inspirations of clinical prospect and potential, WSI has met AI at a road converged where both may continue to a destination of enhanced clinical understanding and optimized patient care. As the night turns and AI embeds itself within the digital bedrock of clinical pathology, Rushmore-esque pillars form to cast monumental gazes of computer vision to an infinitely opportune landscape ahead.

Author Contributions: Conceptualization, A.U.P., S.M. and A.V.P.; writing—original draft preparation, A.U.P.; writing—review and editing, A.U.P., N.S., S.S., S.G. and C.E.; supervision, S.M. and A.V.P. All authors have read and agreed to the published version of the manuscript.

Funding: This research received no external funding.

Institutional Review Board Statement: Not applicable.

Informed Consent Statement: Not applicable.

Data Availability Statement: Not applicable.

Acknowledgments: Thank you to David Kellough, who provided photos of digital pathology integration at the Ohio State University (Columbus, OH, USA).

Conflicts of Interest: The authors declare no conflict of interest.

References

1. Samuelson, M.I.; Chen, S.J.; Boukhar, S.A.; Schnieders, E.M.; Walhof, M.L.; Bellizzi, A.M.; Bellizzi, A.M.; Robinson, R.A.; KD, A.R. Rapid Validation of Whole-Slide Imaging for Primary Histopathology Diagnosis. *Am. J. Clin. Pathol.* **2021**, *155*, 638–648. [CrossRef] [PubMed]
2. Patel, A.; Balis, U.G.J.; Cheng, J.; Li, Z.; Lujan, G.; McClintock, D.S.; Pantanowitz, L.; Parwani, A. Contemporary whole slide imaging devices and their applications within the modern pathology department: A selected hardware review. *J. Pathol. Inform.* **2021**, *12*, 50. [CrossRef]
3. Robboy, S.J.; Weintraub, S.; Horvath, A.E.; Jensen, B.W.; Alexander, C.B.; Fody, E.P.; Crawford, J.M.; Clark, J.R.; Cantor-Weinberg, J.; Joshi, M.G.; et al. Pathologist workforce in the United States: I. Development of a predictive model to examine factors influencing supply. *Arch. Pathol. Lab. Med.* **2013**, *137*, 1723–1732. [CrossRef] [PubMed]
4. Kumar, N.; Gupta, R.; Gupta, S. Whole slide imaging (WSI) in pathology: Current perspectives and future directions. *J. Digit. Imaging* **2020**, *33*, 1034–1040. [CrossRef] [PubMed]
5. Zarella, M.D.; Douglas, B.; Aeffner, F.; Farahani, N.; Xthona, A.; Absar, S.F.; Parwani, A.; Bui, M.; Hartman, D.J. A practical guide to whole slide imaging: A white paper from the digital pathology association. *Arch. Pathol. Lab. Med.* **2019**, *143*, 222–234. [CrossRef] [PubMed]
6. Lujan, G.M.; Savage, J.; Shana'ah, A.; Yearsley, M.; Thomas, D.; Allenby, P.; Otero, J.; Limbach, A.L.; Cui, X.; Scarl, R.T.; et al. Digital Pathology Initiatives and Experience of a Large Academic Institution During the Coronavirus Disease 2019 (COVID-19) Pandemic. *Arch. Pathol. Lab. Med.* **2021**, *145*, 1051–1061. [CrossRef]
7. Mohanty, S.K.; Parwani, A.V. Whole Slide Imaging: Applications. In *Whole Slide Imaging: Current Applications and Future Directions*; Parwani, A.V., Ed.; Springer International Publishing: Cham, Switzerland, 2022; pp. 57–79.
8. Girolami, I.; Pantanowitz, L.; Marletta, S.; Brunelli, M.; Mescoli, C.; Parisi, A.; Barresi, V.; Parwani, A.; Neil, D.; Scarpa, A.; et al. Diagnostic concordance between whole slide imaging and conventional light microscopy in cytopathology: A systematic review. *Cancer Cytopathol.* **2020**, *128*, 17–28. [CrossRef]
9. Bongaerts, O.; Clevers, C.; Debets, M.; Paffen, D.; Senden, L.; Rijks, K.; Ruiten, L.; Sie-Go, D.; Van Diest, P.J.; Nap, M. Conventional Microscopical versus Digital Whole-Slide Imaging-Based Diagnosis of Thin-Layer Cervical Specimens: A Validation Study. *J. Pathol. Inform.* **2018**, *9*, 29. [CrossRef]
10. Eloy, C.; Bychkov, A.; Pantanowitz, L.; Fraggetta, F.; Bui, M.M.; Fukuoka, J.; Zerbe, N.; Hassell, L.; Parwani, A. DPA-ESDIP-JSDP Task Force for Worldwide Adoption of Digital Pathology. *J. Pathol. Inform.* **2021**, *12*, 51. [CrossRef]
11. Pallua, J.D.; Brunner, A.; Zelger, B.; Schirmer, M.; Haybaeck, J. The future of pathology is digital. *Pathol. Res. Pract.* **2020**, *216*, 153040. [CrossRef]
12. Williams, B.J.; Fraggetta, F.; Hanna, M.G.; Huang, R.; Lennerz, J.; Salgado, R.; Sirintrapun, S.J.; Pantanowitz, L.; Parwani, A.; Zarella, M.; et al. The Future of Pathology: What can we Learn from the COVID-19 Pandemic? *J. Pathol. Inform.* **2020**, *11*, 15. [CrossRef] [PubMed]
13. Bacus, J.W.; Belanger, M.G.; Aggarwal, R.K.; Trobaugh, F.E., Jr. Image processing for automated erythrocyte classification. *J. Histochem Cytochem.* **1976**, *24*, 195–201. [CrossRef]
14. Dunn, R.F.; O'Leary, D.P.; Kumley, W.E. Quantitative analysis of micrographs by computer graphics. *J. Microsc.* **1975**, *105*, 205–213. [CrossRef]
15. Van der Poel, H.G.; Schaafsma, H.E.; Vooijs, G.P.; Debruyne, F.M.; Schalken, J.A. Quantitative light microscopy in urological oncology. *J. Urol.* **1992**, *148*, 1–13. [CrossRef]
16. Breiman, L. Random forests. *Mach. Learn.* **2001**, *45*, 5–32. [CrossRef]
17. Abels, E.; Pantanowitz, L. Current state of the regulatory trajectory for whole slide imaging devices in the USA. *J. Pathol. Inform.* **2017**, *8*, 23. [CrossRef]
18. Litjens, G.; Sanchez, C.I.; Timofeeva, N.; Hermsen, M.; Nagtegaal, I.; Kovacs, I.; Hulsbergen-van de Kaa, C.; Bult, P.; Van Ginneken, B.; Van Der Laak, J. Deep learning as a tool for increased accuracy and efficiency of histopathological diagnosis. *Sci. Rep.* **2016**, *6*, 26286. [CrossRef]
19. Somanchi, S.; Neill, D.B.; Parwani, A.V. Discovering anomalous patterns in large digital pathology images. *Stat. Med.* **2018**, *37*, 3599–3615. [CrossRef]
20. Nir, G.; Hor, S.; Karimi, D.; Fazli, L.; Skinnider, B.F.; Tavassoli, P.; Turbin, D.; Villamil, C.F.; Wang, G.; Wilson, R.S.; et al. Automatic grading of prostate cancer in digitized histopathology images: Learning from multiple experts. *Med. Image Anal.* **2018**, *50*, 167–180. [CrossRef]
21. Lucas, M.; Jansen, I.; Savci-Heijink, C.D.; Meijer, S.L.; de Boer, O.J.; van Leeuwen, T.G.; de Bruin, D.M.; Marquering, H.A. Deep learning for automatic Gleason pattern classification for grade group determination of prostate biopsies. *Virchows Arch.* **2019**, *475*, 77–83. [CrossRef]
22. Campanella, G.; Hanna, M.G.; Geneslaw, L.; Miraflor, A.; Werneck Krauss Silva, V.; Busam, K.J.; Brogi, E.; Reuter, V.E.; Klimstra, D.S.; Fuchs, T.J. Clinical-grade computational pathology using weakly supervised deep learning on whole slide images. *Nat. Med.* **2019**, *25*, 1301–1309. [CrossRef] [PubMed]
23. Esteban, A.E.; Lopez-Perez, M.; Colomer, A.; Sales, M.A.; Molina, R.; Naranjo, V. A new optical density granulometry-based descriptor for the classification of prostate histological images using shallow and deep Gaussian processes. *Comput. Methods Programs Biomed.* **2019**, *178*, 303–317. [CrossRef] [PubMed]

24. Kott, O.; Linsley, D.; Amin, A.; Karagounis, A.; Jeffers, C.; Golijanin, D.; Serre, T.; Gershman, B. Development of a deep learning algorithm for the histopathologic diagnosis and gleason grading of prostate cancer biopsies: A pilot study. *Eur. Urol. Focus* **2021**, *7*, 347–351. [CrossRef] [PubMed]
25. Strom, P.; Kartasalo, K.; Olsson, H.; Solorzano, L.; Delahunt, B.; Berney, D.M.; Bostwick, D.G.; Evans, A.J.; Grignon, D.J.; Humphrey, P.A.; et al. Artificial intelligence for diagnosis and grading of prostate cancer in biopsies: A population-based, diagnostic study. *Lancet Oncol.* **2020**, *21*, 222–232. [CrossRef]
26. Raciti, P.; Sue, J.; Ceballos, R.; Godrich, R.; Kunz, J.D.; Kapur, S.; Reuter, V.; Grady, L.; Kanan, C.; Klimstra, D.S.; et al. Novel artificial intelligence system increases the detection of prostate cancer in whole slide images of core needle biopsies. *Mod. Pathol.* **2020**, *33*, 2058–2066. [CrossRef]
27. Pantanowitz, L.; Quiroga-Garza, G.M.; Bien, L.; Heled, R.; Laifenfeld, D.; Linhart, C.; Sandbank, J.; Shach, A.A.; Shalev, V.; Vecsler, M.; et al. An artificial intelligence algorithm for prostate cancer diagnosis in whole slide images of core needle biopsies: A blinded clinical validation and deployment study. *Lancet Digit. Health* **2020**, *2*, e407–e416. [CrossRef]
28. Han, W.; Johnson, C.; Gaed, M.; Gomez, J.A.; Moussa, M.; Chin, J.L.; Pautler, S.; Bauman, G.S.; Ward, A.D. Histologic tissue components provide major cues for machine learning-based prostate cancer detection and grading on prostatectomy specimens. *Sci. Rep.* **2020**, *10*, 9911. [CrossRef]
29. Tolkach, Y.; Dohmgörgen, T.; Toma, M.; Kristiansen, G. High-accuracy prostate cancer pathology using deep learning. *Nat. Mach. Intell.* **2020**, *2*, 411–418. [CrossRef]
30. Nguyen, T.H.; Sridharan, S.; Macias, V.; Kajdacsy-Balla, A.; Melamed, J.; Do, M.N.; Popescu, G. Automatic Gleason grading of prostate cancer using quantitative phase imaging and machine learning. *J. Biomed. Opt.* **2017**, *22*, 36015. [CrossRef]
31. Arvaniti, E.; Fricker, K.S.; Moret, M.; Rupp, N.; Hermanns, T.; Fankhauser, C.; Wey, N.; Wild, P.J.; Rüschoff, J.H.; Claassen, M. Automated Gleason grading of prostate cancer tissue microarrays via deep learning. *Sci. Rep.* **2018**, *8*, 12054. [CrossRef]
32. Nir, G.; Karimi, D.; Goldenberg, S.L.; Fazli, L.; Skinnider, B.F.; Tavassoli, P.; Turbin, D.; Villamil, C.F.; Wang, G.; Thompson, D.J.S.; et al. Comparison of Artificial Intelligence Techniques to Evaluate Performance of a Classifier for Automatic Grading of Prostate Cancer from Digitized Histopathologic Images. *JAMA Netw. Open* **2019**, *2*, e190442. [CrossRef] [PubMed]
33. Tabibu, S.; Vinod, P.K.; Jawahar, C.V. Pan-renal cell carcinoma classification and survival prediction from histopathology images using deep learning. *Sci. Rep.* **2019**, *9*, 10509. [CrossRef] [PubMed]
34. Zhou, M.; Li, J.; Cheng, L.; Egevad, L.; Deng, F.M.; Kunju, L.P.; Magi-Galluzzi, C.; Melamed, J.; Mehra, R.; Mendrinos, S.; et al. Diagnosis of "poorly formed glands" gleason pattern 4 prostatic adenocarcinoma on needle biopsy: An interobserver reproducibility study among urologic pathologists with recommendations. *Am. J. Surg. Pathol.* **2015**, *39*, 1331–1339. [CrossRef] [PubMed]
35. Egevad, L.; Ahmad, A.S.; Algaba, F.; Berney, D.M.; Boccon-Gibod, L.; Comperat, E.; Evans, A.J.; Griffiths, D.; Grobholz, R.; Kristiansen, G.; et al. Standardization of Gleason grading among 337 european pathologists. *Histopathology* **2013**, *62*, 247–256. [CrossRef] [PubMed]
36. Allsbrook, W.C., Jr.; Mangold, K.A.; Johnson, M.H.; Lane, R.B.; Lane, C.G.; Amin, M.B.; Bostwick, D.G.; Humphrey, P.A.; Jones, E.C.; Reuter, V.E.; et al. Interobserver reproducibility of Gleason grading of prostatic carcinoma: Urologic pathologists. *Hum. Pathol.* **2001**, *32*, 74–80. [CrossRef]
37. McKenney, J.K.; Simko, J.; Bonham, M.; True, L.D.; Troyer, D.; Hawley, S.; Newcomb, L.F.; Fazli, L.; Kunju, L.P.; Nicolas, M.M.; et al. The potential impact of reproducibility of Gleason grading in men with early stage prostate cancer managed by active surveillance: A multi-institutional study. *J. Urol.* **2011**, *186*, 465–469. [CrossRef]
38. Kweldam, C.F.; Nieboer, D.; Algaba, F.; Amin, M.B.; Berney, D.M.; Billis, A.; Bostwick, D.G.; Bubendorf, L.; Cheng, L.; Compérat, E.; et al. Gleason grade 4 prostate adenocarcinoma patterns: An interobserver agreement study among genitourinary pathologists. *Histopathology* **2016**, *69*, 441–449. [CrossRef]
39. Van der Kwast, T.H.; van Leenders, G.J.; Berney, D.M.; Delahunt, B.; Evans, A.J.; Iczkowski, K.A.; McKenney, J.K.; Ro, J.Y.; Samaratunga, H.; Srigley, J.R.; et al. ISUP consensus definition of cribriform pattern prostate cancer. *Am. J. Surg. Pathol.* **2021**, *45*, 1118–1126. [CrossRef]
40. Zelic, R.; Giunchi, F.; Lianas, L.; Mascia, C.; Zanetti, G.; Andren, O.; Fridfeldt, J.; Carlsson, J.; Davidsson, S.; Molinaro, L.; et al. Interchangeability of light and virtual microscopy for histopathological evaluation of prostate cancer. *Sci. Rep.* **2021**, *11*, 3257. [CrossRef]
41. Sehn, J.K. Prostate cancer pathology: Recent updates and controversies. *Mo. Med.* **2018**, *115*, 151–155.
42. Ambrosini, P.; Hollemans, E.; Kweldam, C.F.; Leenders, G.; Stallinga, S.; Vos, F. Automated detection of cribriform growth patterns in prostate histology images. *Sci. Rep.* **2020**, *10*, 14904. [CrossRef] [PubMed]
43. Van der Slot, M.A.; Hollemans, E.; den Bakker, M.A.; Hoedemaeker, R.; Kliffen, M.; Budel, L.M.; Goemaere, N.N.T.; van Leenders, G.J.L.H. Inter-observer variability of cribriform architecture and percent Gleason pattern 4 in prostate cancer: Relation to clinical outcome. *Virchows Arch.* **2021**, *478*, 249–256. [CrossRef] [PubMed]
44. Shah, R.B.; Cai, Q.; Aron, M.; Berney, D.M.; Cheville, J.C.; Deng, F.M.; Epstein, J.; Fine, S.W.; Genega, E.M.; Hirsch, M.S.; et al. Diagnosis of "cribriform" prostatic adenocarcinoma: An interobserver reproducibility study among urologic pathologists with recommendations. *Am. J. Cancer Res.* **2021**, *11*, 3990–4001.
45. Singh, M.; Kalaw, E.M.; Jie, W.; Al-Shabi, M.; Wong, C.F.; Giron, D.M.; Chong, K.-T.; Tan, M.; Zeng, Z.; Lee, H.K. Cribriform pattern detection in prostate histopathological images using deep learning models. *arXiv* **2019**, arXiv:1910.04030.

46. Leo, P.; Chandramouli, S.; Farre, X.; Elliott, R.; Janowczyk, A.; Bera, K.; Fu, P.; Janaki, N.; El-Fahmawi, A.; Shahait, M.; et al. Computationally derived cribriform area index from prostate cancer hematoxylin and eosin images is associated with biochemical recurrence following radical prostatectomy and is most prognostic in gleason grade group 2. *Eur. Urol. Focus* **2021**, *7*, 722–732. [CrossRef] [PubMed]
47. Tian, K.; Rubadue, C.A.; Lin, D.I.; Veta, M.; Pyle, M.E.; Irshad, H.; Heng, Y.J. Automated clear cell renal carcinoma grade classification with prognostic significance. *PLoS ONE* **2019**, *14*, e0222641. [CrossRef]
48. Berney, D.M.; Algaba, F.; Camparo, P.; Comperat, E.; Griffiths, D.; Kristiansen, G.; Lopez-Beltran, A.; Montironi, R.; Varma, M.; Egevad, L. The reasons behind variation in Gleason grading of prostatic biopsies: Areas of agreement and misconception among 266 European pathologists. *Histopathology* **2014**, *64*, 405–411. [CrossRef]
49. Nagpal, K.; Foote, D.; Tan, F.; Liu, Y.; Chen, P.C.; Steiner, D.F.; Manoj, N.; Olson, N.; Smith, J.L.; Mohtashamian, A.; et al. Development and validation of a deep learning algorithm for gleason grading of prostate cancer from biopsy specimens. *JAMA Oncol.* **2020**, *6*, 1372–1380. [CrossRef]
50. Bulten, W.; Pinckaers, H.; van Boven, H.; Vink, R.; de Bel, T.; van Ginneken, B.; van der Laak, J.; Hulsbergen-van de Kaa, C.; Litjens, G. Automated deep-learning system for Gleason grading of prostate cancer using biopsies: A diagnostic study. *Lancet Oncol.* **2020**, *21*, 233–241. [CrossRef]
51. Bulten, W.; Balkenhol, M.; Belinga, J.A.; Brilhante, A.; Cakir, A.; Egevad, L.; Eklund, M.; Farré, X.; Geronatsiou, K.; Molinié, V.; et al. Artificial intelligence assistance significantly improves Gleason grading of prostate biopsies by pathologists. *Mod. Pathol.* **2021**, *34*, 660–671. [CrossRef]
52. Bhalla, S.; Chaudhary, K.; Kumar, R.; Sehgal, M.; Kaur, H.; Sharma, S.; Raghava, G.P.S. Gene expression-based biomarkers for discriminating early and late stage of clear cell renal cancer. *Sci. Rep.* **2017**, *7*, 44997. [CrossRef] [PubMed]
53. Fenstermaker, M.; Tomlins, S.A.; Singh, K.; Wiens, J.; Morgan, T.M. Development and validation of a deep-learning model to assist with renal cell carcinoma histopathologic interpretation. *Urology* **2020**, *144*, 152–157. [CrossRef]
54. Giulietti, M.; Cecati, M.; Sabanovic, B.; Scire, A.; Cimadamore, A.; Santoni, M.; Cimadamore, A.; Montironi, R.; Piva, F. The role of artificial intelligence in the diagnosis and prognosis of renal cell tumors. *Diagnostics* **2021**, *11*, 206. [CrossRef] [PubMed]
55. Singh, N.P.; Bapi, R.S.; Vinod, P.K. Machine learning models to predict the progression from early to late stages of papillary renal cell carcinoma. *Comput. Biol. Med.* **2018**, *100*, 92–99. [CrossRef] [PubMed]
56. Singh, N.P.; Vinod, P.K. Integrative analysis of DNA methylation and gene expression in papillary renal cell carcinoma. *Mol. Genet. Genom.* **2020**, *295*, 807–824. [CrossRef] [PubMed]
57. Cheng, J.; Han, Z.; Mehra, R.; Shao, W.; Cheng, M.; Feng, Q.; Ni, D.; Huang, K.; Cheng, L.; Zhang, J. Computational analysis of pathological images enables a better diagnosis of TFE3 Xp11.2 translocation renal cell carcinoma. *Nat. Commun.* **2020**, *11*, 1778.
58. Ginley, B.; Jen, K.-Y.; Rosenberg, A.; Yen, F.; Jain, S.; Fogo, A.; Sarder, P. Neural network segmentation of interstitial fibrosis, tubular atrophy, and glomerulosclerosis in renal biopsies. *arXiv* **2020**, arXiv:200212868.
59. Kannan, S.; Morgan, L.A.; Liang, B.; Cheung, M.G.; Lin, C.Q.; Mun, D.; Nader, R.G.; Belghasem, M.E.; Henderson, J.M.; Francis, J.M.; et al. Segmentation of glomeruli within trichrome images using deep learning. *Kidney Int. Rep.* **2019**, *4*, 955–962. [CrossRef]
60. Hermsen, M.; de Bel, T.; den Boer, M.; Steenbergen, E.J.; Kers, J.; Florquin, S.; Roelofs, J.J.T.H.; Stegall, M.D.; Alexander, M.P.; Smith, B.H. Deep learning-based histopathologic assessment of kidney tissue. *J. Am. Soc. Nephrol.* **2019**, *30*, 1968–1979. [CrossRef]
61. Barisoni, L.; Lafata, K.J.; Hewitt, S.M.; Madabhushi, A.; Balis, U.G.J. Digital pathology and computational image analysis in nephropathology. *Nat. Rev. Nephrol.* **2020**, *16*, 669–685. [CrossRef]
62. Lutnick, B.; Ginley, B.; Govind, D.; McGarry, S.D.; LaViolette, P.S.; Yacoub, R.; Jain, S.; Tomaszewski, J.E.; Jen, K.-Y.; Sarder, P. An integrated iterative annotation technique for easing neural network training in medical image analysis. *Nat. Mach. Intell.* **2019**, *1*, 112–119. [CrossRef] [PubMed]
63. Bukowy, J.D.; Dayton, A.; Cloutier, D.; Manis, A.D.; Staruschenko, A.; Lombard, J.H.; Woods, L.C.S.; Beard, D.A.; Cowley, A.W., Jr. Region-based convolutional neural nets for localization of glomeruli in trichrome-stained whole kidney sections. *J. Am. Soc. Nephrol.* **2018**, *29*, 2081–2088. [CrossRef] [PubMed]
64. Zheng, Y.; Cassol, C.A.; Jung, S.; Veerapaneni, D.; Chitalia, V.C.; Ren, K.Y.M.; Bellur, S.S.; Boor, P.; Barisoni, L.M.; Waikar, S.S.; et al. Deep-learning-driven quantification of interstitial fibrosis in digitized kidney biopsies. *Am. J. Pathol.* **2021**, *191*, 1442–1453. [CrossRef] [PubMed]
65. Marsh, J.N.; Matlock, M.K.; Kudose, S.; Liu, T.C.; Stappenbeck, T.S.; Gaut, J.P.; Swamidass, S.J. Deep learning global glomerulosclerosis in transplant kidney frozen sections. *IEEE Trans. Med. Imaging* **2018**, *37*, 2718–2728. [CrossRef]
66. Ginley, B.; Lutnick, B.; Jen, K.Y.; Fogo, A.B.; Jain, S.; Rosenberg, A.; Walavalkar, V.; Wilding, G.; Tomaszewski, J.E.; Yacoub, R.; et al. Computational segmentation and classification of diabetic glomerulosclerosis. *J. Am. Soc. Nephrol.* **2019**, *30*, 1953–1967. [CrossRef]
67. Kremers, W.K.; Denic, A.; Lieske, J.C.; Alexander, M.P.; Kaushik, V.; Elsherbiny, H.E.; Chakkera, H.A.; Poggio, E.D.; Rule, A.D. Distinguishing age-related from disease-related glomerulosclerosis on kidney biopsy: The Aging Kidney Anatomy study. *Nephrol. Dial. Transplant.* **2015**, *30*, 2034–2039. [CrossRef]
68. Kolachalama, V.B.; Singh, P.; Lin, C.Q.; Mun, D.; Belghasem, M.E.; Henderson, J.M.; Francis, J.M.; Salant, D.J.; Chitalia, V.C. Association of pathological fibrosis with renal survival using deep neural networks. *Kidney Int. Rep.* **2018**, *3*, 464–475. [CrossRef]
69. Untch, M.; Fasching, P.A.; Konecny, G.E.; Hasmüller, S.; Lebeau, A.; Kreienberg, R.; Camara, O.; Müller, V.; Du Bois, A.; Kühn, T.; et al. Pathologic Complete Response After Neoadjuvant Chemotherapy Plus Trastuzumab Predicts Favorable Survival in

Human Epidermal Growth Factor Receptor 2–Overexpressing Breast Cancer: Results from the TECHNO Trial of the AGO and GBG Study Groups. *J. Clin. Oncol.* **2011**, *29*, 3351–3357. [CrossRef]
70. Fournier, M.V.; Goodwin, E.C.; Chen, J.; Obenauer, J.C.; Tannenbaum, S.H.; Brufsky, A.M. A Predictor of Pathological Complete Response to Neoadjuvant Chemotherapy Stratifies Triple Negative Breast Cancer Patients with High Risk of Recurrence. *Sci. Rep.* **2019**, *9*, 14863. [CrossRef]
71. Santonja, A.; Sánchez-Muñoz, A.; Lluch, A.; Chica-Parrado, M.R.; Albanell, J.; Chacón, J.I.; Antolín, S.; Jerez, J.M.; de la Haba, J.; de Luque, V.; et al. Triple negative breast cancer subtypes and pathologic complete response rate to neoadjuvant chemotherapy. *Oncotarget* **2018**, *9*, 26406–26416. [CrossRef]
72. Li, X.B.; Krishnamurti, U.; Bhattarai, S.; Klimov, S.; Reid, M.D.; O'Regan, R.; Aneja, R. Biomarkers Predicting Pathologic Complete Response to Neoadjuvant Chemotherapy in Breast Cancer. *Am. J. Clin. Pathol.* **2016**, *145*, 871–878. [CrossRef] [PubMed]
73. Loi, S.; Sirtaine, N.; Piette, F.; Salgado, R.; Viale, G.; Van Eenoo, F.; Rouas, G.; Francis, P.; Crown, J.P.; Hitre, E.; et al. Prognostic and predictive value of tumor-infiltrating lymphocytes in a phase III randomized adjuvant breast cancer trial in node-positive breast cancer comparing the addition of docetaxel to doxorubicin with doxorubicin-based chemotherapy: BIG 02–98. *J. Clin. Oncol.* **2013**, *31*, 860–867. [CrossRef] [PubMed]
74. Hou, Y.; Nitta, H.; Wei, L.; Banks, P.M.; Parwani, A.V.; Li, Z. Evaluation of Immune Reaction and PD-L1 Expression Using Multiplex Immunohistochemistry in HER2-Positive Breast Cancer: The Association with Response to Anti-HER2 Neoadjuvant Therapy. *Clin. Breast Cancer* **2018**, *18*, e237–e244. [CrossRef]
75. Wimberly, H.; Brown, J.R.; Schalper, K.; Haack, H.; Silver, M.R.; Nixon, C.; Bossuyt, V.; Pusztai, L.; Lannin, D.R.; Rimm, D.L. PD-L1 Expression Correlates with Tumor-Infiltrating Lymphocytes and Response to Neoadjuvant Chemotherapy in Breast Cancer. *Cancer Immunol. Res.* **2015**, *3*, 326–332. [CrossRef] [PubMed]
76. Bhargava, R.; Dabbs, D.J.; Beriwal, S.; Yildiz, I.A.; Badve, P.; Soran, A.; Johnson, R.R.; Brufsky, A.M.; Lembersky, B.C.; McGuire, K.P.; et al. Semiquantitative hormone receptor level influences response to trastuzumab-containing neoadjuvant chemotherapy in HER2-positive breast cancer. *Mod. Pathol.* **2011**, *24*, 367–374. [CrossRef]
77. Li, A.C.; Zhao, J.; Zhao, C.; Ma, Z.; Hartage, R.; Zhang, Y.; Li, X.; Parwani, A.V. Quantitative digital imaging analysis of HER2 immunohistochemistry predicts the response to anti-HER2 neoadjuvant chemotherapy in HER2-positive breast carcinoma. *Breast Cancer Res. Treat.* **2020**, *180*, 321–329. [CrossRef] [PubMed]
78. Kim, H.; Lee, S.J.; Park, S.J.; Choi, I.Y.; Hong, S.H. Machine learning approach to predict the probability of recurrence of renal cell carcinoma after surgery: Prediction model development study. *JMIR Med. Inform.* **2021**, *9*, e25635. [CrossRef]
79. Bulten, W.; Kartasalo, K.; Chen, P.-H.C.; Ström, P.; Pinckaers, H.; Nagpal, K.; Cai, Y.; Steiner, D.F.; van Boven, H.; Vink, R.; et al. Artificial intelligence for diagnosis and Gleason grading of prostate cancer: The PANDA challenge. *Nat. Med.* **2022**, *28*, 154–163. [CrossRef]
80. Ishida, J.; Masuda, T. Surgical case of lung cancer with anomalous right pulmonary vein; Report of a case. *Kyobu Geka* **2020**, *73*, 230–232.
81. Iizuka, O.; Kanavati, F.; Kato, K.; Rambeau, M.; Arihiro, K.; Tsuneki, M. Deep learning models for histopathological classification of gastric and colonic epithelial tumours. *Sci. Rep.* **2020**, *10*, 1504. [CrossRef]
82. FDA. *Authorizes Software that Can Help Identify Prostate Cancer [Press Release]*; U.S. Food and Drug Administration: Silver Spring, MD, USA, 2021.
83. Anaba, E.L.; Cole-Adeife, M.O.; Oaku, R.I. Prevalence, pattern, source of drug information, and reasons for self-medication among dermatology patients. *Derm. Ther.* **2021**, *34*, e14756. [CrossRef] [PubMed]
84. Perincheri, S.; Levi, A.W.; Celli, R.; Gershkovich, P.; Rimm, D.; Morrow, J.S.; Rothrock, B.; Raciti, P.; Klimstra, D.; Sinard, J. An independent assessment of an artificial intelligence system for prostate cancer detection shows strong diagnostic accuracy. *Mod. Pathol.* **2021**, *34*, 1588–1595. [CrossRef] [PubMed]
85. Paige Receives First Ever FDA Approval for AI Product in Digital Pathology. 2021. Available online: https://www.businesswire.com/news/home/20210922005369/en/Paige-Receives-First-Ever-FDA-Approval-for-AI-Product-in-Digital-Pathology (accessed on 24 April 2022).
86. Da Silva, L.M.; Pereira, E.M.; Salles, P.G.; Godrich, R.; Ceballos, R.; Kunz, J.D.; Casson, A.; Viret, J.; Chandarlapaty, S.; Gil Ferreira, C.; et al. Independent real-world application of a clinical-grade automated prostate cancer detection system. *J. Pathol.* **2021**, *254*, 147–158. [CrossRef] [PubMed]
87. Humphrey, P.A. Variants of acinar adenocarcinoma of the prostate mimicking benign conditions. *Mod. Pathol.* **2018**, *31*, S64–S70. [CrossRef]
88. Yang, C.; Humphrey, P.A. False-Negative Histopathologic Diagnosis of Prostatic Adenocarcinoma. *Arch. Pathol. Lab. Med.* **2020**, *144*, 326–334. [CrossRef]
89. Trpkov, K. Benign mimics of prostatic adenocarcinoma. *Mod. Pathol.* **2018**, *31*, S22–S46. [CrossRef]
90. Ibex Medical Analytics. First, U.S. Lab Implements AI-Based Solution for Cancer Detection in Pathology: PR Newswire; 2020 Updated September 1. Available online: https://www.prnewswire.com/il/news-releases/first-us-lab-implements-ai-based-solution-for-cancer-detection-in-pathology-301121728.html (accessed on 22 May 2022).
91. Laifenfeld, D.; Sandbank, J.; Linhart, C.; Bien, L.; Raoux, D. (Eds.) Performance of an AI-based Cancer Diagnosis System in France's Largest Network of Pathology Institutes. In Proceedings of the European Congress of Pathology, Nice, France, 7–11 September 2019.

92. Comperat, E.; Rioux-Leclercq, N.; Levrel, O.; Rouleau, V.; Terrier, J.; Neumann, F.; Raoux, L.; Bien, G.; Decktor, S.; Rossat, M.; et al. Clinical level AI-based solution for primary diagnosis and reporting of prostate biopsies in routine use: A prospective reader study. *Virchows Archiv.* **2021**, *479* (Suppl. S1), S60–S61.
93. Raoux, D.; Sebag, G.; Yazbin, I.; Rouleau, V.; Terrier, J.-P.; Tingaud, C.; Boissy, C.; Carpentier, S.; Neumann, F.; Frieman, T.; et al. Novel AI based solution for supporting primary diagnosis of prostate cancer increases the accuracy and efficiency of reporting in clinical routine. In Proceedings of the USCAP, Palm Springs, CA, USA, 13–18 March 2021.
94. Fraggetta, F.; Caputo, A.; Guglielmino, R.; Pellegrino, M.G.; Runza, G.; L'Imperio, V. A Survival Guide for the Rapid Transition to a Fully Digital Workflow: The "Caltagirone Example". *Diagnostics* **2021**, *11*, 1916. [CrossRef]
95. Evans, A.J.; Salama, M.E.; Henricks, W.H.; Pantanowitz, L. Implementation of Whole Slide Imaging for Clinical Purposes: Issues to Consider from the Perspective of Early Adopters. *Arch. Pathol. Lab. Med.* **2017**, *141*, 944–959. [CrossRef]
96. Andjelkovic, S.; Todorovic, S.; Pavlovic, D.; Littlechild, S.; Mihajlovic, I.; Weston, C.; Laris, C.; Moran, T.; Quick, M.; Mayer, S.; et al. Deep Multi-Instance Learning to Predict Mismatch Repair Deficiency in Colon Biopsies. In Proceedings of the Digital Pathology Association's Annual Pathology Visions Conference, Las Vegas, NV, USA, 17–19 October 2021.
97. Wharton, K.A., Jr.; Wood, D.; Manesse, M.; Maclean, K.H.; Leiss, F.; Zuraw, A. Tissue Multiplex Analyte Detection in Anatomic Pathology—Pathways to Clinical Implementation. *Front. Mol. Biosci.* **2021**, *8*, 672531. [CrossRef]
98. Paxton, A. Quantitative image analysis: In guideline, preliminary rules for pathology's third revolution. *Cap Today* **2019**, *7*, 1–3.
99. Salto-Tellez, M.; Maxwell, P.; Hamilton, P. Artificial intelligence—The third revolution in pathology. *Histopathology* **2019**, *74*, 372–376. [CrossRef] [PubMed]

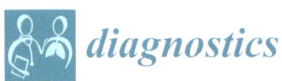 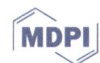

Systematic Review

Virtual Versus Light Microscopy Usage among Students: A Systematic Review and Meta-Analytic Evidence in Medical Education

Sabyasachi Maity [1,†], Samal Nauhria [2,*,†], Narendra Nayak [3], Shreya Nauhria [4], Tamara Coffin [5], Jadzia Wray [5], Sepehr Haerianardakani [5], Ramsagar Sah [6], Andrew Spruce [2], Yujin Jeong [7], Mary C. Maj [8], Abhimanyu Sharma [9], Nicole Okpara [2], Chidubem J. Ike [7], Reetuparna Nath [10], Jack Nelson [11] and Anil V. Parwani [12]

1. Department of Physiology, Neuroscience, and Behavioral Sciences, St. George's University School of Medicine, St. George's, Grenada
2. Department of Pathology, St. Matthews University School of Medicine, Georgetown P.O. Box 30992, Cayman Islands
3. Department of Microbiology, St. Matthews University School of Medicine, Georgetown P.O. Box 30992, Cayman Islands
4. Department of Psychology, University of Leicester, Leicester LE1 7RH, UK
5. Medical Student Research Institute, St. George's University School of Medicine, St. George's, Grenada
6. Department of Public Health, Torrens University, Ultimo, Sydney, NSW 2007, Australia
7. Department of Clinical Medicine, American University of Antigua, St. John's, Antigua and Barbuda
8. Department of Biochemistry, St. George's University School of Medicine, St. George's, Grenada
9. Department of Pathology, Government Medical College, Jammu 180001, India
10. Department of Education Service, St. George's University, St. George's, Grenada
11. Medical Illustrator, The Centre for Biomedical Visualization, St. George's University, St. George's, Grenada
12. Department of Pathology, Wexner Medical Center, The Ohio State University, Cooperative Human Tissue Network (CHTN) Midwestern Division, Columbus, OH 43210, USA
* Correspondence: snauhria@stmatthews.edu
† These authors contributed equally to this work.

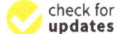

Citation: Maity, S.; Nauhria, S.; Nayak, N.; Nauhria, S.; Coffin, T.; Wray, J.; Haerianardakani, S.; Sah, R.; Spruce, A.; Jeong, Y.; et al. Virtual Versus Light Microscopy Usage among Students: A Systematic Review and Meta-Analytic Evidence in Medical Education. *Diagnostics* **2023**, *13*, 558. https://doi.org/10.3390/diagnostics13030558

Academic Editor: Valerio Gaetano Vellone

Received: 19 July 2022
Revised: 26 January 2023
Accepted: 30 January 2023
Published: 2 February 2023

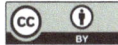

Copyright: © 2023 by the authors. Licensee MDPI, Basel, Switzerland. This article is an open access article distributed under the terms and conditions of the Creative Commons Attribution (CC BY) license (https:// creativecommons.org/licenses/by/ 4.0/).

Abstract: Background: The usage of whole-slide images has recently been gaining a foothold in medical education, training, and diagnosis. Objectives: The first objective of the current study was to compare academic performance on virtual microscopy (VM) and light microscopy (LM) for learning pathology, anatomy, and histology in medical and dental students during the COVID-19 period. The second objective was to gather insight into various applications and usage of such technology for medical education. Materials and methods: Using the keywords "virtual microscopy" or "light microscopy" or "digital microscopy" and "medical" and "dental" students, databases (PubMed, Embase, Scopus, Cochrane, CINAHL, and Google Scholar) were searched. Hand searching and snowballing were also employed for article searching. After extracting the relevant data based on inclusion and execution criteria, the qualitative data were used for the systematic review and quantitative data were used for meta-analysis. The Newcastle Ottawa Scale (NOS) scale was used to assess the quality of the included studies. Additionally, we registered our systematic review protocol in the prospective register of systematic reviews (PROSPERO) with registration number CRD42020205583. Results: A total of 39 studies met the criteria to be included in the systematic review. Overall, results indicated a preference for this technology and better academic scores. Qualitative analyses reported improved academic scores, ease of use, and enhanced collaboration amongst students as the top advantages, whereas technical issues were a disadvantage. The performance comparison of virtual versus light microscopy meta-analysis included 19 studies. Most (10/39) studies were from medical universities in the USA. VM was mainly used for teaching pathology courses (25/39) at medical schools (30/39). Dental schools (10/39) have also reported using VM for teaching microscopy. The COVID-19 pandemic was responsible for the transition to VM use in 17/39 studies. The pooled effect size of 19 studies significantly demonstrated higher exam performance (SMD: 1.36 [95% CI: 0.75, 1.96], $p < 0.001$) among the students who used VM for their learning. Students in the VM group demonstrated significantly higher exam performance than LM in pathology (SMD: 0.85 [95% CI: 0.26, 1.44], $p < 0.01$) and histopathology (SMD: 1.25 [95% CI: 0.71, 1.78], $p < 0.001$).

For histology (SMD: 1.67 [95% CI: −0.05, 3.40], $p = 0.06$), the result was insignificant. The overall analysis of 15 studies assessing exam performance showed significantly higher performance for both medical (SMD: 1.42 [95% CI: 0.59, 2.25], $p < 0.001$) and dental students (SMD: 0.58 [95% CI: 0.58, 0.79], $p < 0.001$). Conclusions: The results of qualitative and quantitative analyses show that VM technology and digitization of glass slides enhance the teaching and learning of microscopic aspects of disease. Additionally, the COVID-19 global health crisis has produced many challenges to overcome from a macroscopic to microscopic scale, for which modern virtual technology is the solution. Therefore, medical educators worldwide should incorporate newer teaching technologies in the curriculum for the success of the coming generation of health-care professionals.

Keywords: digital pathology; dental students; education; medical students; medical school; virtual microscopy; whole-slide imaging; systematic review; meta-analyses

1. Introduction

The advent of the COVID-19 pandemic and physical distancing posed an unprecedented challenge to the world of medical education. How do you teach medicine, a human-centered subject that requires active interaction and engagement with people, without face-to-face contact? In response to this challenge, medical schools worldwide have implemented various changes such as online lectures and virtual classrooms in their education during the last two years to adapt to the new norm [1–3].

1.1. Whole-Slide Imaging (WSI)

Even before the pandemic, however, digital pathology using digital whole-slide imaging (WSI) was steadily gaining a foothold in medical education, training, and diagnosis [4,5]. Cumulative validations of the outstanding diagnostic concordance between WSI and glass-slide diagnoses prompted constant development and establishment of guidelines regarding WSI, thus progressively broadening the scope of its use [6,7]. Following the release of the guideline on the validation of WSI for diagnostic purposes by the Pathology and Laboratory Quality Center for Evidence-Based Guidelines of the College of American Pathologists (CAP) in 2013, WSI later gained approval from the Food and Drug Administration (FDA) for its use in primary diagnosis in 2017 and continues to be updated, the latest being the Guideline Update from the College of American Pathologists in Collaboration with the American Society for Clinical Pathology and the Association for Pathology Informatics in 2022 [6,8].

WSI technology is readily utilized by virtual microscopy (VM), a computerized conversion of light microscopy images in full resolution and their presentation over a computer network [9]. VM software can reproduce a digitized, high-resolution image of a traditional glass slide and allows the users to highlight, annotate, pan, and zoom. With the ease of use, added features, and reliability, interest in the exciting potential of VM continues to be on the rise [7,10,11].

1.2. Virtual Microscopy and COVID-19

Numerous literature reviews and meta-analyses reported the advantages of virtual microscopy before the global wave of digitization from the COVID-19 pandemic in 2019 [12–15]. Researchers have endlessly highlighted advantages of digital pathology using VM in medical practice [16–19]. These advantages include:

1.2.1. General

- No risk of deterioration of staining quality or breakage of slides, no fading or stored slides, shorter sign-out time, access from any device, better flexibility, easy image sharing in clinical communication

1.2.2. Telepathology
- Quick access, elimination of physical slide transfer, better availability of service for remote and understaffed areas

1.2.3. Cost and Efficiency
- Better archiving, sharing, and easy retrieval; faster turnaround times, reduced cost of equipment, lab maintenance, and auxiliary techniques (less immunohistochemistry).

Advantages of VM use for medical educational are observed as well. Learners benefit from VM through remote teaching, multiple user access, the comfort of use amongst the modern "digital native" generation with prior computer knowledge, and better interaction between teachers and students by viewing the same image at the same time [17,20]. A meta-analysis by Wilson et al. also found that learners prefer VM to conventional light microscopy as well [13].

One notable advantage of using VM worth acknowledging is the benefit of access to slide images without restricting time and space. This unique characteristic of VM came into the spotlight upon facing the lockdowns during the coronavirus global health crisis. To ensure undisrupted quality education for students, lecturers adjusted their teaching methods to social distancing and disease-prevention regulations accordingly. In addition, the massive shift in medical education towards remote learning and digitization of the learning materials granted researchers an abundant opportunity and data to investigate VM more deeply. With the already known benefits of using digital slides, additional positive effects such as self-paced learning, improved tissue recognition due to better access to slides, improved understanding, and better academic performance have been reported during COVID-19 lockdown-adapted online classes [2,21,22].

In this review, we aim to compare the academic performance of medical students by using VM technology to learn the microscopic aspect of the disease. In addition, this study intends to include recent data on VM and WSI to present the most updated synthesis on VM and to explore any differences in usage, benefits, and drawbacks of VM that may have been newly discovered during the COVID-19 era.

2. Materials and Methods

This review reports the systematic findings according to the Preferred Reporting Items for Systematic Reviews and Meta-Analysis (PRISMA) guidelines [23]. The systematic review protocol was registered in the prospective register of systematic reviews (PROSPERO; https://www.crd.york.ac.uk/prospero (accessed on 21 September 2020)) with registration number CRD42020205583.

The review questions were "Does virtual or digital microscopy enhance student exam performance?" along with secondary qualitative assessment: "Is virtual microscopy a reliable and a better method for teaching and learning in medical education?" and "What are the student preferences for this newer technology?"

2.1. Literature Review

One author (NN) performed a literature search to identify if any systematic reviews were available or protocols registered as to our study objective. We identified three similar reviews [13,14,24]. However, these reviews had major limitations, such as not including studies that measured the efficacy of VM during or after the COVID-19 pandemic period. One of these previous studies included both medical students and pathology residents [24]. Its literature search was performed in a limited number of databases and failed to report comprehensive search criteria. Furthermore, these studies had narrow selection criteria, including only the pathology course at medical school, despite existing papers demonstrating VM or LM use in cytopathology, anatomy, histology, or hematopathology courses in medical, dental, and veterinary schools.

2.2. Eligibility Criteria

Only original research articles assessing the performance of LM and VM through the process of any data type—academic scores, student feedback, questionnaires, and surveys—were included for this review. Additionally, we included articles assessing the performance or perception of medical or dental students using VM or traditional LM. Articles were included irrespective of use for pathology, histology, anatomy or histopathology. The meta-analysis included comparative studies of LM versus VM or crossover studies. Studies with data on the students' performance measured as a percentage or score on a definitive scale and clear mention of method of evaluating students' perceptions were included. Studies published in English were included (or others if the translation in English was available).

Studies mentioning a VM resource or description of the technology used in medical or dental schools were also included. Along with this information, studies describing VM use due to the transition toward online teaching during COVID-19 were included.

2.3. Exclusion Criteria

Studies that described VM used for pathological diagnosis or involving perceptions of pathology residents were excluded from this review. Literature reviews (systematic, meta-analyses, narrative), editorial letters, book chapters, and case reports were excluded. Publications in which the modality of WSI was unclear/unspecified or no data (qualitative or quantitative) in the form of survey or comparison were available were also excluded.

2.4. Search Criteria and Database

A comprehensive database search was performed on 15 December 2021 and again on 15 March 2022 (to include updates) from the date of inception in Scopus, PubMed, CINAHL, Web of Science, Embase, Cochrane Library and Google Scholar. Various search terms such as "virtual microscopy/microscop*," "digital microscopy/microscop*," "virtual slides," "whole slide imaging," "students," and "medical education" in combinations of Boolean operators and truncation were used to ensure comprehensive inclusion of relevant articles. Search criteria were adjusted to the selected database. In addition, we manually searched recent reviews or eligible studies to identify any potential studies.

2.5. Article Screening and Eligibility Evaluation

For a fair screening process, two teams (SM, SN, and ShN; JW, TC, and SH) of researchers independently performed title and abstract screening based on study inclusion criteria. In addition, we performed a full-text analysis if the potentially relevant article's abstract did not contain sufficient information. The inclusion and exclusion criteria were used to select the eligible studies and access the full-text articles. Zotero software was used as the reference manager to import the search results from the database and exclude duplicates [25]. Google Sheets was used to screen the articles and register a primary reason for exclusion. Disagreements were resolved by collective discussion involving both teams, which ensured that appropriate publications were selected according to the eligibility criteria.

2.6. Extraction of Qualitative and Quantitative Data

One author (SM) independently extracted the available data from the eligible studies, followed by the second author (SN) reviewing the extracted data. Finally, we designed a standardized data collection Google sheet to organize the qualitative and quantitative data.

For each selected study, the following information was extracted (when available): year and country of publication, which variable was analyzed (performance, perception or both), number of participants, students' educational level, type of equipment and software used to assess WSI, types of workstation, digital slide accessibility, equipment training, LM availability and its specification, number and Scope of used samples, and how the students' performance and/or perception were assessed and their results. The outcome of interest for this meta-analysis was focused on estimating overall exam performance based on discipline and subject.

2.7. Quality Assessment

Two authors independently (SM and RN) used the original version of the Newcastle Ottawa Scale (NOS) for the quality appraisal of the included studies [26]. The NOS scale is a star-based system that evaluates the study based on three major perspectives: the selection of the study groups, comparability of the groups, and the ascertainment of either the exposure or outcome of interest for non-RCTs. For case–control studies, a study was awarded a maximum of one star for each numbered item within the selection and exposure categories. A maximum of two stars were given for comparability. For cohort studies, a study was awarded a maximum of one star for each numbered item within the selection and outcome categories. For comparability, a maximum of two stars were given (see Supplementary File S1). Finally, each study was categorized as good, fair or poor quality. A subgroup quantitative analysis of the studies was done after classifying them as good, fair or poor quality according to Agency for Health Research and Quality (AHRQ) standards (see Supplementary File S2). Any discrepancies were resolved by discussion with the third reviewer (SN).

2.8. Statistical Analyses

The Google sheet was cleaned and organized to conduct qualitative and quantitative analysis. Qualitative results were organized and included in the systematic review, whereas the quantitative data were analyzed further to estimate the overall better educational technique (VM versus LM). Review Manager version 5.4 calculated mean differences, pooled effect size, and heterogeneity. Only the studies with data on comparative exam scores went to the quantitative analytical stage (meta-analyses). Since the overall analysis demonstrated considerable heterogeneity, the random effect model to generate forest plots and publication bias was used. The choice of a random effect model was made due to the heterogeneity that was observed for different countries, different year of study, different faculty, different discipline, different teaching technique, different technical setup, and pre/COVID-19. Included studies used different scales to measure the same outcome, i.e., the units for the outcome of interest were different across studies. For such cases, the mean differences (MD) cannot be directly pooled and analyzed. Thus, MD was divided by the respective standard deviations (SDs) to yield a statistic known as the standardized mean difference (SMD) [27]. Therefore, the extracted data were computed and organized as continuous data followed by an inverse variance analysis method to estimate the SMD and 95% confidence interval. The heterogeneity was assessed using Higgins square I^2 or Q-statistic. I^2 can be interpreted as minimal (0–40%), moderate (30–60%), substantial (50–90%) and considerable (75–100%) [28]. Begg and Mazumdar's rank correlation and Egger's test were used to confirm the publication bias [29]. Subgroup analyses according to the subject (pathology, histology or histopathology) and faculty (medical or dental) were also performed.

In the qualitative data review of included articles, themes that referred to the applications, advantages, and disadvantages of VM were identified. In addition, perceptions, surveys, or questionnaire data related to student experiences with VM were extracted from the Google sheet.

3. Results

3.1. Search Results and Study Characteristics

A total of 1627 studies were identified from the selected database search. After removal of 676 duplicates, there were 951 eligible studies, of which those conducted before year 2019 were further excluded. Thus, a final number of 263 articles were screened for title and abstract and 39 full-text articles were reviewed to be included in the systematic review. The meta-analysis of the performance comparison of VM versus LM included 19 studies (see flowchart in Figure 1).

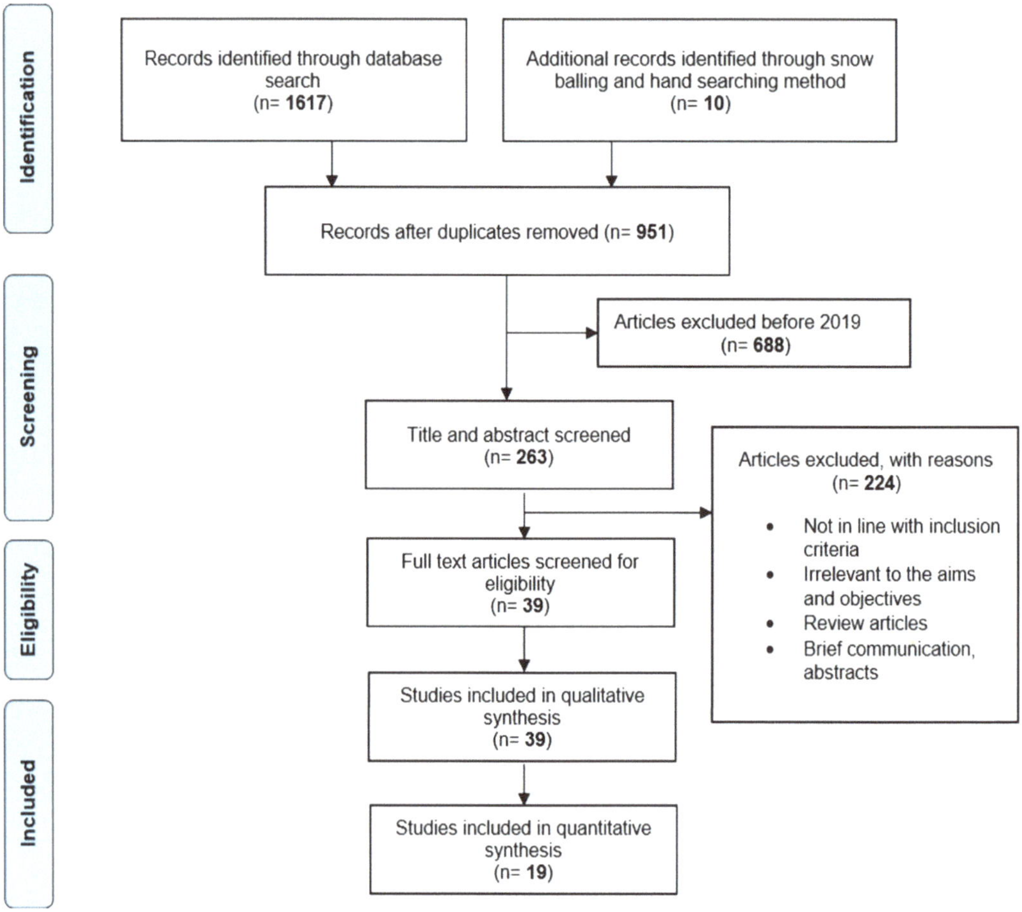

Figure 1. Included 19 studies (PRISMA flow diagram).

The included articles were published from 2019 to 2022, and originated from North America, South America, Europe, Australia, the United Kingdom and Asia. Most (10/39) were from medical universities in the USA. VM was mostly used for teaching pathology (25/39) at medical schools (30/39). Dental schools (10/39) also reported using VM for teaching microscopy. The most commonly used VM software reported by the studies (6/39) was Aperio ImageScope [30]. Only three studies in this review collected data using a randomized controlled trial protocol, whereas most collected data were based on group performance comparison without randomization. COVID-19 was responsible for transition to VM use in 17/39 studies. A detailed synthesis of included studies in this review is provided in Table 1.

Table 1. Characteristics of all included studies.

Author and Year	University and Location	Course Subject/Medical or Dental	Study Design	Total Participants	VM Setup Used	Conclusion/Results
Waugh S, 2022 [31]	Griffith University, Australia	Histopathology, medical students	Observational case–control study	150	BEST slice cloud-based library	A thematic analysis of the qualitative comments strongly indicated that online histopathology teaching was instrumental, more comfortable to engage in and better structured compared to face-to-face teaching. Compared to the prior cohort completing the same curriculum the mean overall mark was significantly improved.
Sakthi-Velavan S, 2022 [32]	Marian University College of Osteopathic Medicine, USA	Histology, medical students	Observational case–control study	477	VM podcast	Most students indicated that the podcasts enabled more efficient study time and improved their confidence in the histology content on examinations. A summary of students' feedback and academic performance supported that integration of the VMPs into Histology teaching improved the learning experience. The findings align with previous studies on the effectiveness of multimedia-based teaching in histology laboratory modules. There was a significant difference between the average histology performance of earlier classes that did not have access to the VMPs versus the average performance of the classes that had access to the VMPs.
Ahmed S, 2022 [33]	Shifa College of Medicine, Pakistan	Pathology, 3rd-year medical students	Randomized crossover control study	111	Not specified	Evidence showed that the microscopic practical skills achieved by virtual microscopy are comparable to or even better than those achieved by light microscopy.
Qing J, 2022 [34]	Wuhan University, China	Histopathology, dental students	Observational case–control study	156	NanoZoomer Digital Pathology sofware	Study compared results of assignments and exams between VM group and LM group and a questionnaire survey was used to collect feedback. Results showed an increase laboratory final test grades increased and the feedback of the questionnaire was positive, indicating that students were satisfied with the system. This study concluded that VM is an efficient and feasible teaching technology and improves students' academic performance.

Table 1. Cont.

Author and Year	University and Location	Course Subject/ Medical or Dental	Study Design	Total Participants	VM Setup Used	Conclusion/Results
Francis DV, 2022 [35]	Christian Medical College, Vellore, India	Histology, medical students	Observational case-control study	100 (cohort one), 99 (cohort 2)	VM software-Open Microscopy Environment Remote Objects (OMERO), University of Dundee, UK. WSI scanner-Digiscan (https://digiscan.co.in/)	Majority students were reported to be enthusiastic about using VM. Some of the benefits of VM as cited by the students were the ease of usage, annotations, the superior quality of images, accessibility to slides outside of lab time, in class internet access to additional learning material, promotion of self-learning and efficient use of their study time. Performance score analysis showed a statistically significant improvement of grades in the VM arm.
Nikas IP, 2021 [36]	School of Medicine, European University, Cyprus	Histology and pathology, medical students	Cross-sectional surveys	173	Websites e.g., Michigan Histology and Virtual Microscopy Learning Resources	Both histology and pathology online delivery was well-accepted by most medical students. Pathology students and students with high final examination scores perceived their virtual education more favorably.
Zhong Y, 2021 [37]	Nanjing Medical University, China	Histopathology, dental students	Comparative cross-sectional	192	NanoZoomer Digital Pathology	The mean scores of the online group (VM) were significantly higher than those of the traditional group (LM). Furthermore, both remote learning and virtual microscopy courses were well accepted by students according to the questionnaire.
Yakin M, 2021 [38]	Adelaide Dental School, University of Adelaide, Australia	Histology, year 1 and year 3, dental students	Comparative prospective cohort study	43	Biomedical Education Skills and Training network (www.best.edu.au)	Students obtained significantly higher scores in experimental exam questions than control exam questions. A significantly larger number of students perceived that the adaptive lessons improved their knowledge of the subject.
Chang JYF, 2021 [39]	National Taiwan University, Taiwan	Oral pathology, dental students	Comparative cross-sectional	38	Dot-slide system developed by Soft Imaging System GmbH (Olympus Deutschland GmbH, Hamburg, Germany)	Results showed a significantly higher acceptance rate and a significantly better histopathological diagnosis ability among dental students using the virtual slide learning than those using the glass-slide learning for the oral pathology laboratory course. VM with digitized virtual slides may gradually replace the real microscopy with glass slides for the learning of oral pathology laboratory course.

Table 1. *Cont.*

Author and Year	University and Location	Course Subject/ Medical or Dental	Study Design	Total Participants	VM Setup Used	Conclusion/Results
Darici D, 2021 [40]	Westfälische-Wilhelms-University, Germany	Histology, preclinical medical students	Cross-sectional cohort study	400	Custom histology software-Virtuelle Mikroskopie	The study concluded that the implementation of a curricular histology course in an online-format is technically realizable, effective and well accepted among students. The study also reported that availability and prior experience with digitized specimen in VM facilitates transition into an online-only setting.
Tanaka KS, 2021 [41]	University of California, USA	Pathology, fourth year medical students	Cross-sectional cohort study	37	Custom UCSF digital library	End-of-rotation data showed the remote pathology course performed well when compared to the traditional in-person pathology elective. Core strengths highlighted in this study include a high educational value, flexibility of content and schedule, organization, tailoring to an individual's learning goals and a positive education environment. Drawbacks were the inability to gross surgical specimens, inadequate observation or feedback about students' skills, and impaired social connections.
Tauber Z, 2021 [42]	Palacky University, Czech Republic	Histology, dental students	Structured questionnaire	82 Dentistry, 192 General medicine	Not mentioned	All students in this study indicated that they prefer the use of VM or the combination of VM together with the examination of glass mounted specimens by microscope.
Guiter GE, 2021 [43]	Weill Cornell Medicine, Qatar	Pathology, medical students	Cross-sectional surveys	29	University of Leeds' Virtual Pathology Library	Students conveyed high levels of satisfaction about the elective's overall quality, their pathology learning and online interactions, with minimal challenges related to the remote nature of the course.
Somera dos Santos F, 2021 [44]	Ribeirao Preto Medical School, Brazil	Histology, medical students	Cross-sectional Cohort study	189	NanoZoomer S60 digital whole slide scanner	The study reported positive subjective feedback related to handling, suitability, learning effectiveness, and pleasure using the tools for VM. Although no statistically significant differences were found between groups for academic performance, VM proved to be adequate to the Brazilian medical education in light of Brazilian social contexts and COVID-19 pandemic.

Table 1. *Cont.*

Author and Year	University and Location	Course Subject/ Medical or Dental	Study Design	Total Participants	VM Setup Used	Conclusion/Results
Cruz M, 2021 [45]	Cooper Medical School of Rowan University, USA	Pathology, medical students	Comparative cross-sectional	44	Web-based program (Aperio)	VM could help first- and second-year medical students understand case-based scenarios and clinical pathology more deeply than photomicrographs, particularly with direct faculty support for navigating virtual slides. Participation in and completion of pathology-VM learning modules enhances student learning of pathology-related topics.
Sharma R, 2021 [46]	School of Medicine, University of Texas Health San Antonio, USA	Histopathology, medical students	Cross-sectional cohort study	215 (MS1); 207 (MS2)	Not specified	Majority students agreed that the VM helped in their learning. Students performed better in module examinations in 2020 than in the previous years.
White MJ, 2021 [47]	Johns Hopkins University, USA	Pathology, medical students	Cross-sectional surveys	43	Leica Aperio AT and Roche iScan HT	Most students provided positive objective feedback related to VM use.
Lakhtakia R, 2021 [48]	Mohammed Bin Rashid University of Medicine and Health Sciences, UAE	Pathology, medical students	Cross-sectional surveys	49	Cirdan PathXL Tutor, Lisburn, Ireland	VM usage was reported as a user-friendly resource that helped students develop a strong clinical foundation and clinico-pathological correlation. High student attendance and improved assessment scores on critical thinking were observed. Easy access was a significant student-centric advantage reported by this study.
Liu Q, 2021 [49]	Shandong First Medical University, China	Histology, embryology and pathology, medical students	Observational case-control study	512	Medical Morphology Digital Teaching System	With regard to the teaching performance of VM based teaching, students demonstrated a high degree of satisfaction. Majority students achieved high scores in the web-based learning group than in the offline learning control group.
Simok AA, 2021 [50]	Universiti Sains, Malaysia	Histology, medical students	Randomized control study	120	Pannoramic viewer VM software by 3DHISTECH Ltd.	The VM group had a significantly higher satisfaction score towards the learning tool than the LM group. The knowledge acquisition of the VM group was equal to the LM group as they were shown to have a similar improvement in the test scores, comprehension level and learning ability. The study revealed a significant improvement in test scores for VM.

Table 1. *Cont.*

Author and Year	University and Location	Course Subject/ Medical or Dental	Study Design	Total Participants	VM Setup Used	Conclusion/Results
Manou E, 2021 [51]	National and Kapodistrian University of Athens, Greece	Pathology, medical students	Observational cohort study	91	e-learning platform HIPON (HistoPathology Online)	The study concluded that further research to enhance understanding of the aspects of the e-learning environment towards the formulation of policies for higher-quality education is needed.
Laohawetwanit T, 2021 [52]	Thammasat University, Thailand	Pathology, second year medical students	Observational case-control study	29	PathPresenter	There was a significant improvement between student pre-test scores and post-test scores. VM was viewed as a preferred learning modality, mainly because of its portability, satisfactory quality of images, permitting learning in less time, and stimulating cooperation between students while improving interaction with teachers.
Uraiby H, 2021 [53]	University Hospitals of Leicester, UK	Histopathology, medical students	Cross-sectional surveys	90	VM software-Philips Xplore, WSI scanner-Hamamatsu NanoZoomer S210	Study showed a significant improvement in interest, confidence and competence in histopathology. The mean performance scores were significantly increased.
Ali SAA, 2020 [54]	King Khalid University, Saudi Arabia	Histology, dental students	Cross-sectional surveys	129	Not specified	Majority students reported that using VM for practical training sessions makes the oral histology course easier and more interesting.
Samueli B, 2020 [22]	Ben Gurion University of the Negev, Israel	Pathology, medical students	Cross-sectional surveys	59	VM software-CaseViewer (3DHistech, Budapest) and Aperio ImageScope (Leica, Illinois). WSI scanner-Pannoramic MIDI automated digital slide scanner (3DHistech, Budapest).	Study reported an overall favorable response on questions relating to course interest and improvement in understanding of the covered diseases. The most significant disadvantage was technical challenges in accessing the slides.
Parker EU, 2020 [55]	University of Washington School of Medicine, USA	Pathology, medical students	Structured questionnaire survey	70	PathPresenter	The study reported an overwhelmingly positive result regarding understanding of pathology concepts as well as attitudes toward pathology.
Dennis JF, 2020 [56]	Kansas City University, USA	Histology and pathology, medical students	Cross-sectional surveys	200	Virtual Microscopy Database (VMD)	VM use improved student attitudes towards histology content and had a positive impact on student-faculty rapport. Students self-reporting an increased comfortability and understanding with differential diagnosis suggested a strengthening of self-efficacy skills.

Table 1. Cont.

Author and Year	University and Location	Course Subject/ Medical or Dental	Study Design	Total Participants	VM Setup Used	Conclusion/Results
Bacha D, 2020 [57]	University of Tunis El Manar, Tunisia	Pathology, medical students	Observational cohort study	45	Not specified	This study reported that performance of the VM is comparable to that of the LM. Thus, VM could serve as an alternative tool to LM in teaching students' general pathological anatomy.
Lee BC, 2020 [58]	National Taiwan University, Taiwan	Histology and pathology, medical and dental students	Observational case–control study	649	EBM Technologies Inc., Taiwan	The study reported a positive effect of the VM platform on laboratory test Grades was associated with prior experience using the VM platform and was synergistic with more interim tests. Both teachers and students agreed that the VM platform enhanced laboratory learning. The incorporation of the VM platform in the context of test-enhanced learning may help more students master microscopic laboratory content.
Amer MG, 2020 [59]	Taif University, Saudi Arabia	Histology, medical students	Cross-sectional surveys	166	VM software-Aperio's ImageScope. WSI scanner-Aperio AT2 High Volume (Leica Biosystems).	The study used VM during online objective structural practical examination (OSPE) of 3rd year medical students. The net students feedback was positive and the students recorded the easy image access at any time and place with VM as the most distinctive feature.
Romeike BFM, 2019 [60]	Jena University Hospital, Germany	Histopathology, medical students	Observational case–control study	140	Not specified	This study reported impact of VM use in collaborative "buzz groups" and showed an overall improvement of the histopathological competencies. The course also increased the appreciation of students for histopathology.
King TS, 2019 [61]	UT-Health, San Antonio, USA	Histology and pathology, medical students	Observational case–control study	220	VM software-Biolucida (MicroBrightField Bioscience), WSI scanner-BLiSSTM-200 (MicroBrightField Bioscience)	The study concluded that VM promoted understanding and encouraged discussion of the topics covered during the week and that group members worked well together and contributed to the completion of the portfolios. Performances on the Histology and Cell Biology and Pathology sections on the United States Medical Licensing Examination (USMLE) remained consistent and in line with national averages.
Husmann PR, 2019 [62]	Indiana University School of Medicine, Indiana, USA	Anatomy, medical students	Cross-sectional surveys	426	Bacus Laboratories (Olympus, 2008)	Statistically significant positive correlations were found with use of VM suggesting that increased use of these resources was more common in students with higher exam scores in the class.

Table 1. *Cont.*

Author and Year	University and Location	Course Subject/ Medical or Dental	Study Design	Total Participants	VM Setup Used	Conclusion/Results
Yohannan DG, 2019 [63]	Government Medical College, Thiruvananthapuram, India	Histopathology, first year medical students	Nonrandomized controlled trial with a crossover design	200	VM software-Aperio's ImageScope	Majority students agreed that VM made them understand histology better than LM. Almost 90% students agreed that they preferred VM for viewing a histology slide. A paired t test indicated that the histology knowledge of the students of both control and test groups significantly improved.
Chen CP, 2019 [64]	University of Pittsburgh School of Medicine, USA	Pathology, medical students	Observational case–control study	123 control group and 164 test group	Tutor (Philips Pathology, Amsterdam, Netherlands), formerly PathXL	The majority students responded positively that the test questions improved their understanding of pediatric diseases (75%) and test questions were helpful in assessing their knowledge of the pediatric pathology (90%), and relative ease of use for the Tutor program (80%).
Nauhria S, 2019 [20]	Windsor University School of Medicine, St. Kitts and Nevis	Pathology, second year medical students	Randomized crossover control study	152	VM software-Aperio's ImageScope. WSI-IOWA Virtual Slide Box	A majority (83%) of the students preferred to use VM over LM. Students who used VM scored significantly higher in the crossover study compared to those who used LM. This study concluded that using VM to learn histopathology significantly increased student learning and performance compared to using LM.
Tauber Z, 2019 [65]	Palacky University, Czech Republic	Histology, dentistry and general medicine students	Observational case–control study	82 dentistry and 126 general medicine students	Not specified	This study reported that a combination of both electronic materials (VM) and textbooks was commonly used by students with electronic resources being used regularly by the majority of students. No statistically relevant differences were found between the approaches of dentistry versus general medicine students. Cooperation amongst students for individual presentations was seen to be beneficial by a majority of dentistry students.

Table 1. Cont.

Author and Year	University and Location	Course Subject/ Medical or Dental	Study Design	Total Participants	VM Setup Used	Conclusion/Results
Felszeghy S, 2019 [66]	University of Eastern Finland, Finland	Histology, medical and dental students	Cross-sectional surveys	160	Whole-slide imaging platform (Aiforia, Fimmic Oy, Finland).	In the open-ended survey, most students viewed collaborative team- and gamification-based learning positively.
Yazid F, 2019 [67]	Universiti Kebangsaan Malaysia, Malaysia	Oral pathology, fourth year dentistry students	Observational case-control study	53	VM software-OlyVIA viewer. WSI-Precipoint M8 microscopescanner.	A majority of students preferred VM over LM and agreed that DM was effective for the course purpose. For the diagnosis exercise, all participants managed to answer correctly using VM compared to LM. Thus, indicating that VM should certainly be integrated as a teaching tool to enhance the learning process within the dental curriculum.

Using Table 1, we performed thematic analyses for the advantages/disadvantages reported by various studies on using VM or LM. Thematic analyses revealed various codes describing the advantages and disadvantages from the included articles (Supplementary Table S1). The top themes highlighting advantages that emerged were improvements in academic performance of the students, ease of use of VM, a positive student perception and acceptability of VM, and enhanced cooperation and student collaboration. In addition, one of the generated themes highlighted a positive impact on the teaching faculty.

Results from various studies revealed significantly improved academic test scores [20,31,32,36–38,46,48,50,52,53,58,62,63] along with improvements in the medical knowledge of students [22,34,38,44–46,48,55,58,61,63,64,67].

Development of diagnostic and practical skills during laboratory sessions was an important finding [33,39,48,53,56,58,59,64]. Studies also reported that VM promotes self-directed learning [31,35,38,41,48,58,59,64] and thus an overall better method of learning for exam preparation for the students [32,38,52,53,56].

Accessibility to the slide images outside classroom [35,44,47–49,52–54,59,64,67], ability to annotate slides [20,35] and availability of ample free resources led to a more efficient and feasible method of learning [20,34,40,41,44,48,54,67].

An overall positive acceptance for VM with a higher student satisfaction for VM-based teaching in addition to increased levels of subject interest was another reported advantage [20,22,35–37,39,41,47,49,50,53–55,59,60,64,66,67].

Improved student and faculty rapport [33,34,42,45,51,52,56,60] as well as better cooperation and participation amongst students was another interesting finding [20,31–34,36,43,52,57,60,61,66,67].

The teaching faculty also reported higher levels of satisfaction with VM use [20,35,42,57,59] and also reported VM as a time-saving and cost-effective teaching method [20,31–33,35,36,42,57,67].

Technical and internet issues while accessing the slides were the main disadvantages [22,33,38,41,44,57,67]. Few studies reported less interaction and impaired social connections along with a lack of faculty feedback as main disadvantages [22,41,44].

3.2. Quality Assessment of Included Studies Using NOS

The final included articles were predominantly of cross-sectional design, and thus an adapted version of the NOS scale was applied for quality assessment of cross-sectional studies. Others were evaluated using the original NOS scale. To evaluate each study, a n asterisk was assigned to any of the fulfilled criteria in the selected scale parameter. Table 2 represents the summary of quality assessment using the NOS scale for cohort studies.

Table 3 represents the summary of quality assessment using the NOS scale for cross-sectional studies (total nine articles).

Table 4 represents the summary of quality assessment using the NOS scale for randomized controlled studies (total three articles).

Table 5 represents the summary of quality assessment using the NOS scale for case–control studies (total seven articles).

The pooled effect size of 19 studies significantly demonstrated higher exam performance (SMD: 1.36 [95% CI: 0.75, 1.96], $p < 0.001$) among the students who studied by VM method than the LM method with considerable heterogeneity (I^2: 100%, p-value <0.001) as shown in Figure 2.

Students in the VM group demonstrated significantly higher exam performance than LM in pathology (SMD: 0.85 [95% CI: 0.26, 1.44], $p < 0.01$) and histopathology (SMD: 1.25 [95% CI: 0.71, 1.78], $p < 0.001$). For histology (SMD: 1.67 [95% CI: −0.05, 3.40], $p = 0.06$), the result was insignificant (Figure 3).

The overall analysis of 15 studies assessing exam performance showed significantly higher performance for both medical (SMD: 1.42 [95% CI: 0.59, 2.25], $p < 0.001$) and dental students (SMD: 0.58 [95% CI: 0.58, 0.79], $p < 0.001$) under VM learning than the conventional method (Figure 4).

Table 2. Summary of quality assessment of cohort studies using NOS scale.

Author, Year	Selection							Comparability		Outcomes				
	Representation of Sample		Selection of the Non-Exposed Cohort	Ascertainment of Exposure			Demonstration That Outcome of Interest was not Present at Start of Study	Comparability of Cohorts on the Basis of the Design or Analysis Controlled for Confounders		Assessment of Outcome		Was Follow-up Long Enough for Outcomes to Occur	Adequacy of Follow-up of Cohorts	
	Truly representative	Somewhat representative	Drawn from the same community as the exposed cohort	Drawn from a different source	Secure record (e.g., surgical record)	Structured interview	Yes	The study controls for age, sex and marital status	Study controls for other factors	Independent blind assessment	Record linkage	Yes	Complete follow up all subject accounted for	Subjects lost to follow-up unlikely to introduce bias; number lost less than or equal to 20% or description of those lost suggested no different from those followed
Darici D, 2021 [40]	*		*		*		*							
Tauber Z, 2021 [42]		*	*	*			*							
Somera dos Santos F, 2021 [44]	*		*	*			*							
Cruz M, 2021 [45]		*					*	*	*	*		*	*	
Sharma R, 2021 [46]		*					*		*	*		*	*	
Liu Q, 2021 [49]	*		*				*					*	*	
Lee BC, 2020 [58]	*		*			*	*					*	*	
Yohannan DG, 2019 [63]		*	*			*	*	*	*		*	*	*	
Sakthi-Velavan S, 2022 [32]		*	*		*		*				*	*	*	*

Table 3. Summary of quality assessment of cross-sectional studies using the NOS scale.

Author, Year	Selection						Comparability		Outcome		
	Sample Representation		Sample Size Justified	Non-Respondents	Ascertainment of the Exposure		Important Confounding Factors Controlled	Study Control for any Additional Factors	Outcome Assessment		Statistical Test
	All Subjects/ Random Sampling	Non-Random Sampling			Validated Measurement Tool. **	Non-Validated Measurement Tool, but the Tool is Available or Described. *			Independent Blind Assessment/ Record Linkage. **	Self-Report *	
Nikas IP, 2021 [36]		*			**				**		*
Chang JYF, 2021 [39]				*				*	**		*
Tanaka KS, 2021 [41]				*				*		*	*
Guiter GE, 2021 [43]		*		*		*		*			
White MJ, 2021 [47]		*				*				*	
Yakin M, 2021 [38]		*								*	
Lakhtakia R, 2021 [48]		*				*				*	
Uraiby H, 2021 [53]		*								*	
Samueli B, 2020 [22]		*								*	
Bacha D, 2020 [57]		*		*						*	*
Amer M, 2020 [59]		*		*	**			*	**		*
Ali SAA, 2020 [54]	*			*		*				*	*
Romeike BFM, 2019 [60]		*	*	*	**				**		
Tauber Z, 2019 [65]		*		*		*				*	*
King TS, 2019 [61]				*		*			**		
Husmann PR, 2019 [62]				*		*	*			*	
Felszeghy S, 2019 [66]		*		*					**		
Manou E, 2021 [51]				*		*				*	
Yazid F, 2019 [67]				*						*	
Laohawetwanit T, 2021 [52]				*		*		*	**		

Table 4. The summary of quality assessment of randomized controlled studies using NOS scale.

Author, Year	Selection				Comparability		Exposure		
	Adequate Case Definition	Case Representativeness	Selection of Control	Definition of Control	Important Study Control	Study Controls for any Additional Factors	Ascertainment of Exposure	Same Method of Ascertainment for Cases and Controls	Non-Response Rate
Nauhria S, 2019 [20]	*	*	*	*			*	*	*
Simok, A.A. 2021 [50]	*	*	*	*		*	*	*	*
Ahmed S, 2022 [33]		*	*		*		*	*	*

Table 5. Summary of quality assessment of case–control studies using the NOS scale.

Author, Year	Selection				Comparability		Exposure		
	Adequate Case Definition (Yes, with Independent Validation)	Case representativeness (Consecutive or Obviously Representative Series of Cases)	Selection of Control (Community Controls)	Definition of Control: no History of Disease (Endpoint)	Important Study Control	Study Controls for any Additional Factors	Ascertainment of Exposure	Same Method of Ascertainment for Cases and Controls	Non-Response Rate
Waugh S, 2022 [31]	*	*	*				*	*	*
Zhong Y, 2021 [37]	*	*	*		*		*	*	*
Chen CP, 2019 [64]			*	*		*	*	*	*
Sakthi-Velavan S, 2022 [32]	*						*		
Yazid F, 2019 [67]	*	*	*		*		*	*	*
Qing J, 2022 [34]	*			*				*	*
Francis DV, 2022 [35]	*	*		*		*	*	*	*

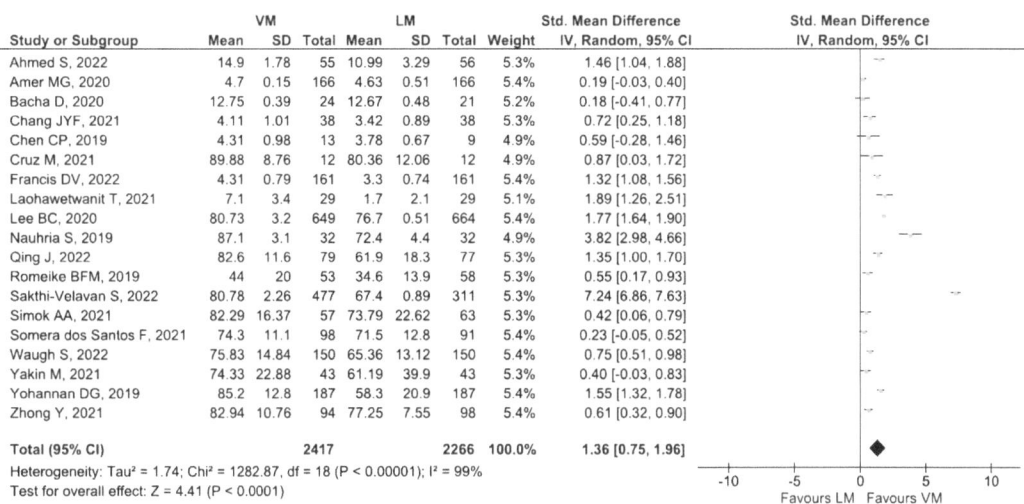

Figure 2. Pooled effect size of 19 studies [20,31–35,37–39,44,45,50,52,57–60,63,64].

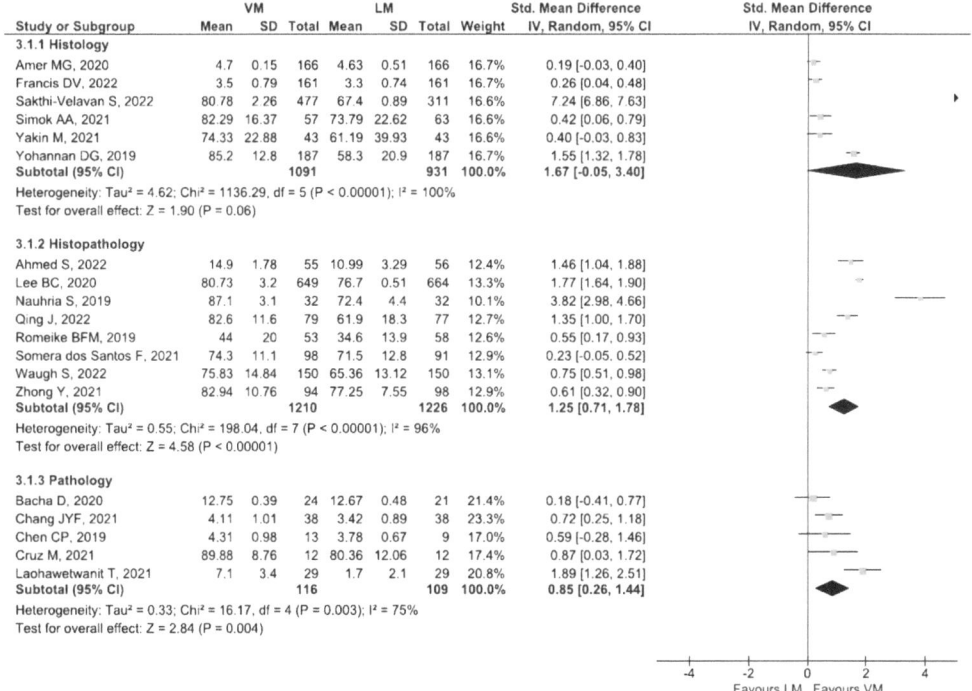

Figure 3. Analysis of studies assessing subject-wise exam performance of students [20,31–35,37–39,44,45,50,52,57–60,63,64].

A subgroup analysis on studies of low risk or bias compared to higher risk of bias was also performed based on the results of the NOS scale (Figure 5).

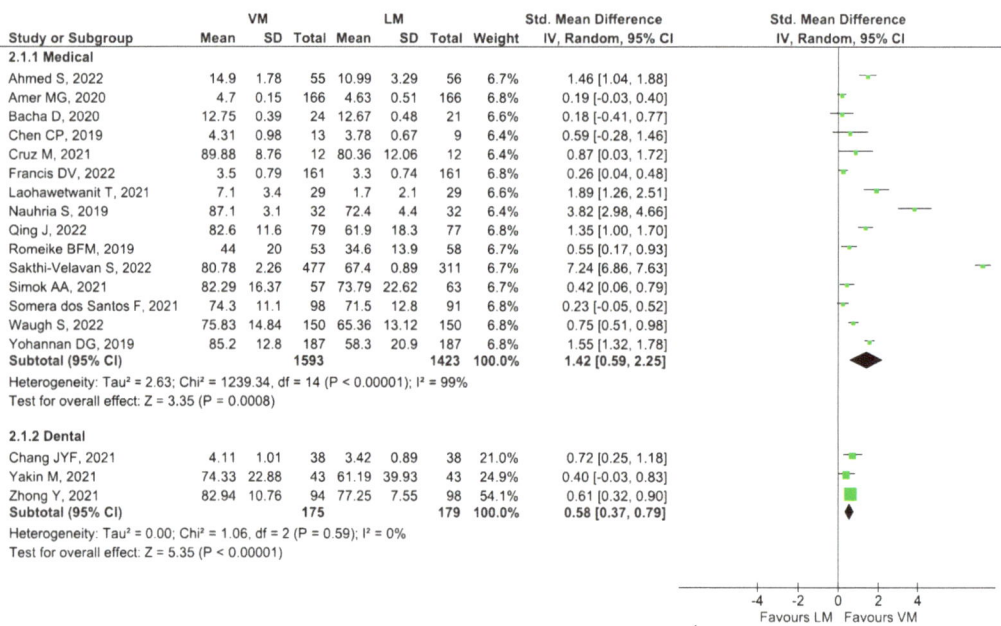

Figure 4. Overall analysis of 15 studies assessing exam performance among medical students [20,31–33,35,44,45,50,52,57,59,60,63,64].

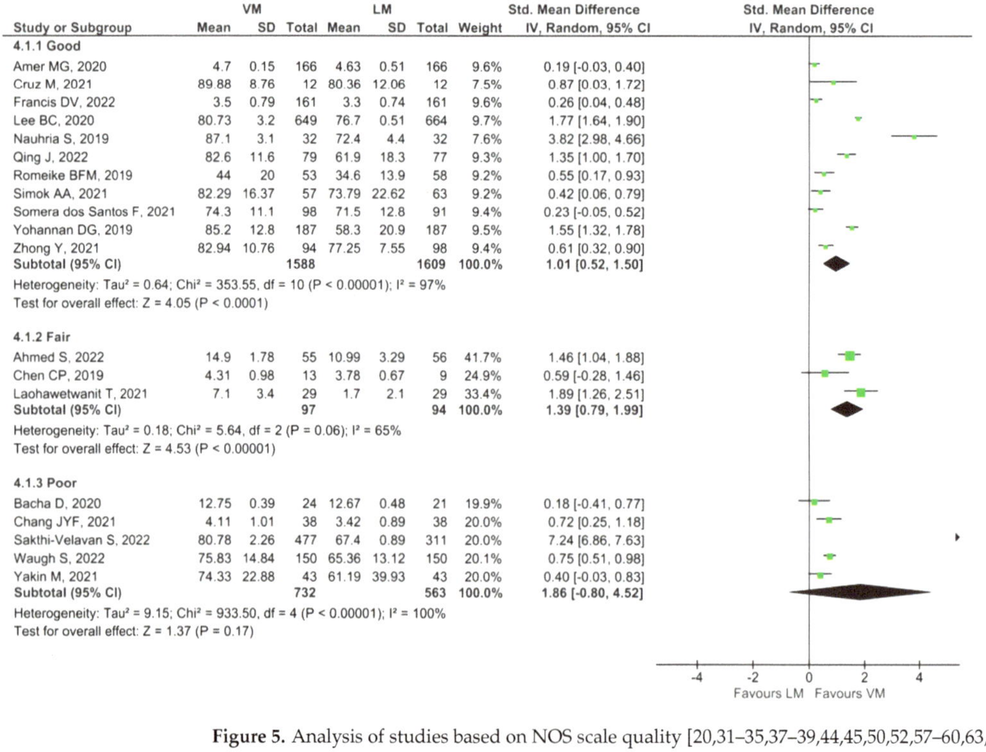

Figure 5. Analysis of studies based on NOS scale quality [20,31–35,37–39,44,45,50,52,57–60,63,64].

In sum, 11/19 studies were categorized as good quality, whereas 3/19 were fair and 5/19 were of poor quality. The result showed a clear significance for the "good" subgroup (SMD: 1.01 [95% CI: 0.52, 1.50], $p < 0.001$) as well as the "fair" subgroup (SMD: 1.39 [95% CI: 0.79, 1.99], $p < 0.001$). The result was not significant for the "poor" rated studies (SMD: 1.86 [95% CI: −0.80, 4.52], $p = 0.17$).

The studies in the funnel plot are distributed asymmetrically, which suggests publication bias. Begg's and Mazumdar's for rank correlation have a p-value of 0.19, suggesting publication bias. Eggers test for a regression intercept of 10.36 resulted in p-value (one-tailed) of 0.06, which confirms the presence of publication bias (Figure 6).

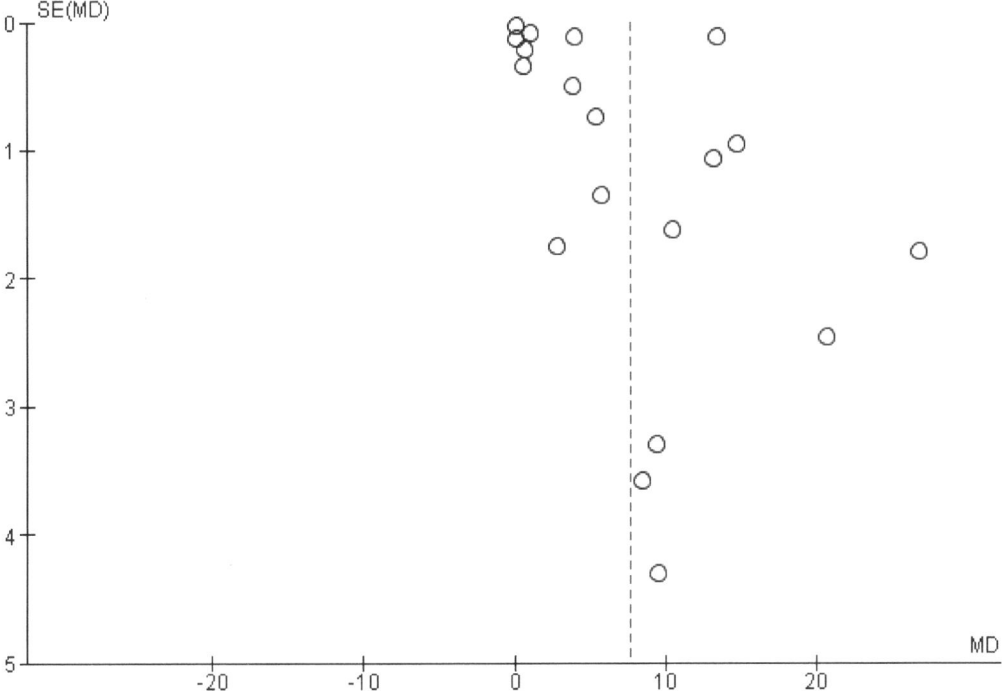

Figure 6. Publication bias (funnel plot).

4. Discussion

In this review article, the authors compared the utility of VM for teaching medical subjects in medical and dental schools. The results of our qualitative and quantitative analyses show a comparison of student performance after using VM technology. The digitization of glass slides undoubtedly enhances the ease of teaching and learning of microscopic aspects of disease. Additionally, the COVID-19 global health crisis has produced many challenges to overcome from a macroscopic to microscopic scale, for which modern virtual technology has been the solution [1].

The authors performed a systematic review considering how to remove existing literature limitations. A well-designed study criterion to include more studies, including the articles published during COVID-19 pandemic to analyze available evidence on the usage of VM for the learning process for medical and dental school learners compared to the traditional LM, was developed.

The results from the systematic review clearly show a preference for using VM. In contrast, the meta-analysis results statistically prove that overall student performance on the examination is better when using such technology for learning.

As the use of virtual learning platforms and virtual meeting spaces proliferated, educators of undergraduate and preclinical sciences adapted to using VM with remote students [2]. The use of VM in education is not unprecedented, of course, but its application and scope has significantly expanded over the last two years [21,32,36,68,69]. Much like modern students are more likely to have experience editing a digital photograph than developing an analogue photograph, the technology offers a more intuitive experience to the novice user. Clinical medicine, too, has shown VM to be a ready solution for histopathology diagnosis, supported by double-blind evidence of no inferiority to traditional modalities of diagnosis [70–72].

Various researchers around the globe have highlighted the advantages of such digital technologies when used for histopathology diagnosis, including diagnosis for such specialties as dermatology, neurology, gastrointestinal, cancer pathology and hematological diagnosis [73–78]. The advent of newer artificial intelligence (AI) and machine learning technologies that are being embedded into digital pathology and VM software have extended a pathologist's diagnostic capabilities beyond the scope of the tissue section on a glass slide [79].

The newer applications and ever-increasing usage of VM software and WSI systems propel the need to integrate such technologies for medical education, especially at the undergraduate level, as students may encounter such technology during their residency years and during medical practice.

VM has gained increasing interest in the last four decades. The benefits over traditional LM include the practical, such as storage and maintenance of slides on a hard drive with backup, and the user experience, where an entire classroom can work with a single slide. For many years, however, this resource had severe limitations due to limited data storage and image magnification technology. Using WSI technology, starting in the early 2000s, VM has allowed the user to choose the magnification of the image with the stroke of a mouse and with less technical skill than traditional LM [9,17].

Results of this systematic review highlighted findings with a focus on advantages of VM use for both students and medical teachers. Most of the included articles mentioned various advantages, such as ease of use of digital slides. Easy access and constant availability with online access were the top advantages, whereas cost of implementation was the most discussed disadvantage of VM. The current COVID-19 pandemic has clearly given a boost to the field, so more robust real-world data from larger-scale VM implementations can be expected soon.

While students have largely returned to in-person learning in the pandemic's third year, many of the innovations and remote learning adaptations of the pandemic are being integrated rather than discarded [80]. Prevailing tides of change in the digital era were already moving academic histopathology away from traditional LM in favor of a modern approach [19]. Digitizing the workspace has been a welcome improvement for learners. In one survey of pathology students utilizing VM in a remote clerkship, respondents reported greater interest and understanding of the material [22]. While some larger organizations have been able to produce and maintain their own VM database, smaller organizations have been able to benefit from the free access many institutions have offered.

An interesting aspect of the review findings in this study were the areas of VM use in medical education. Various VM-based learning activities have been employed by medical educators. Such activities include active learning activities such as group discussions, collaborative discussions, podcasts and clinical case discussions. In this review, the results show an overall positive impact of VM in a digitized learning environment and evidence indicates high acceptability and adaptability by medical learners.

Educators at the University of Eastern Finland initiated a curricular reform for histology education focused on development of a student-centered WSI platform [66]. A "gamification" histology learning model was developed that is based on incorporation of game mechanics and game theory into education [81,82].

Introduction of such a learning system into dental and medical histology courses stimulated learning and improved student satisfaction [66].

Another interesting application of VM by Sakthi-Velavan et al. involved the blending of histology content using podcasts into an integrated curriculum [32]. VM-based podcasts are narrative recordings of digital histology images. Results of the study showed a positive association between podcast viewing and improved overall class performance. The students reported a better learning experience after using the podcast-based VM. The findings align with the current review and previous studies on exploring the effectiveness of VM podcast-based teaching in medical schools [83].

During the COVID-19 pandemic, educators were forced to transition to an online distance learning pedagogy. Westfälische-Wilhelms-University, Germany and the University of California San Francisco are a couple of many such universities that successfully transitioned the entire VM-based courses to a completely online distance learning histology and pathology curriculum. Researchers at these universities used customized VM university databases and reported that the implementation of a curricular histology course in an online format was technically realizable, effective and well accepted among students. While distance learning models are insufficient for career progression in pathology, VM can still be adapted to enhance collaboration and microscopic learning of disease [40,41].

High costs of WSI scanners and VM software pose a significant challenge for adoption of digital microscopy in medical schools. Ample alternative options are available for implementation of VM for teaching and learning microscopy. Such resources include free online websites or cloud-based servers that can be accessed via the internet freely for educational purpose. Results from the analysis of the studies included in this review highlight the use of such free websites and cloud-based servers for VM resources [20,31,36,38,43].

One of the most used VM apps in this review was Aperio ImageScope, which allows viewing online or local network WSI [30]. The Biolucida viewer [84] is another such VM viewer that connects to the digital slide cloud library at the University of Iowa and can be viewed freely worldwide without any cost involved. The University of Michigan Virtual Slide Box [85] and Virtual Pathology at the University of Leeds [86] offer many WS images that can be viewed over the internet by any available web browser.

Another interesting aspect of VM implementation in medical education is the development of competence in students. American accreditation agencies such as the Accreditation Council for Graduate Medical Education (ACGME) [87] and Liaison Committee on Medical Education (LCME) [88] have outlined core skills that need to be addressed by medical schools to meet the required educational standards, including medical knowledge, patient care, communication skills, professionalism, lifelong learning and social context of health care [89]. Due to the accreditation body requirements along with the ongoing transition towards remote or distance learning, implementation of VM can help in addressing such competence and ensuring development of competent physicians for the society [9,20].

Limitations of this Review

A significant limitation of our study is the presence of a considerable level of heterogeneity. This could be due to the methodological (differences in study design, risk of bias, etc.) and statistical (variation in intervention effects or results) differences from the diverse geographical population with different cultures. For example, Lee et al. (2020) reported academic scores as percentages to compare LM and VM groups. However, Chen et al. (2019) reported academic scores on a five point scale to compare the academic improvement by using the VM. The quality of published articles can be further improved by standardizing of the research design and methodology for such an educational intervention. The NOS scale resulted in only four studies with a high score (six or seven stars) and 15 studies had a score above three stars. A total of 24 out of 39 studies had poor research design according to the NOS scale. As most educators and medical schools around the world use a wide spectrum of teaching methods along with diverse curricular designs, results for educational intervention impact will continue to be heterogeneous.

Nonetheless, this meta-analysis provides strong evidence that students prefer VM over LM (although it cannot be replaced completely) and exam performance also increased by using VM. The heterogeneity of results and different outcomes posed could be resolved in the future by introducing more subgroup analysis that would still need some homogeneous data set to work on.

5. Conclusions

This review highlights various advantages of VM compared to traditional LM for medical education. Most studies in this meta-analysis were pilot projects and first-time implementation of digital technology at various medical universities. Globally, VM and WSI technology have undoubtedly reshaped pathology teaching and learning in medical and dental schools. Use of VM in medical education has provided a venue for stimulated learning, improved student satisfaction and an overall better learning experience. Easy access to educational content and constant availability with online access are amongst the top advantages, whereas cost of implementation and access to the internet are still the most discussed disadvantages of such technology.

Availability of numerous free online VM resources has fueled global access to educational materials geared towards learning microscopy of normal tissue and pathological features of various human diseases. The ongoing COVID-19 pandemic has further fueled the need for digitization of teaching methods, particularly increased use of VM in medical education worldwide. As much of the current work on VM usage outcomes is from early technology implementation, a certain degree of enthusiastic bias in favor of VM is inevitable.

Funding: This research received no external funding.

Supplementary Materials: The following supporting information can be downloaded at https://www.mdpi.com/article/10.3390/diagnostics13030558/s1. Table S1: Themes depicting advantages/disadvantages of VM in comparison to LM; File S1: Newcastle—Ottawa Quality assessment scale case control studies; File S2: Thresholds for converting the Newcastle-Ottawa scales to AHRQ standards.

Conflicts of Interest: The authors declare no conflict of interest.

References

1. Camargo, C.P.; Tempski, P.Z.; Busnardo, F.F.; de Arruda Martins, M.; Gemperli, R. Online learning and COVID-19: A meta-synthesis analysis. *Clinics* **2020**, *75*, e2286. [CrossRef] [PubMed]
2. Caruso, M.C. Virtual Microscopy and Other Technologies for Teaching Histology During COVID-19. *Anat. Sci. Educ.* **2020**, *14*, 19–21. [CrossRef] [PubMed]
3. Cheng, X.; Chan, L.K.; Cai, H.; Zhou, D.; Yang, X. Adaptions and perceptions on histology and embryology teaching practice in China during the COVID-19 pandemic. *Transl. Res. Anat.* **2021**, *24*, 100115. [CrossRef]
4. Retamero, J.A.; Aneiros-Fernandez, J.; del Moral, R.G. Complete Digital Pathology for Routine Histopathology Diagnosis in a Multicenter Hospital Network. *Arch. Pathol. Lab. Med.* **2019**, *144*, 221–228. [CrossRef]
5. Volynskaya, Z.; Chow, H.; Evans, A.; Wolff, A.; Lagmay, T.C.; Asa, S.L. Integrated Pathology Informatics Enables High-Quality Personalized and Precision Medicine: Digital Pathology and Beyond. *Arch. Pathol. Lab. Med.* **2017**, *142*, 369–382. [CrossRef]
6. Evans, A.J.; Brown, R.W.; Bui, M.M.; Chlipala, E.A.; Lacchetti, C.; Milner, D.A.; Pantanowitz, L.; Parwani, A.V.; Reid, K.; Riben, M.W.; et al. Validating Whole Slide Imaging Systems for Diagnostic Purposes in Pathology. *Arch. Pathol. Lab. Med.* **2022**, *146*, 440–450. [CrossRef]
7. Jahn, S.W.; Plass, M.; Moinfar, F. Digital Pathology: Advantages, Limitations and Emerging Perspectives. *J. Clin. Med.* **2020**, *9*, 3697. [CrossRef]
8. FDA Allows Marketing of First Whole Slide Imaging System for Digital Pathology. Available online: https://www.fda.gov/news-events/press-announcements/fda-allows-marketing-first-whole-slide-imaging-system-digital-pathology (accessed on 22 January 2022).
9. Nauhria, S.; Hangfu, L. Virtual microscopy enhances the reliability and validity in histopathology curriculum: Practical guidelines. *MedEdPublish* **2019**, *8*, 28. [CrossRef]
10. Boyce, B.F. An update on the validation of whole slide imaging systems following FDA approval of a system for a routine pathology diagnostic service in the United States. *Biotech. Histochem.* **2017**, *92*, 381–389. [CrossRef] [PubMed]

11. Kumar, N.; Gupta, R.; Gupta, S. Whole Slide Imaging (WSI) in Pathology: Current Perspectives and Future Directions. *J. Digit. Imaging* **2020**, *33*, 1034–1040. [CrossRef]
12. Araújo, A.L.D.; Arboleda, L.P.A.; Palmier, N.R.; Fonsêca, J.M.; de Pauli Paglioni, M.; Gomes-Silva, W.; Ribeiro, A.C.P.; Brandão, T.B.; Simonato, L.E.; Speight, P.M.; et al. The performance of digital microscopy for primary diagnosis in human pathology: A systematic review. *Virchows Arch.* **2019**, *474*, 269–287. [CrossRef] [PubMed]
13. Wilson, A.B.; Taylor, M.A.; Klein, B.A.; Sugrue, M.K.; Whipple, E.C.; Brokaw, J.J. Meta-analysis and review of learner performance and preference: Virtual versus optical microscopy. *Med. Educ.* **2016**, *50*, 428–440. [CrossRef] [PubMed]
14. Kuo, K.H.; Leo, J.M. Optical Versus Virtual Microscope for Medical Education: A Systematic Review. *Anat. Sci. Educ.* **2018**, *12*, 678–685. [CrossRef]
15. Joaquim, D.C.; Hortsch, M.; Silva, A.S.R.d.; David, P.B.; Leite, A.C.R.d.M.; Girão-Carmona, V.C.C. Digital information and communication technologies on histology learning: What to expect?—An integrative review. *Anat. Histol. Embryol.* **2021**, *51*, 180–188. [CrossRef] [PubMed]
16. Indu, M.; Rathy, R.; Binu, M.P. "Slide less pathology": Fairy tale or reality? *J. Oral Maxillofac. Pathol.* **2016**, *20*, 284–288. [CrossRef]
17. Saco, A.; Bombi, J.A.; Garcia, A.; Ramírez, J.; Ordi, J. Current Status of Whole-Slide Imaging in Education. *Pathobiology* **2016**, *83*, 79–88. [CrossRef] [PubMed]
18. Sasongko, W.D.; Widiastuti, I. Virtual lab for vocational education in Indonesia: A review of the literature. In Proceedings of the The 2nd International Conference on Science, Mathematics, Environment, and Education; AIP Publishing: Long Island, NY, USA, 2019.
19. Lujan, G.M.; Savage, J.; Shana'ah, A.; Yearsley, M.; Thomas, D.; Allenby, P.; Otero, J.; Limbach, A.L.; Cui, X.; Scarl, R.T.; et al. Digital Pathology Initiatives and Experience of a Large Academic Institution During the Coronavirus Disease 2019 (COVID-19) Pandemic. *Arch. Pathol. Lab. Med.* **2021**, *145*, 1051–1061. [CrossRef] [PubMed]
20. Nauhria, S.; Ramdass, P. Randomized cross-over study and a qualitative analysis comparing virtual microscopy and light microscopy for learning undergraduate histopathology. *Indian J. Pathol. Microbiol.* **2019**, *62*, 84–90. [CrossRef]
21. Balseiro, A.; Pérez-Martínez, C.; de Paz, P.; García Iglesias, M.J. Evaluation of the COVID-19 Lockdown-Adapted Online Methodology for the Cytology and Histology Course as Part of the Degree in Veterinary Medicine. *Vet. Sci.* **2022**, *9*, 51. [CrossRef]
22. Samueli, B.; Sror, N.; Jotkowitz, A.; Taragin, B. Remote pathology education during the COVID-19 era: Crisis converted to opportunity. *Ann. Diagn. Pathol.* **2020**, *49*, 151612. [CrossRef]
23. Page, M.J.; McKenzie, J.E.; Bossuyt, P.M.; Boutron, I.; Hoffmann, T.C.; Mulrow, C.D.; Shamseer, L.; Tetzlaff, J.M.; Akl, E.A.; Brennan, S.E.; et al. The PRISMA 2020 statement: An updated guideline for reporting systematic reviews. *BMJ* **2021**, *372*, n71. [CrossRef] [PubMed]
24. Rodrigues-Fernandes, C.I.; Speight, P.M.; Khurram, S.A.; Araújo, A.L.D.; Perez, D.E.d.C.; Fonseca, F.P.; Lopes, M.A.; de Almeida, O.P.; Vargas, P.A.; Santos-Silva, A.R. The use of digital microscopy as a teaching method for human pathology: A systematic review. *Virchows Arch.* **2020**, *477*, 475–486. [CrossRef] [PubMed]
25. Mueen Ahmed, K.K.; Dhubaib, B.E.A. Zotero: A bibliographic assistant to researcher. *J. Pharm. Pharm.* **2022**, *2*, 304–305. [CrossRef]
26. Luchini, C.; Stubbs, B.; Solmi, M.; Veronese, N. Assessing the quality of studies in meta-analyses: Advantages and limitations of the Newcastle Ottawa Scale. *World J. Meta-Anal.* **2017**, *5*, 80–84. [CrossRef]
27. Andrade, C. Mean Difference, Standardized Mean Difference (SMD), and Their Use in Meta-Analysis. *J. Clin. Psychiatry* **2020**, *81*, 20f13681. [CrossRef]
28. Higgins, J.P.T.; Thomas, J.; Chandler, J.; Cumpston, M.; Li, T.; Page, M.J.; Welch, V.A. *Cochrane Handbook for Systematic Reviews of Interventions*; Wiley: Hoboken, NJ, USA, 2019.
29. Van Enst, W.A.; Ochodo, E.; Scholten, R.J.P.M.; Hooft, L.; Leeflang, M.M. Investigation of publication bias in meta-analyses of diagnostic test accuracy: A meta-epidemiological study. *BMC Med. Res. Methodol.* **2014**, *14*, 70. [CrossRef]
30. Aperio ImageScope—Pathology Slide Viewing Software. Available online: https://www.leicabiosystems.com/digital-pathology/manage/aperio-imagescope/ (accessed on 14 December 2022).
31. Waugh, S.; Devin, J.; Lam, A.K.-Y.; Gopalan, V. E-learning and the virtual transformation of histopathology teaching during COVID-19: Its impact on student learning experience and outcome. *BMC Med. Educ.* **2022**, *22*, 22. [CrossRef]
32. Sakthi-Velavan, S.; Zahl, S. Integration of virtual microscopy podcasts in the histology discipline in osteopathic medical school: Learning outcomes. *Anat. Sci. Educ.* **2022**, *16*, 157–170. [CrossRef]
33. Ahmed, S.; Habib, M.; Naveed, H.; Mudassir, G.; Bhatti, M.M.; Ahmad, R.N. Improving Medical Students' Learning Experience of Pathology by Online Practical Sessions through Virtual Microscopy. *J. Rawalpindi Med. Coll.* **2022**, *26*, 122–127. [CrossRef]
34. Qing, J.; Cheng, G.; Ni, X.-Q.; Yang, Y.; Zhang, W.; Li, Z. Implementation of an interactive virtual microscope laboratory system in teaching oral histopathology. *Sci. Rep.* **2022**, *12*, 5492. [CrossRef]
35. Francis, D.V.; Charles, A.S.; Jacob, T.M.; Ruban, A.; Premkumar, P.S.; Rabi, S. Virtual microscopy as a teaching–learning tool for histology in a competency-based medical curriculum. *Med. J. Armed India* **2022**. [CrossRef]
36. Nikas, I.P.; Lamnisos, D.; Meletiou-Mavrotheris, M.; Themistocleous, S.C.; Pieridi, C.; Mytilinaios, D.G.; Michaelides, C.; Johnson, E.O. Shift to emergency remote preclinical medical education amidst the COVID-19 pandemic: A single-institution study. *Anat. Sci. Educ.* **2022**, *15*, 27–41. [CrossRef] [PubMed]
37. Zhong, Y.; Sun, W.; Zhou, L.; Tang, M.; Zhang, W.; Xu, J.; Jiang, Y.; Liu, L.; Xu, Y. Application of remote online learning in oral histopathology teaching in China. *Med. Oral Patol. Oral Cir. Bucal* **2021**, *26*, e533–e540. [CrossRef]

38. Yakin, M.; Linden, K. Adaptive e-learning platforms can improve student performance and engagement in dental education. *J. Dent. Educ.* **2021**, *85*, 1309–1315. [CrossRef]
39. Chang, J.Y.-F.; Lin, T.-C.; Wang, L.-H.; Cheng, F.-C.; Chiang, C.-P. Comparison of virtual microscopy and real microscopy for learning oral pathology laboratory course among dental students. *J. Dent. Sci.* **2021**, *16*, 840–845. [CrossRef] [PubMed]
40. Darici, D.; Reissner, C.; Brockhaus, J.; Missler, M. Implementation of a fully digital histology course in the anatomical teaching curriculum during COVID-19 pandemic. *Ann. Anat.-Anat. Anz.* **2021**, *236*, 151718. [CrossRef]
41. Tanaka, K.S.; Ramachandran, R. Perceptions of a Remote Learning Pathology Elective for Advanced Clinical Medical Students. *Acad. Pathol.* **2021**, *8*, 23742895211006846. [CrossRef]
42. Tauber, Z.; Lacey, H.; Lichnovska, R.; Erdosova, B.; Zizka, R.; Sedy, J.; Cizkova, K. Students' preparedness, learning habits and the greatest difficulties in studying Histology in the digital era: A comparison between students of general and dental schools. *Eur. J. Dent. Educ.* **2020**, *25*, 371–376. [CrossRef]
43. Guiter, G.E.; Sapia, S.; Wright, A.I.; Hutchins, G.G.A.; Arayssi, T. Development of a Remote Online Collaborative Medical School Pathology Curriculum with Clinical Correlations, across Several International Sites, through the COVID-19 Pandemic. *Med. Sci. Educ.* **2021**, *31*, 549–556. [CrossRef]
44. Somera dos Santos, F.; Osako, M.K.; Perdoná, G.d.S.C.; Alves, M.G.; Sales, K.U. Virtual Microscopy as a Learning Tool in Brazilian Medical Education. *Anat. Sci. Educ.* **2021**, *14*, 408–416. [CrossRef]
45. Cruz, M.; Murphy, M.; Gentile, M.M.; Stewart, K.; Barroeta, J.E.; Carrasco, G.A.; Kocher, W.D.; Behling, K.C. Assessment of Pathology Learning Modules With Virtual Microscopy in a Preclinical Medical School Curriculum. *Am. J. Clin. Pathol.* **2021**, *156*, 794–801. [CrossRef] [PubMed]
46. Sharma, R.; King, T.S.; Hanson, E.R.; Fiebelkorn, K. Medical Histopathology Laboratories: Remote Teaching in Response to COVID-19 Pandemic. *Acad. Pathol.* **2021**, *8*, 2374289521998049. [CrossRef] [PubMed]
47. White, M.J.; Birkness, J.E.; Salimian, K.J.; Meiss, A.E.; Butcher, M.; Davis, K.; Ware, A.D.; Zarella, M.D.; Lecksell, K.; Rooper, L.M.; et al. Continuing Undergraduate Pathology Medical Education in the Coronavirus Disease 2019 (COVID-19) Global Pandemic: The Johns Hopkins Virtual Surgical Pathology Clinical Elective. *Arch. Pathol. Lab. Med.* **2021**, *145*, 814–820. [CrossRef] [PubMed]
48. Lakhtakia, R. Virtual Microscopy in Undergraduate Pathology Education. *Sultan Qaboos Univ. Med. J. SQUMJ* **2021**, *21*, 428–435. [CrossRef] [PubMed]
49. Liu, Q.; Sun, W.; Du, C.; Yang, L.; Yuan, N.; Cui, H.; Song, W.; Ge, L. Medical Morphology Training Using the Xuexi Tong Platform During the COVID-19 Pandemic: Development and Validation of a Web-Based Teaching Approach. *JMIR Med. Inform.* **2021**, *9*, e24497. [CrossRef]
50. Simok, A.A.; Kasim, F.; Hadie, S.N.H.; Abdul Manan@Sulong, H.; Yusoff, M.S.B.; Mohd Noor, N.F.; Asari, M.A. Knowledge Acquisition and Satisfaction of Virtual Microscopy Usage Among Medical Students of Universiti Sains Malaysia. *Educ. Med. J.* **2021**, *13*, 43–55. [CrossRef]
51. Manou, E.; Lazari, E.-C.; Thomopoulou, G.-E.; Agrogiannis, G.; Kavantzas, N.; Lazaris, A.C. Participation and Interactivity in Synchronous E-Learning Pathology Course During the COVID-19 Pandemic. *Adv. Med. Educ. Pract.* **2021**, *12*, 1081–1091. [CrossRef]
52. Laohawetwanit, T. The use of virtual pathology in teaching medical students: First experience of a medical school in Thailand. *MedEdPublish* **2020**, *9*, 116. [CrossRef]
53. Uraiby, H.; Grafton-Clarke, C.; Gordon, M.; Sereno, M.; Powell, B.; McCarthy, M. Fostering intrinsic motivation in remote undergraduate histopathology education. *J. Clin. Pathol.* **2021**, *75*, 837–843. [CrossRef]
54. Ali, S.A.A.; Syed, S. Teaching and Learning Strategies of Oral Histology Among Dental Students. *Int. J. Morphol.* **2020**, *38*, 634–639. [CrossRef]
55. Parker, E.U.; Chang, O.; Koch, L. Remote Anatomic Pathology Medical Student Education in Washington State. *Am. J. Clin. Pathol.* **2020**, *154*, 585–591. [CrossRef] [PubMed]
56. Dennis, J.F. The HistoHustle: Supplemental Histology Sessions to Enrich Student Learning and Self-Efficacy. *Med. Sci. Educ.* **2020**, *30*, 1725–1726. [CrossRef] [PubMed]
57. Bacha, D.; Ferjaoui, W.; Charfi, L.; Rejaibi, S.; Gharbi, L.; ben Slama, S.; Njim, L.; Lahmar, A. The interest of virtual microscopy as a means of simulation learning in pathological anatomy and cytology. *Oncol. Radiother.* **2020**, *14*, 23–29.
58. Lee, B.C.; Hsieh, S.T.; Chang, Y.L.; Tseng, F.Y.; Lin, Y.J.; Chen, Y.L.; Wang, S.H.; Chang, Y.F.; Ho, Y.L.; Ni, Y.H.; et al. A Web-Based Virtual Microscopy Platform for Improving Academic Performance in Histology and Pathology Laboratory Courses: A Pilot Study. *Anat. Sci. Educ.* **2020**, *13*, 743–758. [CrossRef] [PubMed]
59. Amer, M.; Nemenqani, D. Successful use of virtual microscopy in the assessment of practical histology during pandemic COVID-19: A descriptive study. *J. Microsc. Ultrastruct.* **2020**, *8*, 156–161. [CrossRef] [PubMed]
60. Romeike, B.F.M.; Fischer, M. Buzz groups facilitate collaborative learning and improve histopathological competencies of students. *Clin. Neuropathol.* **2019**, *38*, 285–293. [CrossRef]
61. King, T.S.; Sharma, R.; Jackson, J.; Fiebelkorn, K.R. Clinical Case-Based Image Portfolios in Medical Histopathology. *Anat. Sci. Educ.* **2019**, *12*, 200–209. [CrossRef]
62. Husmann, P.R.; O'Loughlin, V.D. Another Nail in the Coffin for Learning Styles? Disparities among Undergraduate Anatomy Students' Study Strategies, Class Performance, and Reported VARK Learning Styles. *Anat. Sci. Educ.* **2019**, *12*, 6–19. [CrossRef]

63. Yohannan, D.G.; Oommen, A.M.; Umesan, K.G.; Raveendran, V.L.; Sreedhar, L.S.L.; Anish, T.S.N.; Hortsch, M.; Krishnapillai, R. Overcoming Barriers in a Traditional Medical Education System by the Stepwise, Evidence-Based Introduction of a Modern Learning Technology. *Med. Sci. Educ.* **2019**, *29*, 803–817. [CrossRef]
64. Chen, C.P.; Clifford, B.M.; O'Leary, M.J.; Hartman, D.J.; Picarsic, J.L. Improving Medical Students' Understanding of Pediatric Diseases through an Innovative and Tailored Web-based Digital Pathology Program with Philips Pathology Tutor (Formerly PathXL). *J. Pathol. Inform.* **2019**, *10*, 18. [CrossRef]
65. Tauber, Z.; Cizkova, K.; Lichnovska, R.; Lacey, H.; Erdosova, B.; Zizka, R.; Kamarad, V. Evaluation of the effectiveness of the presentation of virtual histology slides by students during classes. Are there any differences in approach between dentistry and general medicine students? *Eur. J. Dent. Educ.* **2019**, *23*, 119–126. [CrossRef] [PubMed]
66. Felszeghy, S.; Pasonen-Seppänen, S.; Koskela, A.; Nieminen, P.; Härkönen, K.; Paldanius, K.M.A.; Gabbouj, S.; Ketola, K.; Hiltunen, M.; Lundin, M.; et al. Using online game-based platforms to improve student performance and engagement in histology teaching. *BMC Med. Educ.* **2019**, *19*, 273. [CrossRef] [PubMed]
67. Yazid, F.; Ghazali, N.; Rosli, M.S.A.; Apandi, N.I.M.; Ibrahim, N. The Use of Digital Microscope in Oral Pathology Teaching. *J. Int. Dent. Med. Res.* **2019**, *12*, 1095–1099.
68. Lionetti, K.A.; Townsend, H. Teaching Microscopy Remotely: Two Engaging Options. *J. Microbiol. Biol. Educ.* **2022**, *23*, 1–3. [CrossRef]
69. Clarke, E.; Doherty, D.; Randell, R.; Grek, J.; Thomas, R.; Ruddle, R.A.; Treanor, D. Faster than light (microscopy): Superiority of digital pathology over microscopy for assessment of immunohistochemistry. *J. Clin. Pathol.* **2022**. [CrossRef] [PubMed]
70. Samuelson, M.I.; Chen, S.J.; Boukhar, S.A.; Schnieders, E.M.; Walhof, M.L.; Bellizzi, A.M.; Robinson, R.A.; Rajan, K.D.A. Rapid Validation of Whole-Slide Imaging for Primary Histopathology Diagnosis. *Am. J. Clin. Pathol.* **2021**, *155*, 638–648. [CrossRef]
71. Liscia, D.S.; Bellis, D.; Biletta, E.; D'Andrea, M.; Croci, G.A.; Dianzani, U. Whole-Slide Imaging Allows Pathologists to Work Remotely in Regions with Severe Logistical Constraints Due to COVID-19 Pandemic. *J. Pathol. Inform.* **2020**, *11*, 20. [CrossRef]
72. Blum, A.E.; Murphy, G.F.; Lee, J.J. Digital dermatopathology: The time is now. *J. Cutan. Pathol.* **2021**, *48*, 469–471. [CrossRef] [PubMed]
73. Alassiri, A.; Almutrafi, A.; Alsufiani, F.; Al Nehkilan, A.; Al Salim, A.; Musleh, H.; Aziz, M.; Khalbuss, W. Whole slide imaging compared with light microscopy for primary diagnosis in surgical neuropathology: A validation study. *Ann. Saudi Med.* **2020**, *40*, 36–41. [CrossRef]
74. Ammendola, S.; Bariani, E.; Eccher, A.; Capitanio, A.; Ghimenton, C.; Pantanowitz, L.; Parwani, A.; Girolami, I.; Scarpa, A.; Barresi, V. The histopathological diagnosis of atypical meningioma: Glass slide versus whole slide imaging for grading assessment. *Virchows Arch.* **2020**, *478*, 747–756. [CrossRef]
75. Babawale, M.; Gunavardhan, A.; Walker, J.; Corfield, T.; Huey, P.; Savage, A.; Bansal, A.; Atkinson, M.; Abdelsalam, H.; Raweily, E.; et al. Verification and Validation of Digital Pathology (Whole Slide Imaging) for Primary Histopathological Diagnosis: All Wales Experience. *J. Pathol. Inform.* **2021**, *12*. [CrossRef] [PubMed]
76. Borowsky, A.D.; Glassy, E.F.; Wallace, W.D.; Kallichanda, N.S.; Behling, C.A.; Miller, D.V.; Oswal, H.N.; Feddersen, R.M.; Bakhtar, O.R.; Mendoza, A.E.; et al. Digital Whole Slide Imaging Compared With Light Microscopy for Primary Diagnosis in Surgical Pathology. *Arch. Pathol. Lab. Med.* **2020**, *144*, 1245–1253. [CrossRef] [PubMed]
77. Lam, A.K.; Leung, M. Whole-Slide Imaging for Esophageal Adenocarcinoma. In *Esophageal Adenocarcinoma*; Methods in Molecular Biology; Springer: Berlin/Heidelberg, Germany, 2018; pp. 135–142.
78. Wang, C.; Wei, X.-L.; Li, C.-X.; Wang, Y.-Z.; Wu, Y.; Niu, Y.-X.; Zhang, C.; Yu, Y. Efficient and Highly Accurate Diagnosis of Malignant Hematological Diseases Based on Whole-Slide Images Using Deep Learning. *Front. Oncol.* **2022**, *12*, 879308. [CrossRef] [PubMed]
79. Niazi, M.K.K.; Parwani, A.V.; Gurcan, M.N. Digital pathology and artificial intelligence. *Lancet Oncol.* **2019**, *20*, e253–e261. [CrossRef] [PubMed]
80. Frazier, P.I.; Cashore, J.M.; Duan, N.; Henderson, S.G.; Janmohamed, A.; Liu, B.; Shmoys, D.B.; Wan, J.; Zhang, Y. Modeling for COVID-19 college reopening decisions: Cornell, a case study. *Proc. Natl. Acad. Sci. USA* **2022**, *119*, e2112532119. [CrossRef] [PubMed]
81. Van Gaalen, A.E.J.; Brouwer, J.; Schönrock-Adema, J.; Bouwkamp-Timmer, T.; Jaarsma, A.D.C.; Georgiadis, J.R. Gamification of health professions education: A systematic review. *Adv. Health Sci. Educ.* **2020**, *26*, 683–711. [CrossRef]
82. Bai, S.; Hew, K.F.; Gonda, D.E.; Huang, B.; Liang, X. Incorporating fantasy into gamification promotes student learning and quality of online interaction. *Int. J. Educ. Technol. High. Educ.* **2022**, *19*, 29. [CrossRef]
83. Roth, J.; Chang, A.; Ricci, B.; Hall, M.; Mehta, N. Why Not a Podcast? Assessing Narrative Audio and Written Curricula in Obstetrical Neurology. *J. Grad. Med. Educ.* **2020**, *12*, 86–91. [CrossRef]
84. Biolucida. Available online: https://www.mbfbioscience.com/biolucida (accessed on 14 December 2022).
85. University of Michigan Virtual Slide Box. Available online: https://www.pathology.med.umich.edu/apps/slides/ (accessed on 14 December 2022).
86. Virtual Pathology at the University of Leeds. Available online: https://www.virtualpathology.leeds.ac.uk/ (accessed on 10 October 2022).
87. The Milestones Guidebook. Available online: https://www.acgme.org/globalassets/MilestonesGuidebook.pdf (accessed on 25 December 2021).

88. Standards, Publications, & Notification Forms. Available online: https://lcme.org/publications/ (accessed on 10 January 2021).
89. Hassell, L.A.; Fung, K.-M.; Chaser, B. Digital slides and ACGME resident competencies in anatomic pathology: An altered paradigm for acquisition and assessment. *J. Pathol. Inform.* **2011**, *2*, 27. [CrossRef]

Disclaimer/Publisher's Note: The statements, opinions and data contained in all publications are solely those of the individual author(s) and contributor(s) and not of MDPI and/or the editor(s). MDPI and/or the editor(s) disclaim responsibility for any injury to people or property resulting from any ideas, methods, instructions or products referred to in the content.

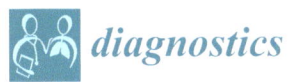

Review

Virtual Pathology Education in Medical Schools Worldwide during the COVID-19 Pandemic: Advantages, Challenges Faced, and Perspectives

Angela Ishak [1,†], Mousa M. AlRawashdeh [1,†], Maria Meletiou-Mavrotheris [2] and Ilias P. Nikas [1,*]

1 School of Medicine, European University Cyprus, Nicosia 2404, Cyprus; angela.ishak.10@gmail.com (A.I.); mousa99mahmoud@gmail.com (M.M.A.)
2 Department of Education Sciences, European University Cyprus, Nicosia 2404, Cyprus; m.mavrotheris@euc.ac.cy
* Correspondence: i.nikas@euc.ac.cy
† These authors contributed equally to this work.

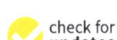

Citation: Ishak, A.; AlRawashdeh, M.M.; Meletiou-Mavrotheris, M.; Nikas, I.P. Virtual Pathology Education in Medical Schools Worldwide during the COVID-19 Pandemic: Advantages, Challenges Faced, and Perspectives. *Diagnostics* **2022**, *12*, 1578. https://doi.org/10.3390/diagnostics12071578

Academic Editor: Catarina Eloy

Received: 8 June 2022
Accepted: 27 June 2022
Published: 29 June 2022

Publisher's Note: MDPI stays neutral with regard to jurisdictional claims in published maps and institutional affiliations.

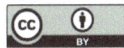

Copyright: © 2022 by the authors. Licensee MDPI, Basel, Switzerland. This article is an open access article distributed under the terms and conditions of the Creative Commons Attribution (CC BY) license (https://creativecommons.org/licenses/by/4.0/).

Abstract: The COVID-19 pandemic shifted pathology education in medical schools worldwide towards online delivery. To achieve this goal, various innovative platforms were used by pathology educators and medical students, facilitating both synchronous and asynchronous learning. The aim of this study was to review the published evidence regarding remote pathology teaching at the medical school level during this period, present our own experience, and provide some perspectives regarding the best mode of pathology teaching post-pandemic. Among its advantages, virtual pathology education was considered among students and educators as convenient, flexible, and engaging, while learning outcomes were met and students' academic performance was in general satisfactory. However, several challenges were faced. For instance, suboptimal internet connection compromised the flow of classes and was even associated with a lower academic performance. The lack of hands-on laboratory activities, such as operating the light microscope and tissue grossing, and the reduced student interactions among themselves and their instructors, were also pointed out as significant drawbacks of remote pathology education. Whereas online education has multiple advantages, experiencing the physical university environment, in-person interactions and teamwork, exposure to the "hidden curriculum", and hands-on activities are vital for medical school education and future student development. In conclusion, the implementation of a blended approach in pathology education—where online and face-to-face sessions are jointly used to promote students' engagement, interaction with their instructors and peers, and learning—could be the most optimal approach to pathology teaching in medical schools post-pandemic.

Keywords: digital pathology; online education; laboratory medicine; histopathology; medical students; distance learning; emergency remote teaching; e-learning; virtual microscopy; anatomy and histology

1. Introduction

Pathology teaching in medical schools worldwide focuses on the study of disease, being the bridge between basic science and clinical practice [1]. Medical students learn the basics of pathology through various teaching modalities including lectures, small group sessions, and assignments as well as traditional and/or virtual microscopy. Recently, there has been a tendency to include more case studies and exercises highlighting clinicopathological correlations into pathology teaching, in order to integrate with other courses within the medical school curriculum and emphasize pathology's clinical significance in medicine's multidisciplinary setting [1–3]. In general, pathology courses run for a whole semester or more when designed for preclinical medical students [3–6]. Notably, in some medical schools, senior medical students can additionally choose to attend a more advanced pathology elective which could be 2- to 4- weeks duration. In such electives and in contrast to the preclinical pathology courses, participants are exposed more to pathology as a profession, in addition to the role of pathologists in today's medical practice, by shadowing residents and attendings, attending grand rounds, and participating in daily sign-out sessions [7–11].

In the pre-pandemic era, most pathology teachings were performed conventionally within the medical schools' premises [12,13]. However, due to the unprecedented challenges to medical schools worldwide induced by the COVID-19 pandemic, pathology teaching around the world largely shifted towards remote delivery, and whole courses needed to be re-designed to fit the online environment. In addition, pathology educators had to adjust their teaching style, learn novel technologies, and create new material suitable to teach remotely during the unprecedented period they were facing [4,8,11,14,15]. Various innovative platforms were used, designed to facilitate both synchronous and asynchronous learning, as well as small group sessions. Examples of such platforms include Zoom (Zoom Video Communications, Inc., San Jose, CA, USA), Blackboard Learn (Blackboard Inc., Washington, DC, USA), Microsoft Teams (Microsoft Corporation, Albuquerque, NM, USA), Google Classroom (Google LLC., Mountain View, CA, USA), and Google Meet (Google LLC., Mountain View, CA, USA) [8,11,14,16]. Notably, digital pathology was exclusively utilized for the microscopic slide sessions [8,11]. In our pathology sessions and during this period, we used a combination of modalities such as synchronous interactive lectures, laboratory sessions with static images (gross and microscopic) and digital pathology, asynchronous assignments highlighting clinicopathological correlations, and quizzes providing immediate feedback to the students. Furthermore, our exams were administered online using proctoring software [3].

As several pathology educators worldwide have published their experience teaching pathology online to medical students during the pandemic period as well as the reported learning experience of their students, the aims of this review were to:

- Summarize the existing evidence in the literature regarding the advantages and challenges of remote pathology education in medical schools;
- Describe our students' experience with online pathology education and compare it with what has been reported in the literature;
- Provide some perspectives regarding the best mode of pathology teaching post-pandemic in medical schools.

2. Methods

This was a combined study, including both a review of the literature and our own experience regarding remote pathology education—at the medical school level—during the COVID-19 period.

2.1. Literature Review

The PubMed database was searched for studies describing changes in pathology education at medical schools worldwide during the pandemic. The following search algorithm was applied: (Pathology OR Histopathology OR Histology) AND medical education AND COVID-19. Initially, the database was searched on 28 January 2022, yet the search was updated on 21 June 2022. Studies describing the pathology education of residents or fellows, pathology practice implications in general, or focusing solely on histology education were outside the scope of this review and were excluded. The article selection was first performed in a title-abstract fashion, followed by a full-text evaluation of articles that fitted the selection criteria. Data extraction was performed by three authors (I.P.N, A.I., and M.M.A.), while any disagreement was resolved by reaching a consensus.

2.2. Our Own Experience

To describe our own experience, we mostly used data from our recent survey in addition to a few personal observations from our remote sessions. This anonymous e-survey was delivered to our medical students via Google Forms (Google LLC, Mountain View, CA, USA). The survey was kept open for four weeks, and following its completion, we received and analyzed the answers from 173/255 (68%) of the enrolled students (100 females and 73 males) that participated. Although its quantitative results (including the complete demographic data, predictors of the virtual learning experience, and perceived stress) have recently been published by our team [3], this survey also included some unpublished qualitative data derived from the students' answers to its five open-ended questions (Table 1) which we aimed to include in the current study and evaluate together with the literature review findings. Analysis of these qualitative data followed a thematic analysis approach [17,18], during which, data were coded and clustered as themes.

Table 1. Open-ended questions of the survey delivered to our students.

- Were there any aspects of virtual learning that you found better than campus-based learning?
- Were there any aspects of virtual learning which were impossible or impractical to follow?
- What was your biggest concern/worry related to COVID-19 and its impact on your performance in this course?
- What particular difficulties emerged in relation to the remote attendance of this course?
- What opportunities for improving the teaching and learning of this course have emerged as a result of it being offered at-distance?

Regarding the following chapters of this study, the "Results" section presents the advantages and challenges of virtual pathology education, giving a brief "literature review" coupled with "our own experience" while teaching pathology remotely during the COVID-19 period. "Our own experience" chapters begin by briefly describing the main quantitative findings published in our previous study [3], followed by a summary of the unpublished qualitative data derived from the survey in addition to a few of our personal observations while teaching pathology remotely. The "Discussion" section attempts to interpret the findings presented in the "Results" and provide some perspectives regarding the best mode of pathology teaching post-pandemic in medical schools.

3. Results

3.1. Literature Search

Figure 1 shows the flowchart of our study, following the PRISMA guidelines [19]. A search of the PubMed database revealed 988 articles, the title and abstract of which were screened for eligibility with the objectives of our study. This screening step resulted in 37 articles, and their full text was evaluated by three authors of this study (I.P.N., A.I., and M.M.A.). At this step, 14 articles were additionally excluded; 10 of them described training at the level of residents, fellows, or implications in pathology practice, while 4 focused only on histology education. Subsequently, 23 studies were included in our literature review, and their findings are discussed in the following chapters.

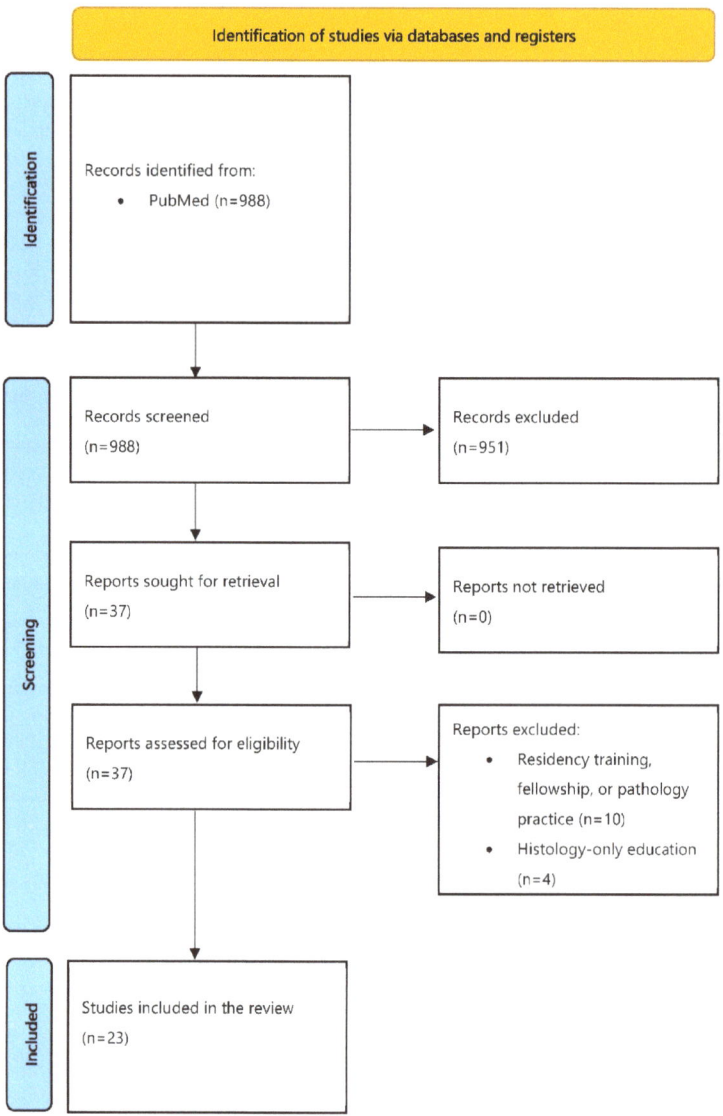

Figure 1. Flowchart of our literature search.

3.2. Advantages of Virtual Pathology Education: Literature Review

Our literature review revealed that the remote delivery of pathology courses worldwide was generally followed by highly positive student evaluations, as reported by several authors [3,5,9,10]. Notably, evaluation scores were often improved, compared to the previous years when traditional on-site delivery had taken place [5,9]. Medical students regarded the remote delivery of classes as flexible and less time-consuming, while they appreciated that teaching materials (e.g., session recordings and virtual slides) were available to access anytime and from anywhere [4,10]. On this subject, a group reported creating a YouTube channel containing all the high-quality recordings from their pathology sessions, which was very much appreciated by their students [20]. Furthermore, virtual small group teaching using digital pathology slides was considered a very convenient, engaging, and effective teaching modality by the learners [9]. Similarly, instructors also reported that virtual laboratory sessions were effective in a recent study [21]. Of interest, some students often found the online sessions more interactive, engaging, and better structured compared to the conventional ones, finding it easier to participate and ask questions [4,6]. A study by Rodrigues et al. reported that, although both sexes were asking more questions during virtual classes, female students felt significantly more comfortable doing so than males (48.9 vs. 33%, $p < 0.03$) [4]. Our recent study also showed that the female sex was an independent predictor associated with an enhanced virtual learning experience [3]. Apart from student satisfaction, pathology instructors often addressed that their teaching and even diagnostic skills were improved during the unprecedented period of the COVID-19 pandemic [9]. Furthermore, many of them reported creating new materials and innovative tools to fit their students' needs while shifting to virtual classes [8]. For instance, Tóth et al. successfully developed 3D autopsy models, using photogrammetry, for their online forensic pathology sessions [22].

In addition to pathology teaching early on in the preclinical medical school curriculum, a number of pathology electives—designed for more senior medical students—were successfully organized around the world during the pandemic period. Parker et al. pointed out the high number of students enrolling in their virtual elective, especially when compared to its conventional equivalent in the previous years (nearly a 10-fold increase); they also addressed the improved attitude of their students towards pathology, as well as their understanding of pathology basics, after they finished this elective [23]. Fu et al. commented on the flexibility of virtual electives to host more students compared to the traditional ones, enhancing their exposure to pathology as a potential future specialization and their understanding of pathology's crucial role in patient care [8]. In addition, in their survey which was administered pre- and post-rotation, participants claimed they were significantly more likely to choose pathology as their future medical specialty, and reported an improved understanding of what pathologists do or confidence to ask specific questions to them, when their post-rotation survey answers were compared with their pre-rotation answers [8]. Similarly, as shown in another study, students expressed an increased interest in pursuing forensic pathology as their future profession after completing a relevant elective [24]. Of interest, in a study published by Tanaka and Ramachandran [25], their virtual pathology elective received higher evaluation scores than the conventional on-campus elective (4.88 vs. 4.73/5), even from all advanced clinical clerkships (mean = 4.51; range 2.63–5.00), implying that pathology may be a discipline more suitable to virtual learning than other courses. Another elective, organized by the pathology faculty at Weill Cornell Medicine-Qatar, highlighted the virtual elective's flexibility in place and time, allowing synchronous and asynchronous interactions among students and faculty from multiple institutions and countries, while it was praised by the participants for its high overall quality and versatility [10]. White et al. addressed that their virtual pathology elective was more intensive than their traditional in-person one, and their students got exposed to the same representative cases per rotation regardless of the department's workload, emphasizing the standardization of teaching, feedback, and student assessment with virtual electives [11]. Lastly, a new website (PathElective; https://www.pathelective.com/, accessed on 7 June 2022) was developed to facilitate pathology e-learning. With PathElective, medical students worldwide can enroll in an organized virtual pathology elective at their own time and pace; multiple modules are included on the website and each contains its objectives, a to-do list, videos, recommended study resources, assignments, and assessments. PathElective received excellent reviews from participants taking this course in a recent survey delivered by its creators [26].

To evaluate a new teaching model, and despite students' perceptions and virtual experience, a very important parameter is to assess if the learning outcomes are fulfilled and if students' academic performance is satisfactory. The latter is most commonly assessed by evaluating the examination scores and contrasting them with a gold standard (e.g., examination scores in an already established teaching model). Although the literature is still limited, pathology learning outcomes' acquisition and academic performance at the medical school level were found to be satisfactory during the pandemic-induced remote course delivery, compared to the gold standard of on-campus teaching. A study by Waugh et al. compared two student cohorts completing the same pathology curriculum, one with remote delivery (during the pandemic) and a prior one taught face-to-face; there was a significant improvement in the mean practical examination overall mark (65.36% ± 13.12% to 75.83% ± 14.84%, $p < 0.05$) for the online student cohort [6]. Likewise, in another study, pathology students attending a virtual pathology course performed significantly better in their practical questions devoid of images (96.5 ± 7.0 vs. 91.2 ± 15.2; $p = 0.004$) and on questions coupled with gross pathology images (88.4 ± 7.5 vs. 84.4 ± 10.3; $p = 0.007$), as compared to students completing the on-campus course the previous year [5]. Lastly, Krasowski et al. reported similar examination scores among three consecutive years of preclinical pathology teaching, the last of which was conducted virtually [27].

3.3. Advantages of Virtual Pathology Education: Our Own Experience

The shift to virtual classes was perceived very positively by our medical students who were satisfied by the organization, lecture and laboratory session delivery, the resources provided, and the overall support they received. They also claimed they appreciated the value of histology and/or pathology to understand disease and that the knowledge obtained was crucial for their future profession. Female sex, better performance in the final exam, lower stress levels, and previous degree-holders were all independent predictors associated with an enhanced virtual learning experience [3].

Unpublished results, resulting from our students' answers to the open-ended questions of the survey delivered to them, revealed that many enjoyed the virtual pathology sessions, as there was "a lot less fuss" and "fewer distractions" compared to the on-campus sessions. This made it easier for the instructor to lecture without being "constantly disrupted by the noises made by fellow students" and for students to concentrate on the lecture without "any disturbances". Students could "regulate the volume" and thus could listen clearly to everything the instructor was saying. In addition, many of them found the virtual sessions more engaging and interactive than the face-to-face ones. They argued that the various technological tools used (e.g., virtual laboratory sessions, electronic voting, chats, and discussion forums) enhanced their active participation and learning during the online sessions, while they also made it easier to interact with their instructors and with one another. Others stressed the flexibility accompanying virtual learning, noting that attending courses via online platforms was more convenient and less time-consuming, since "there was no need for time wasted traveling back and forth from the university". This enabled them to better organize their studying schedule ("we were gaining time").

Similar to the study by Samueli et al. [28], several of our students stressed the value of the available session recordings (the latter were unavailable during our on-campus sessions), a modality that students found to be extremely useful for study purposes. Of interest, our histology students more often appreciated access to the online recordings and their impact on their studying, compared to the pathology ones, exhibiting a stronger need to re-check the materials after their online delivery. In addition, whereas pathology students reported more commonly that virtual learning was convenient, flexible, and time-efficient, histology students more often claimed that they preferred on-campus than online laboratory sessions, emphasizing the importance of microscopy hands-on exercises and the use of glass slides. Lastly, in accordance with the literature previously presented [4], we also personally observed that some of our students were asking more questions (especially using the chat function) during our virtual, compared to the on-campus, sessions the previous years, often making our sessions lengthier and more interactive. A selection of our students' comments regarding the advantages of virtual education is shown in Table 2.

Table 2. Selection of comments from our students regarding the advantages of virtual education during the COVID-19 pandemic.

More engaging and interactive
- "Participation was easier for all students during online sessions as well as asking questions."
- "I could engage more during the lectures and search fast the net."
- "Polls made the experience more engaging."
- "In the virtual labs although they were not in the microscope the professor explained us and we could see all the things he was describing much clearer."
- " . . . . being able to type any questions in the chat was definitely helpful for students who are more shy or find it difficult to speak in front of the whole . . . ."

Fewer distractions/Easier to concentrate
- "We could listen more clearly and concentrate to what the professor was saying. . . . "
- "It was easier in the sense of having less distractions since friends weren't there to distract nor was there excess sound from the class."

Flexibility, comfort, and improved time management
- "Attending from home is very convenient and less time-consuming."
- "Less time consuming overall as we were able to divide the time to study/focus for each class according to our personal needs."
- "The freedom of not having to be formal when attending class was nice, meaning we could be in pyjamas and no one would have a clue."

Access to high-quality recordings
- "Being able to go back to previous lecture recordings was one of the biggest pros with online classes."
- "While studying for exams, it was EXTREMELY useful to have access to the recordings."

First-hand experience that high-quality online teaching is feasible
- "You showed that you can do it remotely, keep it and don't go back to stone age!!"

Adaptability skills
- "Learned to be flexible in respect of a pandemic."

3.4. Challenges Faced during Virtual Pathology Education: Literature Review

A number of studies reported the presence of technical issues hindering the online delivery of pathology classes, such as the suboptimal internet connection. A high internet speed and bandwidth are necessary, especially while examining digital pathology slides [5,9,10,21,29]. Notably, our recent study revealed that a suboptimal internet connection was associated with a worse final examination performance ($p = 0.04$), while the former was also independently associated with enhanced perceived stress levels [3]. Samueli et al. reported that a few of their students reported technical issues while evaluating the digital pathology slides [28]. In some countries, limited access to computers was also addressed [29]. Considering other challenges, students often found it hard to stay attentive during the online classes [6], facing difficulty in separating work from home [4], or experiencing anxiety [21]. Furthermore, others found remote education hampered peer-to-peer teaching and their motivation in general [4,5].

Regarding remote laboratory sessions, and as shown in various studies, a high number of students expressed their preference to return to their on-campus pathology activities the soonest. A common complaint was the lack of conventional microscopy exercises, and many emphasized the importance of learning how to operate the light microscope [2]. Others mentioned their inability to participate in surgical pathology grossing or the laboratory facilities in general, due to the social distancing measures induced by the pandemic [11,25]. Another drawback of virtual education reported was the decrease in interactions and collaborative work among students and instructors during pathology sessions and the teachers' inability to observe, interact, and provide feedback the same way, compared to what was happening during the on-site delivery [21,25]. Lastly, organizing and conducting virtual laboratory activities and small-group teaching sessions were reported to occupy a significant amount of time for the educators involved [9,11].

3.5. Challenges Faced during Virtual Pathology Education: Our Own Experience

In accordance with the literature, the results of our recent study also pointed out that the internet connection quality was also a significant issue for a few of our students while attending the virtual pathology and histology classes. As stated before, a suboptimal internet connection was associated with a worse final examination performance ($p = 0.04$), while the former was found to be an independent predictor of elevated perceived stress [3].

Based on unpublished data resulting from the participant's answers to the open-ended questions of our survey, a few of our students addressed the concentration issues they faced during the remote sessions. Specifically, they pointed out that "it was tiring to always be sitting in front of the laptop", and that this had a negative effect on their focus span and their physical wellbeing (e.g., tiredness, headaches, and eye fatigue). They found it "impossible to concentrate on the screen the whole day" and, as a result, they "couldn't follow the lecture, as much as in the on-campus classes". In addition, others reported a few technical issues hampering their learning experiences, such as a weak internet connection or sound problems. According to them, these issues were "tiring" and "particularly frustrating", or even a "really big problem", since it led them to be frequently "kicked out of sessions" or even their online exams. Some felt that it was more difficult to ask questions during the virtual sessions, while others did not find virtual labs as useful as those conducted on campus. These particular students noted that virtual labs were "uncomfortable and less useful", stressing that "the microscope part of lab" cannot be replaced virtually. Lastly, a few participants noted that, due to the lack of face-to-face interaction, engagement in online sessions and communication among each other and with their instructors were much more challenging compared to the on-campus sessions.

In addition, our students often listed various sources of concern they experienced during remote learning, which could have a direct impact on their perceived stress levels. Some mentioned anxiety about exams as a major issue. At the beginning of the lockdown, these students had been worried about the format and procedure of the examinations, and whether these would be different from the type of exams previously administered on-campus. The possibility of proctoring issues during the online exams, falsely perceiving a movement (e.g., looking outside the window) as an attempt to cheat, had also been a source of anxiety for some of them. The possibility of technical issues, not only during the exams, but also during the teaching sessions, was a constant source of concern for a few students, while others reported emotional issues stemming from the COVID-19 pandemic itself, such as anxiety about family members' health and well-being, uncertainty about family members' jobs, and lack of motivation to study. Lastly, some participants addressed their concerns regarding the impact of the COVID-19 lockdown on their overall academic progress and performance. A selection of our students' comments, regarding the challenges faced during the remote delivery of our pathology and histology courses during the COVID-19 pandemic, is shown in Table 3.

Table 3. Selection of comments from our students regarding the challenges faced while attending the virtual classes during the COVID-19 pandemic.

Technical issues
- "Sometimes, it was particularly frustrating when my internet would disconnect in the middle of a session."
- "And of course, any technical issues during important classes . . . ."
- "The stress during the examinations because of possible technical problems."
- "That based on my poor internet connection, my online exams would crash."

Laboratory sessions and lack of hands-on training
- "The lab sessions weren't as helpful as they were on campus."
- "I think the microscope part of lab is really important and I think it can't be replaced."

Table 3. *Cont.*

Difficulties in asking questions during the online sessions
- "I felt it was difficult to ask questions during the online labs and lectures."
- ".... it's much easier in real life since I can easily raise my hand and just ask or quickly go find you upstairs in your office/after lab."

Screen fatigue and concentration issues
- "Focusing for a long period of time in front of a screen was difficult."
- "It was impossible being in front of a screen literally all day; my eyes were hurting, I constantly had headache, I couldn't study on my computer more hours etc."
- "It's just too comfortable at home and I need the university area to concentrate properly."
- "Long hours in front of a laptop made it unbearable to focus after some point."
- "I lived in a place full of family so sometimes it was hard to concentrate."

Missing interaction with instructors and peers
- "The lack of personal interaction makes it really hard to focus and listen to classes."
- "Not having interaction and discussions with my classmates and professors."
- "The absence of a face-to-face, more "human" relationship with my instructors."

4. Discussion

Both the "literature review" and our "own experience" showed that virtual pathology education during the COVID-19 period exhibited some advantages, yet significant challenges in its implementation as well. A summary of this information is shown in Table 4.

Table 4. A summary of advantages, challenges faced, and perspectives regarding virtual pathology education, as shown in the "literature review" and "our own experience".

Advantages:
- Flexibility and improved time management
- Sessions/teaching materials are available anywhere and anytime
- Interactivity, more questions asked by some students
- High-quality recordings
- Use of innovative teaching platforms
- New teaching materials and technologies
- Instructors improving their teaching skills
- Enhanced enrolment rates in pathology electives
- Improved attitude towards pathology
- Enhanced consideration of pathology as a future medical specialty
- Satisfactory academic performance

Challenges Faced:
- Technical issues
- Screen fatigue
- Reduced engagement by some students during classes
- Instructors' difficulty in appraising students' engagement
- Hard to separate work from home
- No light microscopy exercises and/or grossing during laboratory sessions
- Reduced student interactions with instructors and peers
- Reduced student exposure to the "hidden curriculum" (e.g., role modeling and professionalism)

Perspectives:
- Shift towards a blended approach

As briefly described in the aforementioned chapters and outlined in Tables 2 and 4, the pandemic-induced virtual pathology education exhibited many advantages for both students and faculty. In general, online education was considered to be very convenient, flexible, and engaging, allowing lectures, both big and small group/breakout room sessions, and virtual microscopy labs, while supporting both synchronous and asynchronous teaching modalities [3,8,16]. Several free pathology teaching resources exist online which could be directly implemented into virtual education—for example, the PathElective, Path-

Presenter, Iowa Virtual Slidebox, Leeds Virtual Pathology Library, and Virtual Microscopy Database (VMD)—while educators worldwide have constantly been creating new material, particularly during the pandemic [3,10,26,30,31]. Especially through the chat function, we and others noticed that some students engage and ask more questions in general [4]; this may result in more interactive and lengthier sessions. Notably, virtual pathology education resulted in students' satisfactory learning outcomes acquisition and overall academic performance, as shown by comparing pathology exam scores before and during the pandemic in a few published studies [5,9]. However, as evidence is still sparse and these findings could be the result of confounding factors (e.g., different exam structure, level of difficulty, and online setting) other than the virtual teaching itself, more studies are needed to reach reliable conclusions on this matter.

Regarding the use of digital pathology in medical school education, various studies have pointed out its advantages over traditional microscopy, including its flexibility, versatility, efficiency, standardization of both laboratory sessions and exams using high-quality slides, and cost-effectiveness. These support a switch to virtual microscopy, at least for the medical school level [11,31–34]. Of importance, digital pathology seems to enhance student engagement and collaboration among one another [23,32,33]. In addition, multiple authors have stated that the use of virtual over traditional microscopy does not negatively affect the academic performance of students; in fact, it has been shown to boost it in several studies [35–39]. One common disadvantage of using exclusively digital pathology in medical school education is that students do not learn how to operate the conventional light microscope [32]; this was also pointed out by a few of our students. However, the vast majority of medical students will never have to operate optical microscopy after the first years of medical school or as future physicians. For the ones that exhibit special interest, pathology electives or clerkships could be an alternative option. Consequently, educators and students may best focus on the content (acquisition of pathology knowledge), rather than the tool itself, during pathology sessions [32].

Apart from the advantages of remote pathology education, the implementation of the latter was also followed by several challenges for the stakeholders, including technical problems, screen fatigue, and diminished student interactions among themselves and their instructors, besides their limited exposure to the "hidden curriculum" (Tables 3 and 4). Regarding remote education, others emphasized the lack of hands-on practical sessions (e.g., traditional microscopy exercises, as mentioned before), specific issues regarding online examinations in general, and the reduced engagement of some of them during the virtual classes [40,41]. Notably, both enhanced and reduced engagement was reported within student surveys in different studies as well as our own [4,6,40,41]. We suspect it could be a matter of learning preference among the medical student community, yet cofounding factors (especially during the COVID-19 period) may have also played a significant role. Parker et al. attempted to enhance student engagement during their online classes by encouraging them to turn on their cameras and speak up throughout the sessions or by providing the session handouts only after the end of the sessions [23]. Others prompted the use of interactive polling software such as Mentimeter (Mentimeter AB, Stockholm, Sweden) and Slido (Slido s.r.o., Bratislava, Slovakia), or gaming applications such as Kahoot! (Kahoot! A.S., Oslo, Norway) in their online sessions [24,42]. However, the benefits of participating in traditional on-campus pathology education in this regard may be impossible to reach simply by its remote delivery while experiencing the physical university environment, in-person interactions, and hands-on activities are undoubtedly crucial for medical school education [43,44].

Given the aforementioned evidence, a few authors have proposed the implementation of a blended approach regarding pathology education in medical schools, attempting to incorporate the best practices of both remote and on-campus teaching. This way, the advantages offered by both could be maximized and the challenges minimized [3,10,45]. Notably, a recent meta-analysis within the spectrum of health education supported blended learning which was reported to result in superior learning outcomes [46]. In a blended model, online learning would complement face-to-face learning rather than replace it, enhancing medical students' learning experience and academic performance [45]. Bryant et al. utilized a blended approach to teach gross pathology during the COVID-19 pandemic, which was positively welcomed by medical students and staff. In their flipped model, short videos were provided before the laboratory sessions to students, familiarizing them with the teaching material. Then, laboratory sessions took place using small student cohorts, where students rotated through different stations to examine the gross specimens, emphasizing active learning [47]. A few authors have recently pointed out the preference of students for blended learning. For instance, Manou et al. stated in their recent study that most pathology students in their institute exhibited a preference for the integration of e-learning into their conventional on-campus teaching post-pandemic [48]. Similarly, when our students were asked about the best delivery mode of the pathology course as soon as the pandemic finishes, the majority preferred a blended rather than an entirely on-campus or online approach [3]. It is clear to us that all the knowledge and experience gained throughout this pandemic period should not be considered just a short-term adaptation and get discarded to go back to the way things were; they can be used post-pandemic, as they have proved to be beneficial for both learners and instructors. For instance, a few of our students noted in our survey that the at-distance offering of the course provided first-hand experience on how high-quality online teaching and learning is feasible in case the need for at-distance instruction arises again or even as a permanent change. Others saw a great opportunity for a more constructive use of technology in pathology education, noting that the technological tools and applications that had been utilized in our online course (e.g., high-quality session recordings, digital pathology, online polls and quizzes, online case studies, discussion forums, and chat) could also be used in the future to enhance students' participation, communication, collaboration, and learning [3].

In a pathology teaching blended approach, online learning could focus, for example, on delivering the introductory material and digital slide sessions; this could offer flexibility, innovative teaching solutions, and high-quality recordings, boosting students' academic performance [3,39,49,50]. On the other hand, on-campus sessions could focus on small group teaching, hands-on exercises, and teamwork, in addition to exposure to the "hidden curriculum" (role modeling and professionalism) [27,51]. Selected tools could also be used for on-campus exercises, for example, gross dissection or fine-needle aspiration biopsy simulation models [52,53]. Our opinion is that student assessment also needs to be conducted on-campus rather than online whenever possible. A few studies dealing with medical or non-medical education have shown that, with online examinations, the prevalence of cheating may increase among students [54,55]. Various institutions, therefore, asked their students to sign academic integrity documents before exams and used certain proctoring programs; however, potential cheating attempts may still be very hard to detect, whereas students often report such programs increase their stress levels [6,55,56]. Lastly, as evidence has so far shown the overwhelmingly positive impact of virtual pathology electives worldwide [8,11,23,26], which are typically conducted later on during medical studies, we believe they should keep their current form with potential minor modifications on a case-by-case basis, according to the feedback instructors receive from their students.

5. Conclusions

This study summarizes the existing evidence regarding the advantages of remote pathology education in medical schools worldwide during the COVID-19 pandemic, the challenges faced, and opportunities that have arisen for future implementation. As both online and on-campus pathology education have pros and cons, a blended approach could highlight the best practices of both and minimize the challenges in order to offer the best pathology education to the medical student community. Whereas online education is convenient, flexible, and efficient, experiencing the physical university environment, in-person interactions and teamwork, exposure to the "hidden curriculum", and hands-on activities are vital for medical school education and future student development. The main challenge in the post-COVID medical education era would be to re-design our pathology courses—including the structure, didactic methodology, and resources—and offer a mixture of student-centered activities, maximizing our students' engagement, interaction with their instructors and peers, and learning. The technologies employed and experience gained from teaching remotely during the COVID-19 period would need to continue being used and shared among educators worldwide, rather than being discarded and simply returning to the pre-pandemic era and the way things were. The application of state-of-the-art technological tools that promote engagement (e.g., simulations, gaming, and interactive polling) would need to be emphasized in modern medical schools, in addition to the implementation of social media to encourage both on-campus and remote interactions whenever possible [24,42,52,53,57,58]. A number of challenges related to online learning, such as the lack of reliable electronic devices or internet connection for some students, could be potentially overcome with the support of Universities themselves, for instance, by ensuring each student with accessibility issues is provided with a suitable computing device and/or by investing in their library services (e.g., physical space with adequate hardware infrastructure and a reliable internet connection and access to variable e-resources). Lastly, pathology educators would also have to transform themselves digitally, become familiar with novel interactive tools, and develop a creative mindset to teach efficiently and effectively in the challenging post-COVID medical school education era.

Author Contributions: Writing, review, and editing, A.I., M.M.A., M.M.-M. and I.P.N. All authors have read and agreed to the published version of the manuscript.

Funding: This research received no external funding.

Institutional Review Board Statement: The Cyprus National Bioethics Committee approved the protocol of the research of which some data are used in this manuscript (reference number: 2020.01.139; 24 June 2020).

Informed Consent Statement: All participants gave their informed consent to participate in the research, some data of which are used in this manuscript.

Data Availability Statement: Data are contained within the article.

Conflicts of Interest: Ilias P. Nikas is a content reviewer at Kenhub GmbH. All other authors declare no conflict of interest.

References

1. Humphreys, H.; Stevens, N.; Leddin, D.; Callagy, G.; Burke, L.; Watson, R.W.; Toner, M. Pathology in Irish Medical Education. *J. Clin. Pathol.* **2020**, *73*, 47–50. [CrossRef] [PubMed]
2. Somera Dos Santos, F.; Osako, M.K.; Da Perdoná, G.S.C.; Alves, M.G.; Sales, K.U. Virtual Microscopy as a Learning Tool in Brazilian Medical Education. *Anat. Sci. Educ.* **2021**, *14*, 408–416. [CrossRef] [PubMed]
3. Nikas, I.P.; Lamnisos, D.; Meletiou-Mavrotheris, M.; Themistocleous, S.C.; Pieridi, C.; Mytilinaios, D.G.; Michaelides, C.; Johnson, E.O. Shift to Emergency Remote Preclinical Medical Education amidst the COVID-19 Pandemic: A Single-Institution Study. *Anat. Sci. Educ.* **2021**, *15*, 27–41. [CrossRef] [PubMed]
4. Rodrigues, M.A.M.; Zornoff, D.; Kobayasi, R. Remote Pathology Teaching under the COVID-19 Pandemic: Medical Students' Perceptions. *Ann. Diagn. Pathol.* **2022**, *56*, 151875. [CrossRef] [PubMed]
5. Hernandez, T.; Fallar, R.; Polydorides, A.D. Outcomes of Remote Pathology Instruction in Student Performance and Course Evaluation. *Acad. Pathol.* **2021**, *8*, 23742895211061824. [CrossRef]
6. Waugh, S.; Devin, J.; Lam, A.; Gopalan, V. E-Learning and the Virtual Transformation of Histopathology Teaching during COVID-19: Its Impact on Student Learning Experience and Outcome. *BMC Med. Educ.* **2022**, *22*, 1–7. [CrossRef]
7. Hartsough, E.M.; Arries, C.; Amin, K.; Powell, D. Designing and Implementing a Virtual Anatomic Pathology Elective during the COVID-19 Pandemic. *Acad. Pathol.* **2021**, *8*, 23742895211010264. [CrossRef]
8. Fu, L.; Swete, M.; Selgrade, D.; Chan, C.W.; Rodriguez, R.; Wolniak, K.; Blanco, L.Z., Jr. Virtual Pathology Elective Provides Uninterrupted Medical Education and Impactful Pathology Education during the COVID-19 Pandemic. *Acad. Pathol.* **2021**, *8*, 23742895211010276. [CrossRef]
9. Koch, L.K.; Correll-Buss, A.; Chang, O.H. Implementation and Effectiveness of a Completely Virtual Pathology Rotation for Visiting Medical Students. *Am. J. Clin. Pathol.* **2022**, *157*, 406–412. [CrossRef]

10. Guiter, G.E.; Sapia, S.; Wright, A.I.; Hutchins, G.G.A.; Arayssi, T. Development of a Remote Online Collaborative Medical School Pathology Curriculum with Clinical Correlations, across Several International Sites, through the COVID-19 Pandemic. *Med. Sci. Educ.* **2021**, *31*, 1–8. [CrossRef]
11. White, M.J.; Birkness, J.E.; Salimian, K.J.; Meiss, A.E.; Butcher, M.; Davis, K.; Ware, A.D.; Zarella, M.D.; Lecksell, K.; Rooper, L.M.; et al. Continuing Undergraduate Pathology Medical Education in the Coronavirus Disease 2019 (COVID-19) Global Pandemic: The Johns Hopkins Virtual Surgical Pathology Clinical Elective. *Arch. Pathol. Lab. Med.* **2021**, *145*, 814–820. [CrossRef] [PubMed]
12. Gopalan, V.; Kasem, K.; Pillai, S.; Olveda, D.; Ariana, A.; Leung, M.; Lam, A.K.Y. Evaluation of Multidisciplinary Strategies and Traditional Approaches in Teaching Pathology in Medical Students. *Pathol. Int.* **2018**, *68*, 459–466. [CrossRef] [PubMed]
13. Herrmann, F.E.M.; Lenski, M.; Steffen, J.; Kailuweit, M.; Nikolaus, M.; Koteeswaran, R.; Sailer, A.; Hanszke, A.; Wintergerst, M.; Dittmer, S.; et al. A Survey Study on Student Preferences Regarding Pathology Teaching in Germany: A Call for Curricular Modernization. *BMC Med. Educ.* **2015**, *15*, 94. [CrossRef] [PubMed]
14. Koch, L.K.; Chang, O.H.; Dintzis, S.M. Medical Education in Pathology: General Concepts and Strategies for Implementation. *Arch. Pathol. Lab. Med.* **2021**, *145*, 1081–1088. [CrossRef]
15. Cuschieri, S.; Calleja Agius, J. Spotlight on the Shift to Remote Anatomical Teaching during COVID-19 Pandemic: Perspectives and Experiences from the University of Malta. *Anat. Sci. Educ.* **2020**, *13*, 671–679. [CrossRef]
16. Torda, A. How COVID-19 Has Pushed Us into a Medical Education Revolution. *Intern. Med. J.* **2020**, *50*, 1150–1153. [CrossRef] [PubMed]
17. Braun, V.; Clarke, V. Using Thematic Analysis in Psychology. *Qual. Res. Psychol.* **2006**, *3*, 77–101. [CrossRef]
18. Guest, G.; MacQueen, K.; Namey, E. *Applied Thematic Analysis*; SAGE Publications, Inc.: Thousand Oaks, CA, USA, 2012; ISBN 978-1-4129-7167-6.
19. Page, M.J.; McKenzie, J.E.; Bossuyt, P.M.; Boutron, I.; Hoffmann, T.C.; Mulrow, C.D.; Shamseer, L.; Tetzlaff, J.M.; Akl, E.A.; Brennan, S.E.; et al. The PRISMA 2020 Statement: An Updated Guideline for Reporting Systematic Reviews. *BMJ* **2021**, *372*, n71. [CrossRef]
20. Manou, E.; Lazari, E.-C.; Thomopoulou, G.-E.; Agrogiannis, G.; Kavantzas, N.; Lazaris, A.C. Participation and Interactivity in Synchronous E-Learning Pathology Course during the COVID-19 Pandemic. *Adv. Med. Educ. Pract.* **2021**, *12*, 1081–1091. [CrossRef]
21. Sharma, R.; King, T.S.; Hanson, E.R.; Fiebelkorn, K. Medical Histopathology Laboratories: Remote Teaching in Response to COVID-19 Pandemic. *Acad. Pathol.* **2021**, *8*, 2374289521998049. [CrossRef]
22. Tóth, D.; Petrus, K.; Heckmann, V.; Simon, G.; Poór, V.S. Application of Photogrammetry in Forensic Pathology Education of Medical Students in Response to COVID-19. *J. Forensic Sci.* **2021**, *66*, 1533–1537. [CrossRef] [PubMed]
23. Parker, E.U.; Chang, O.; Koch, L. Remote Anatomic Pathology Medical Student Education in Washington State. *Am. J. Clin. Pathol.* **2020**, *154*, 585–591. [CrossRef] [PubMed]
24. Jones, R.M. Online Teaching of Forensic Medicine and Pathology during the COVID-19 Pandemic: A Course Evaluation. *J. Forensic Leg. Med.* **2021**, *83*, 102229. [CrossRef] [PubMed]
25. Tanaka, K.S.; Ramachandran, R. Perceptions of a Remote Learning Pathology Elective for Advanced Clinical Medical Students. *Acad. Pathol.* **2021**, *8*, 23742895211006850. [CrossRef] [PubMed]
26. Lilley, C.M.; Arnold, C.A.; Arnold, M.; Booth, A.L.; Gardner, J.M.; Jiang, X.S.; Loghavi, S.; Mirza, K.M. The Implementation and Effectiveness of PathElective.Com. *Acad. Pathol.* **2021**, *8*, 23742895211006828. [CrossRef] [PubMed]
27. Krasowski, M.D.; Blau, J.L.; Chen, S.J.; Jones, K.A.; Schmidt, T.J.; Bruch, L.A. Teaching Pathology in an Integrated Preclinical Medical School Curriculum and Adaptations to COVID-19 Restrictions. *Acad. Pathol.* **2021**, *8*, 23742895211015336. [CrossRef]
28. Samueli, B.; Sror, N.; Jotkowitz, A.; Taragin, B. Remote Pathology Education during the COVID-19 Era: Crisis Converted to Opportunity. *Ann. Diagn. Pathol.* **2020**, *49*, 151612. [CrossRef]
29. Mukhopadhyay, S.; Joshi, D.; Goel, G.; Singhai, A.; Kapoor, N. Evolution of Pathology Teaching for MBBS Students during COVID-19 Pandemic Lockdown: Moving from a Real to a Virtual Classroom. *Indian J. Pathol. Microbiol.* **2021**, *64*, 524–527. [CrossRef]
30. Lee, L.M.J.; Goldman, H.M.; Hortsch, M. The Virtual Microscopy Database-Sharing Digital Microscope Images for Research and Education. *Anat. Sci. Educ.* **2018**, *11*, 510–515. [CrossRef]
31. Dee, F.R. Virtual Microscopy in Pathology Education. *Hum. Pathol.* **2009**, *40*, 1112–1121. [CrossRef]
32. Saco, A.; Bombi, J.A.; Garcia, A.; Ramírez, J.; Ordi, J. Current Status of Whole-Slide Imaging in Education. *Pathobiology* **2016**, *83*, 79–88. [CrossRef] [PubMed]
33. Braun, M.W.; Kearns, K.D. Improved Learning Efficiency and Increased Student Collaboration through Use of Virtual Microscopy in the Teaching of Human Pathology. *Anat. Sci. Educ.* **2008**, *1*, 240–246. [CrossRef] [PubMed]
34. Holaday, L.; Selvig, D.; Purkiss, J.; Hortsch, M. Preference of Interactive Electronic versus Traditional Learning Resources by University of Michigan Medical Students during the First Year Histology Component. *Med. Sci. Educ.* **2013**, *23*, 607–619. [CrossRef]
35. Rodrigues-Fernandes, C.I.; Speight, P.M.; Khurram, S.A.; Araújo, A.L.D.; Da Perez, D.E.C.; Fonseca, F.P.; Lopes, M.A.; De Almeida, O.P.; Vargas, P.A.; Santos-Silva, A.R. The Use of Digital Microscopy as a Teaching Method for Human Pathology: A Systematic Review. *Virchows Arch.* **2020**, *477*, 475–486. [CrossRef] [PubMed]

36. Kuo, K.-H.; Leo, J.M. Optical Versus Virtual Microscope for Medical Education: A Systematic Review. *Anat. Sci. Educ.* **2019**, *12*, 678–685. [CrossRef]
37. Selvig, D.; Holaday, L.W.; Purkiss, J.; Hortsch, M. Correlating Students' Educational Background, Study Habits, and Resource Usage with Learning Success in Medical Histology. *Anat. Sci. Educ.* **2015**, *8*, 1–11. [CrossRef]
38. Lee, B.-C.; Hsieh, S.-T.; Chang, Y.-L.; Tseng, F.-Y.; Lin, Y.-J.; Chen, Y.-L.; Wang, S.-H.; Chang, Y.-F.; Ho, Y.-L.; Ni, Y.-H.; et al. A Web-Based Virtual Microscopy Platform for Improving Academic Performance in Histology and Pathology Laboratory Courses: A Pilot Study. *Anat. Sci. Educ.* **2020**, *13*, 743–758. [CrossRef]
39. Caruso, M.C. Virtual Microscopy and Other Technologies for Teaching Histology during COVID-19. *Anat. Sci. Educ.* **2021**, *14*, 19–21. [CrossRef]
40. Longhurst, G.J.; Stone, D.M.; Dulohery, K.; Scully, D.; Campbell, T.; Smith, C.F. Strength, Weakness, Opportunity, Threat (SWOT) Analysis of the Adaptations to Anatomical Education in the United Kingdom and Republic of Ireland in Response to the COVID-19 Pandemic. *Anat. Sci. Educ.* **2020**, *13*, 301–311. [CrossRef]
41. Kalidindi, S. Training and Education in the Pathology and Cytopathology Sphere. *Cancer Cytopathol.* **2018**, *126*, 445–446. [CrossRef]
42. Pather, N.; Blyth, P.; Chapman, J.A.; Dayal, M.R.; Flack, N.A.M.S.; Fogg, Q.A.; Green, R.A.; Hulme, A.K.; Johnson, I.P.; Meyer, A.J.; et al. Forced Disruption of Anatomy Education in Australia and New Zealand: An Acute Response to the COVID-19 Pandemic. *Anat. Sci. Educ.* **2020**, *13*, 284–300. [CrossRef] [PubMed]
43. Franchi, T. The Impact of the COVID-19 Pandemic on Current Anatomy Education and Future Careers: A Student's Perspective. *Anat. Sci. Educ.* **2020**, *13*, 312–315. [CrossRef] [PubMed]
44. Patra, A.; Chaudhary, P.; Ravi, K.S. Adverse Impact of COVID-19 on Anatomical Sciences Teachers of India and Proposed Ways to Handle This Predicament. *Anat. Sci. Educ.* **2021**, *14*, 163–165. [CrossRef] [PubMed]
45. Singh, J.; Steele, K.; Singh, L. Combining the Best of Online and Face-to-Face Learning: Hybrid and Blended Learning Approach for COVID-19, Post Vaccine, & Post-Pandemic World. *J. Educ. Technol. Syst.* **2021**, *50*, 140–171. [CrossRef]
46. Vallée, A.; Blacher, J.; Cariou, A.; Sorbets, E. Blended Learning Compared to Traditional Learning in Medical Education: Systematic Review and Meta-Analysis. *J. Med. Internet Res.* **2020**, *22*, e16504. [CrossRef]
47. Bryant, R.J.; Wilcox, R.; Zhang, B. Engage in Exploration: Pathology Gross Laboratory in the COVID-Era. *Acad. Pathol.* **2021**, *8*, 23742895211002844. [CrossRef] [PubMed]
48. Manou, E.; Lazari, E.-C.; Lazaris, A.C.; Agrogiannis, G.; Kavantzas, N.G.; Thomopoulou, G.-E. Evaluating E-Learning in the Pathology Course during the COVID-19 Pandemic. *Adv. Med. Educ. Pract.* **2022**, *13*, 285–300. [CrossRef]
49. Khalil, M.K.; Abdel Meguid, E.M.; Elkhider, I.A. Teaching of Anatomical Sciences: A Blended Learning Approach. *Clin. Anat.* **2018**, *31*, 323–329. [CrossRef]
50. Chen, J.; Zhou, J.; Wang, Y.; Qi, G.; Xia, C.; Mo, G.; Zhang, Z. Blended Learning in Basic Medical Laboratory Courses Improves Medical Students' Abilities in Self-Learning, Understanding, and Problem Solving. *Adv. Physiol. Educ.* **2020**, *44*, 9–14. [CrossRef]
51. Smith, C.F.; Pawlina, W. A Journey like No Other: Anatomy 2020! *Anat. Sci. Educ.* **2021**, *14*, 5–7. [CrossRef]
52. Alcaraz-Mateos, E.; Jiang, X.S.; Mohammed, A.A.R.; Turic, I.; Hernández-Sabater, L.; Caballero-Alemán, F.; Párraga-Ramírez, M.J.; Poblet, E. A Novel Simulator Model and Standardized Assessment Tools for Fine Needle Aspiration Cytology Training. *Diagn. Cytopathol.* **2019**, *47*, 297–301. [CrossRef] [PubMed]
53. Alcaraz-Mateos, E.; Mirza, K.M.; Molina-Valverde, S.; Togkaridou, M.; Caballero-Alemán, F.; Poblet, E. The Utility of a Gross Dissection Anatomical Model for Simulation-Based Learning in Pathology. *Rev. Española Patol.* **2022**, *in press*. [CrossRef]
54. Comas-Forgas, R.; Lancaster, T.; Calvo-Sastre, A.; Sureda-Negre, J. Exam Cheating and Academic Integrity Breaches during the COVID-19 Pandemic: An Analysis of Internet Search Activity in Spain. *Heliyon* **2021**, *7*, e08233. [CrossRef] [PubMed]
55. Khan, S.; Kambris, M.E.K.; Alfalahi, H. Perspectives of University Students and Faculty on Remote Education Experiences during COVID-19—A Qualitative Study. *Educ. Inf. Technol.* **2022**, *27*, 4141–4169. [CrossRef] [PubMed]
56. Egarter, S.; Mutschler, A.; Brass, K. Impact of COVID-19 on Digital Medical Education: Compatibility of Digital Teaching and Examinations with Integrity and Ethical Principles. *Int. J. Educ. Integr.* **2021**, *17*, 1–19. [CrossRef]
57. Balakrishnan, R.; Singh, K.; Harigopal, M.; Fineberg, S. A Novel "Google Classroom"-Based Pathology Education Tool for Trainees during the COVID-19 Pandemic: Impactful Learning While Social Distancing. *Arch. Pathol. Lab. Med.* **2020**, *144*, 1445b–11447. [CrossRef]
58. Kalleny, N. Advantages of Kahoot! Game.Based Formative Assessments along with Methods of Its Use and Application during the COVID-19 Pandemic in Various Live Learning Sessions. *J. Microsc. Ultrastruct.* **2020**, *8*, 175. [CrossRef]

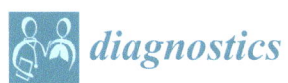

Systematic Review

Deep Learning on Histopathological Images for Colorectal Cancer Diagnosis: A Systematic Review

Athena Davri [1,*], Effrosyni Birbas [2], Theofilos Kanavos [2], Georgios Ntritsos [3,4], Nikolaos Giannakeas [4,*], Alexandros T. Tzallas [4] and Anna Batistatou [1]

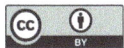

Citation: Davri, A.; Birbas, E.; Kanavos, T.; Ntritsos, G.; Giannakeas, N.; Tzallas, A.T.; Batistatou, A. Deep Learning on Histopathological Images for Colorectal Cancer Diagnosis: A Systematic Review. *Diagnostics* **2022**, *12*, 837. https://doi.org/10.3390/diagnostics12040837

Academic Editor: Catarina Eloy

Received: 28 February 2022
Accepted: 25 March 2022
Published: 29 March 2022

Publisher's Note: MDPI stays neutral with regard to jurisdictional claims in published maps and institutional affiliations.

Copyright: © 2022 by the authors. Licensee MDPI, Basel, Switzerland. This article is an open access article distributed under the terms and conditions of the Creative Commons Attribution (CC BY) license (https://creativecommons.org/licenses/by/4.0/).

[1] Department of Pathology, Faculty of Medicine, School of Health Sciences, University of Ioannina, 45500 Ioannina, Greece; abatista@uoi.gr
[2] Faculty of Medicine, School of Health Sciences, University of Ioannina, 45500 Ioannina, Greece; faybirbas@gmail.com (E.B.); kanavosus@gmail.com (T.K.)
[3] Department of Hygiene and Epidemiology, Faculty of Medicine, University of Ioannina, 45500 Ioannina, Greece; gntritsos@uoi.gr
[4] Department of Informatics and Telecommunications, University of Ioannina, 47100 Arta, Greece; tzallas@uoi.gr
* Correspondence: athinaadav@outlook.com (A.D.); giannakeas@uoi.gr (N.G.)

Abstract: Colorectal cancer (CRC) is the second most common cancer in women and the third most common in men, with an increasing incidence. Pathology diagnosis complemented with prognostic and predictive biomarker information is the first step for personalized treatment. The increased diagnostic load in the pathology laboratory, combined with the reported intra- and inter-variability in the assessment of biomarkers, has prompted the quest for reliable machine-based methods to be incorporated into the routine practice. Recently, Artificial Intelligence (AI) has made significant progress in the medical field, showing potential for clinical applications. Herein, we aim to systematically review the current research on AI in CRC image analysis. In histopathology, algorithms based on Deep Learning (DL) have the potential to assist in diagnosis, predict clinically relevant molecular phenotypes and microsatellite instability, identify histological features related to prognosis and correlated to metastasis, and assess the specific components of the tumor microenvironment.

Keywords: colorectal cancer; CRC; histopathology; microscopy images; deep learning; DL; convolutional neural networks; CNN

1. Introduction

Colorectal cancer (CRC) is one of the most common types of gastrointestinal cancer, the second most common cancer in women and the third in men [1]. Despite existing variations, such as geographical distribution, age and gender differences, the CRC incidence, overall, is estimated to increase by 80% in the year 2035, worldwide [2]. This rising incidence of CRC is mainly due to changes in lifestyle, particularly dietary patterns [3]. Most CRCs are sporadic (70–80%), while approximately one third have a hereditary component [4]. Within the term CRC, a wide range of carcinoma subtypes is included, characterized by different morphological features and molecular alterations.

The cornerstone of CRC diagnosis is the pathologic examination (biopsy or surgical excision) [5]. With the advent of screening methods, many precursor lesions are also detected and biopsied. Consequently, a wide range of pre-malignant lesions have been identified, and occasionally, a differential diagnosis between pre-malignant and malignant lesions is quite challenging [6]. The histopathological examination of the tissue remains the "gold standard" for diagnosis, with the first step being the optimal preparation of the histological section, stained with Hematoxylin and Eosin (H&E) [7]. Further examination with special in situ methods, such as immunohistochemistry (IHC) and in situ hybridization (ISH), and other molecular techniques follows [8]. There are published guidelines for pre-analytical, analytical and post-analytical procedures in a pathology laboratory [9]. As expected, due to the high incidence of CRC, the diagnostic load in a routine pathology laboratory is very heavy and the introduction of an ever-growing list of morpho-molecular features to be examined and noted has made the diagnosis a time-consuming process [10]. All these factors, in combination with the shortage of pathologists worldwide, have led to delays in diagnosis, with consequences to the optimal healthcare of the patient.

It has been shown that pathologists make a diagnosis based mainly on image-based pattern recognition [6]. With this strategy, architectural and cellular characteristics conform to already known features of a disease [11]. In several instances, an accurate diagnosis or estimation of prognostic and predictive factors is subject to personal interpretations, leading to inter- and intra-observer variability [12,13]. In a continuous effort to improve the accuracy of the pathology diagnosis, combined with the timely delivery of all vital information for optimal patient treatment, the new and breakthrough technologies can be of great value. Thus, in the last 5 years, the development of reliable computational approaches, using machine learning based on pattern recognition, has exponentially increased, as reflected in the plethora of published papers [14,15].

The recent World Health Organization (WHO) classification for malignant epithelial tumors of the colorectum includes four main categories: adenocarcinoma (ADC) not otherwise specified (NOS), neuroendocrine tumor NOS, neuroendocrine carcinoma NOS and mixed neuroendocrine-non-neuroendocrine neoplasm (MiMEN) [16]. Of these, colorectal ADC is the most common (90%) and, by definition, it shows glandular and mucinous differentiation. Colorectal ADC has several histopathological subtypes, with specific morphologic, clinical, and molecular characteristics, i.e., serrated ADC, adenoma-like ADC, micropapillary ADC, mucinous ADC, poorly cohesive carcinoma, signet-ring cell carcinoma, medullary ADC, adenosquamous carcinoma, carcinoma undifferentiated NOS and carcinoma with sarcomatoid component.

The diagnosis of CRC is only the first step for a complete pathology report. According to best-practice guidelines, the specific histologic subtype, the histologic grade, the TNM staging system, the lymphovascular and perineural invasion, and the tumor budding should be reported [9,16]. In recent years, the molecular pathological classification of CRC has been proposed, aiming to compliment the traditional histopathologic classification [4]. An integrated molecular analysis performed by the Cancer Genome Atlas Network, has classified CRC into three groups, including highly mutated tumors (~13%), ultra-mutated tumors (~3%) and chromosomal instability (CIN) tumors (~84%). In 2015, an expression-signature-based classification was proposed with four consensus molecular subtype (CMS) groups: CMS1 subtype (MSI-immune, 14%), CMS2 subtype (canonical, 37%), CMS3 subtype (metabolic, 13%) and CMS4 subtype (mesenchymal, 23%). In addition, molecular alterations are prevalent in CRC, consisting of Chromosomal Instability (CIN), Microsatellite Instability (MSI) and a CpG Island Methylator phenotype (CIMP). Defective mismatch repair (MMR) DNA mechanisms lead to increased mutations and, consequently, to MSI [17,18]. The majority of sporadic CRCs are characterized by CIN (~84%), and ~13–16% are hypermutated with an MSI status. The immunohistochemical detection of either an abnormal expression or a loss of expression of the mismatch repair proteins, MLH1, MSH2, MSH6, and PMS2, is of significant diagnostic and prognostic value in CRC, as well as for the detection of hereditary nonpolyposis colorectal cancer (HNPCC), also known as Lynch syndrome, which constitutes approximately 2% to 3% of all colorectal carcinomas [19–21].

Histopathology image generations start with the standard procedure of tissue preparation. Biopsy or surgical specimens (representative sections) are formalin-fixed and paraffin-embedded. Then, the 4μm tissue sections are prepared and stained with H&E dye [22]. The images are extracted after a scanning procedure. Several scanning systems can be used to digitize the whole slide [23], such as the Hamamatsu NanoZoomer series, the Omnyx scanner, the Zeiss scanners, the Pannoramic 250 Flash II, and the Leica Biosystems Aperio systems [24]. Most of the above scanners provide two optical magnifications, 20× and 40×, however, the user can also digitally undersample the image in different magnifications.

A scanner needs several minutes for the scanning of the whole slide, while most of the system can deal with tens or hundreds of slides that are scanned automatically one-by-one. According to the digitalization, each pixel of a Whole Slide Image (WSI) corresponds to a physical area of several decades nm². For example, in the 40× magnification mode, a Hamamatsu NanoZoomer scanner extracts an image, where the size of each pixel edge corresponds to 227 nm [25]. The latter image digitization provides an appropriate resolution for most of the histological findings, which presents a physical size of microns [26]. In most of the cases, the extracting images are storage either in a compressed JPEG-based format or an uncompressed TIFF format. Figure 1 presents the resolution of a WSI, scanned by a Hamamatsu NanoZoomer 210.

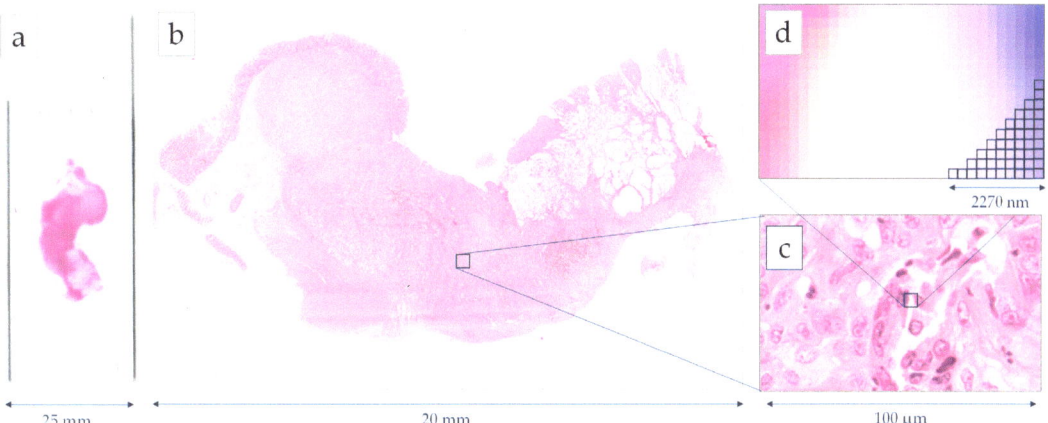

Figure 1. Image generation using a Hamamatsu NanoZoomer whole slide scanner: (**a**) histological slide 75 mm × 25 mm, (**b**) Whole Slide Image (WSI), (**c**) cell level in 40× magnification, (**d**) pixel level in 40× magnification digitizing images 227 nm per pixel.

Machine learning is a branch of AI which is based on the concept that machines could have access to data and be able to learn on their own. AI has a broader scope and involves machines that are capable of carrying out tasks requiring intelligence. Machine learning techniques focus on the creation of intelligent software using statistical learning methods and require access to data for the learning procedure [27]. A branch of machine learning, which has drawn a lot of attention over the last few years, is DL. DL involves training artificial neural networks (ANNs) with multiple layers of artificial neurons (nodes). Neural networks are inspired from the human physiology of the brain, comprising a simplified artificial model of the human neural network. An ANN is a collection of connected artificial neurons. The simplest ANN architecture is the single layer feed forward neural network. In these types of networks, the information moves in one direction only, from the inputs' nodes to the hidden layer nodes and then to the output nodes. The success and wide acceptance of ANNs relies on their capability to solve complex mathematical problems, nonlinear or stochastic, by using very simple computational operations. In contrast to a conventional algorithm, which needs complex mathematical and algorithmic operations and could only apply to one problem, an ANN is computationally and algorithmically very simple and its structure allows it to be applied in a wide range of problems [28].

DL has rapidly developed during the last decade due to the significant increase in processing power and to the fact that, for the first time, artificial models are able to achieve more accurate results than humans in classification tasks [29]. Both DL and machine learning techniques in general affect our everyday life in various ways. From the simple-looking face recognition program used in Facebook, to the classification of abnormal/normal human cells in bioinformatics. For image analysis problems, such as the histological lesions' detections, prognosis and diagnosis, DL approaches mainly employ Convolutional Neural Networks (CNNs) for segmentation and classification, while few studies employ another DL approach, called Generative Adversarial Networks (GANs), to improve the training set of images before classification.

CNNs have produced high classification rates in modern computer vision applications. The term "convolutional" suggests that a deep neural network applies the mathematical convolution operation to at least one of its multiple hidden layers. Many CNN model variations have been implemented in recent years, which are based on a common layer pattern: (a) 1 input layer, (b) L-1 convolution layers and (c) 1 classification layer. The key feature of a sequential CNN is that it transforms the input data through neurons that are connected to neurons of the previous convolution layer. Initially, the raw image is loaded at the input layer, which is usually set to accept a three-dimensional spatial form of an image file (width × height × depth), with the depth, in this case, indicating the RGB (Red, Green, Blue) color channels. More technically, each of the convolution layers calculates the dot product between the area of the neurons in the input layer and the weights in a predetermined size of a filtering kernel (e.g., 3 × 3). In this way, local features can be detected through K declared kernels. As a result, all nodes (neurons) of each convolution layer calculate their activation value based on only one subset of spatially adjacent nodes on the filtered feature maps of each previous convolution layer. The most common deep network architectures, such as AlexNet and GoogleNet, use the same neuron type at each hidden layer [30,31]. These architectures achieve very high accuracy in classification problems, while their training is a computationally intensive and time-consuming process. Currently, many different architectures, such as VGG, DenseNet, ResNet, Inception.v3, etc., have been proposed, performing well under different conditions and problem parameters [31–33].

GANs are also a DL approach applied on digital image analysis [34]. GANs are a smart way to train a model as a supervised learning problem, even if based on their principles they are unsupervised machine learning procedures. A typical GAN consists of two sub-models: (a) the generator network, where the training generates new samples with similar characteristics to the real ones and (b) the discriminator network, which provides a binary classification of the generating samples, discriminating the real (approved) samples from the fake ones. GANs have been rapidly evolved, especially in image processing and classification, providing a sophisticated approach to simulate images for CNN training, avoiding overtraining and overfitting. It is an alternative method of image augmentation which extracts simulated images using simple transformations such as rotation, shearing, stretching, etc.

In this paper, a systematic review for the application of DL in colorectal cancer, using digital image analysis in histopathological images, is presented. The aim of the manuscript focuses on the investigation from both medical and technical viewpoints. The innovative contribution of this systematic review is the combination of the two viewpoints provided, presenting a more comprehensive analysis of AI-based models in CRC diagnosis. A deeper understanding on both medical and technical aspects of DL will better reveal the opportunities of implementing DL-based models in clinical practice, as well as overcome several challenges occurring for the optimal performance of the algorithms. According to the PRISMA guidelines [35], an expanded algorithm was used for searching the literature works. Specific inclusion and exclusion criteria have been defined to result in the final studies of interest, which have been categorized for both medical and technical points of views. In the next sections, significant backgrounds for both the clinical practice and the details about DL in image analysis are outlined, the method for the study selection is analyzed, and results are extensively discussed.

2. Materials and Methods

2.1. Search Strategy

We systematically searched PubMed from inception to 31 December 2021 for primary studies developing a DL model for the histopathological interpretation of large bowel biopsy tissues and CRC. For this purpose, we used the following algorithm: (convolutional neural networks OR CNN OR deep learning) AND ((cancer AND (colon OR colorectal OR intestin* OR bowel)) OR (adenocarcinoma AND (colon OR colorectal OR intestin* OR bowel)) OR (carcinoma AND (colon OR colorectal OR intestin* OR bowel)) OR (malignan* AND (colon OR colorectal OR intestin* OR bowel))) AND (biop* OR microscop* OR histolog* OR slide* OR eosin OR histopatholog*). The search was conducted on 14 January 2022.

2.2. Study Eligibility Criteria

The study was conducted according to the PRISMA guidelines and registered to PROSPERO 2020. Eligible articles were considered based on the following criteria. We included studies presenting the development of at least one DL model for the histopathological assessment of large bowel slides and CRC. Eligible applications of the DL models included diagnosis, tumor tissue classification, tumor microenvironment analysis, prognosis, survival and metastasis risk evaluation, tumor mutational burden characterization and, finally, microsatellite instability detection. We excluded articles that presented in vitro models, used endoscopic or radiological images instead of histological sections, and involved non-photonic microscopy. Furthermore, eligible articles should report original studies and not reviews/meta-analyses, concern humans and be written in English. Additionally, articles referring to organs other than the large bowel and benign entities were deemed ineligible.

2.3. Study Selection

All citations collected by the previously mentioned methodology were independently screened by four researchers, who were properly trained before the process started, using the online software Rayyan. Three of the researchers were scientifically capable of evaluating the medical aspect of the query and one of them was a CNN expert, able to assess the technical part. During the screening period, the researchers would meet regularly to discuss disagreements and continue training. Conflicts were resolved by consensus. The full texts of potentially eligible articles were later retrieved for further evaluation.

2.4. Data Extraction

To facilitate the data extraction process, we specially designed a spreadsheet form, which all researchers could access to import data from all the eligible articles. From each paper, we extracted information on first author, year and journal of publication, PubMed ID, title, aim of medical research, technical method, classification details, dataset and performance metrics.

3. Results

Our systematic search returned 166 articles, 92 of which were selected for full-text screening. Finally, 82 articles were considered eligible for our systematic review according to our criteria of eligibility. A detailed description of the study selection process can be found in the PRISMA flow-chart presented in Figure 2. The selected works are presented both through the medical and technical point of view (Figure 3), while Table 1 includes the characteristics of each study, regarding the medical scope, the technical approach, the employed datasets, and finally, the performance of the proposed method.

3.1. Medical Viewpoint

According to the medical scope of view, there are five categories: (a) studies for diagnostic purposes, (b) the classification of the tumor tissue, (c) the investigation of the tumor microenvironment, (d) the role of histological features to prognosis, metastasis and survival, and finally, (e) the identification of microsatellite instability.

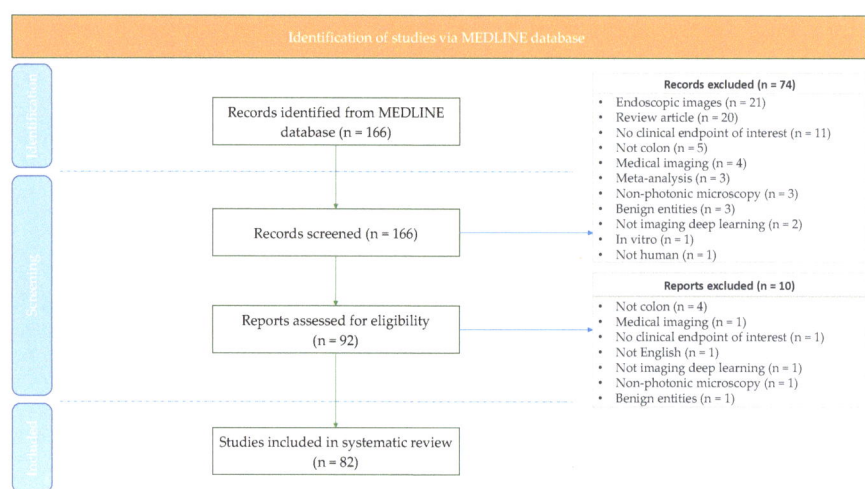

Figure 2. Systematic review flow-chart illustrating systematic search and screening strategy, including number of studies meeting eligibility criteria and number of excluded studies. Last search carried out on 14 January 2022.

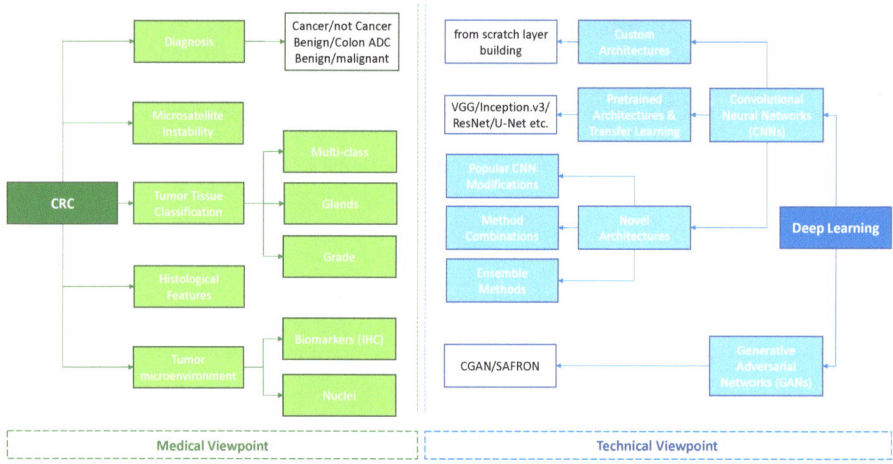

Figure 3. Tree diagram for the categorization of the studies.

3.1.1. Diagnosis

DL techniques can assist in the process of pathology diagnosis [14]. The algorithms perform a binary classification, for instance, cancer/non-cancer, colon benign tissue/colon ADC.

The classification of the tumor regions in WSIs by AI-based models could assist in the time-consuming process of a microscopical examination. The suggested models in the study by Gupta et al. classified normal and abnormal tissue in CRC slides and localized the cancer regions with good performance metrics [36]. Zhou et al. used global labels for tumor classification and localization without the need for annotated images [37]. In the same framework, DL algorithms performed a binary classification of CRC images for detecting cancerous from non-cancerous regions, achieving good performance metrics and supporting the potential for use in clinical practice [38–42]. A recent study evaluating the segmentation performance of different DL models, showed that AI-patch-based models had great advantages, although this segmentation approach could result in lower accuracy when more challenging tumor images are included [43]. Moreover, AI-based models could be combined to persistent homology profiles (PHPs) and effectively identify normal from tumor tissue regions, evaluating the nuclear characteristics of tumor cells [44]. A patch-cluster-based aggregation model, including a great number of WSIs developed by Wang et al., performed the classification of CRC images (cancer, not cancer) assessing the clustering of tumor cells, and the results were comparable to pathologists' diagnosis, revealing no statistical difference [45]. The acceleration of tumor detection by CNNs could be obtained by reducing the number of patches, taking care to select the most representative regions of interest [46]. Both proposed methods in the study of Shen et al. performed with good accuracy and efficiency in detecting negative cases. Lastly, Yu et al., using a large dataset, demonstrated that SSL, with large amounts of unlabeled data, performed well at patch-level recognition and had a similar AUC as pathologists [47].

Colon benign tissue and colon ADC were classified with good accuracy by DL models developed by Toğaçar et al. and Masud et al. [48,49]. The study of Song et al. showed that the DL model and the pathologists' estimation were in agreement in diagnosing CRC [50]. However, the binary classification algorithm for adenoma and non-cancerous (including mucosa or chronic inflammation) tiles showed a proportion of false predictions in challenging tiles consisting of small adenomatous glands.

The accurate identification of benign from malignant tissues achieved a sensitivity of 0.8228 and specificity of 0.9114 by a DL model trained with Multiphoton microscopy (MPM) images, although images were lacking biomarkers such as colonic crypts and goblet cells [51]. Holland et al. used the same classification model and 7 training datasets consisting of a descending number of images [52]. The mean generalization accuracy appeared to rely on the number of images within the different training sets and CNNs, although the larger datasets did not result in a higher mean generalization accuracy, as expected.

3.1.2. Tumor Tissue Classification (Non-Neoplastic, Benign, Malignant, Grade, Architecture and Cellular Characteristics)

Lizuka et al. conducted a classification of CRC into adenocarcinoma, adenoma or normal tissue on three different test sets, revealing great performance metrics and promising results for clinical practice [53]. The progression of CRC could be assessed by CNN, designed to identify benign hyperplasia, intraepithelial neoplasia, and carcinoma using multispectral images, however, the contribution of the pathologist's assessment and a bigger dataset were required [54]. Another study demonstrated that colorectal histological images could be classified into normal mucosa, an early preneoplastic lesion, adenoma and cancer with good accuracy, although these four classes may occasionally overlap and result in uncertainty in labeling [55]. Moreover, the ARA-CNN model was designed for an accurate, reliable and active tumor classification in the histopathological slides, aiming to minimize the uncertainty of mislabeled samples [56]. The model achieved great performance metrics not only in the binary, but also in the multiclass tumor classification, such as the proposed CNN by Xu et al. and Wang et al. [57,58]. Three studies by Papadini et al., Jiao et al. and Ben Hamida et al. proposed CNN approaches for multi-class colorectal tissue classification in a large dataset number, underlining the great potential of AI-based methods to efficiently perform multiple classifications of tumor regions [59–61]. Repurposing a stomach model trained in poorly differentiated cases of gastric ADC using a transfer learning method, DL algorithms could perform the classification of poorly differentiated adenocarcinoma in colorectal biopsy WSIs, benefiting from histological similarities between gastric and colon ADC [62].

The challenging task of gland segmentation was approached by Xu et al. and Graham et al., developing CNNs for gland segmentation and achieving a good performance in statistical metrics as well as generalization capability [63,64]. In addition, Kainz et al. trained two networks to recognize and separate glands which achieved 95% and 98% classification accuracy in two test sets [65]. Further research, both in H&E-stained and IHC images of colorectal tissue, was performed for glandular epithelium segmentation [66].

Grading into normal, low-grade and high-grade CRC was approached by Awan et al. and Shaban et al. with 91% and 95.7% accuracy, respectively, using the same dataset [67,68]. Lastly, the grading of colorectal images was performed by an unsupervised feature extractor via DL, showing great accuracy, although, as expected, the subcategorization of low-grade tissue images had reduced the accuracy [69].

3.1.3. Tumor Microenvironment

An automated assessment of the CRC tumor microenvironment was carried out, including the stroma, necrosis and lymphocytes associated with progression-free intervals (PFI) [70]. Jiao et al. demonstrated that a higher tumor–stroma ratio was a risk factor, whilst high levels of necrosis and lymphocytes features were associated with a low PFI. Pham's et al. proposed a DL model for binary and 8-class tumor classification in CRC images, as well as, for the prediction and prognosis of the protein marker, DNp73 in IHC rectal cancer images provided perfect results and outperformed other CNNs [71]. Pai et al. conducted a tumor microenvironment analysis in colorectal TMAs [72]. The algorithm efficiently detected differences between MMRD and MMRP slides based on inflammatory stroma, tumor infiltrating lymphocytes (TILs) and mucin, and the quantified proportion of tumor budding (TB), and poorly differentiated clusters (PDCs) associated with lymphatic, venous and perineural invasion. A Desmoplastic Reaction (DR) could be also classified by DL algorithms in CRC histopathological slides containing the deepest tumor invasion area [73]. The classification of a DR based on a myxoid stroma could be a significant prognostic marker for patients' survival.

Comprehensive analysis of the tumor microenvironment proved to show a great performance by the ImmunoAIzer, a DL model for cell distribution description and tumor gene mutation status detection in CRC images, proposed by Bian et al. [74]. Optimal results were achieved in accuracy and precision for biomarker prediction, including CD3, CD20, TP53 and DAPI. Additionally, the suggested DL framework could effectively quantify TILs, PD-1 expressing TILs in anti-PD-1 immunofluorescence staining images, as well as detect APC and TP53. Lymphocytes could be detected in colorectal IHC images stained positive for CD3 and CD8 biomarkers by 4 different CNNs, with U-Net showing the best performance according to the F1 score [75]. In the same framework, Xu et al. proposed a DL model for the quantification of the immune infiltration (CD3 and CD8 T-cells' density) within the stroma region using IHC slides [76]. The CNN-IHC model performed with high accuracy and was efficient in predicting survival probability, which was increased when patients had a higher stromal immune score. Predictions of genetic mutation genes, such as APC, KRAS, PIK3CAM SMAD4, TP53 and BRAF, could be followed through the DL algorithms to support the clinical diagnosis and better stratify patients for targeted therapies [77,78]. Schrammen et al. proposed the Slide-Level Assessment Model (SLAM) for simultaneously tumor detection and predictions of genetic alterations [79]. In a 2017 study, recognizing the molecular tumor subtype based on histopathology image data, Popovici et al. proposed a challenging approach utilizing a DCNN, which was effective in predicting relapse-free survival [80]. Xu et al. compared a DCNN to handcraft feature representation in IHC slides of CRC, stained for an Epidermal Growth Factor Receptor (EGFR), and demonstrated that the DCNN showed a better performance versus the handcrafted features in classifying epithelial and stromal regions [81]. In addition, Sarker et al. developed a DL approach for the identification and characterization of an Inducible T-cell COStimulator (ICOS) biomarker, which achieved high accuracy in the ICOS density estimation and showed potential as a prognostic factor [82]. Tumor budding could be quantified in CRC IHC slides stained for pan-cytokeratin, whereas a high tumor budding score was correlated to a positive nodal status [83].

Analysis for cell nuclei types (epithelial, inflammatory, fibroblasts, "other") by a CNN model trained on 853 annotated images showed a 76% classification accuracy [26]. All four cell types were associated with clinical variables, for instance, fewer inflammatory cells were related to mucinous carcinoma, while metastasis, residual tumors, as well as venous invasion were related to lower numbers of epithelial cells. A similar study, by Sirinukunwattana et al., described a CNN method for the detection and classification of four cell nuclei types (epithelial, inflammatory, fibroblast and miscellaneous) in histopathological images of CRC [84]. Höfener et al. used the same dataset as Sirinukunwattana et al. for nuclei detection from Cthe NNs based on the PMap approach [85]. A novel CNN architecture, Hover-net, was proposed by Graham et al. for the simultaneous segmentation and classification of nuclei, as well as for the prediction of 4 different nuclear types [86]. In 2017, the deep contour-aware network (DCAN) was developed by Chen et al. for accurate gland and nuclei segmentations on histological CRC images [87].

3.1.4. Histological Features Related to Prognosis, Metastasis and Survival

A peri-tumoral stroma (PTS) score evaluated by CNNs was significantly higher in patients with positive lymph nodes compared to the Lymph Node Metastasis (LNM)-negative group [88]. However, due to the small dataset and the selection of classes used, the PTS score for LNM and extramural tumor deposits in early-stage CRC was not detected. Kiehl et al. and Brockmoeller et al. showed that LNM could be predicted by DL models with a good performance [89,90]. Furthermore, the incidence of metastasis in histologic slides with one or more lymph nodes was predicted by CNN, with good accuracy, both for micro- and macro-metastases [91].

Bychkov et al., using TMAs of the most representative tumor area of CRC, proved the efficiency of a DL model to predict the 5-year disease-specific survival (DSS), while Skrede et al. reported data for the prediction of cancer-specific survival [92,93]. Similarly, DSS was predicted by a DL model and clinicopathological features, such as poorly differentiated tumor cell clusters, were associated with high DL risk scores [94]. A Crohn-like lymphoid reaction (CLR) density at the invasive front of the tumor was a good predictor of prognosis in patients with advanced CRC, independent of the TNM stage and tumor–stroma ratio [95]. Determining the ratio of the desmoplastic and inflamed stroma in histopathological slides by DL models could be of great value in predicting the recurrence of disease after rectal excision and a lower desmoplastic to inflamed stroma ratio was associated with a good prognosis [96]. Tumor–stroma ratio (TSR) measures could be an important prognostic factor and, as shown by Zhao et al. and Geesink et al., a stroma-high score was associated with reduced overall survival [97,98]. The "deep stroma score" by Kather et al., a combination of non-tumor components of the tissue, could be an independent prognostic factor for overall survival, especially in patients with advanced CRC [99]. IHC slides stained for pan-cytokeratin from patients with pT3 and pT4 colon ADC were used to train a DCNN to predict the occurrence of distant metastasis based on tumor architecture [100]. Another study showed that IHC-stained images of the amplified breast cancer 1 (AIB1) protein from CRC patients could operate as a predictive 5-year survival marker [101].

3.1.5. Microsatellite Instability

Deploying the dataset of the MSIDETECT consortium, Echle et al. developed a DL detector for the identification of MSI in histopathological slides [102]. High MSI scores were accompanied by the presence of a poorly differentiated tumor tissue, however, false MSI scores were also noted in necrotic and lymphocyte infiltrated areas. The binary classification of DL algorithms for predicting MSI and MSS status in CRC images was performed in studies by Wang, Yamashita, Bustos and Cao et al., with the latter study associating MSI with genomic and transcriptomic profiles [103–106]. Another MSS/MSI-H classifier model was trained on tumor-rich patch images for better classification results, although some images were misclassified indicating that a larger dataset was required [107]. Generating synthesized histology images could also be utilized by DL models for detecting MSI in

CRC, as demonstrated by Krause et al. [108]. A synthetic dataset achieved an almost similar AUC in predicting MSI compared to real images, although the best performance was noted when a combination of synthetic and real images was generated. Image-based consensus molecular subtype (CMS) classification in CRC histological slides from 3 datasets showed a good performance, and the slides having the highest prediction confidence were in concordance with the histological image features [109]. In another study, CMS classification was associated with mucin-to-tumor area quantification, and revealed that CMS2 CRC had no mucin and MUC5AC protein expression was an indication for worse overall survival [110]. Lastly, a CNN for predicting tumor mutational burden-high (TMB-H) in H&E slides was developed by Shimada et al. and showed an AUC of 0.91, while high AUC scores were also noted in the validation cohorts [111]. TMB-H was associated with TILs, although further development is important for this CNN model to be included in clinical practice.

3.2. Technical Viewpoint

The presented DL methods for image analysis in colorectal histopathology images could follow a categorization close to the one presented, which is presented in the background section. The systematic review indicates a rapid implementation of the field, presenting DL applications that cover many technical approaches. Most of the presented works in the literature employ a Convolution Neural Network in different segmentation and classification problems (i.e., binary classification for the diagnosis or prognosis of cancer, multiclass problems to characterize different tissue types, segmentation problems for the detection of the microenvironment of the tissue). According to the scope of the study, the authors proposed an appropriate architecture, providing the performance of their method and perhaps comparing with other already developed CNNs. Few studies used GANs to improve the training of the network, while several of them extended architectures for encoding and decoding, such as U-Net. Recent studies took the advantage of a high classification performance, developing retrospective or cohort studies based on the DL results. Technically, almost all the studies utilized popular machine learning environments, such as PyTorch, TensorFlow, Keras, Fastai, etc., which provided robust implementations of DL approaches. The main category of CNN application can be divided into three subcategories: (i) custom CNN architectures, (ii) popular architectures with transfer learning, and finally, (iii) novel architectures, ensemble CNNs or frameworks.

3.2.1. Custom CNN Architecture

Custom CNN architectures denote those approaches where the authors built, from scratch, all the layers of the network, visualizing in detail the feature extraction layers, the fully connected layers of the classifier, as well as all the layers between of them. Commonly, these architectures consisted of few layers and a small number of parameters, instead of the well-known architectures where the networks expanded and were deeper than custom ones. In several cases, custom CNNs performed well for typical simple problems, where it was probably meaningful to avoid complex architectures and networks with a high consuming computational effort. Several proposed custom CNNs were constructed, containing up to 4 convolution layers for feature extraction and up to 2 fully connected layers for the classifier [38,45,53,66,80]. For example, one of the first presented methods by Xu et al. classified the regions of the image as the epithelium or stroma, employing a simple CNN within a total of 4 layers (2 convolution and 2 fully connected) [81]. Other research teams implemented deeper architectures than the latter, including at least 8 layers [40,83,98]. For example, one of the most recent studies used a custom architecture of 15 layers (12 convolutional and 3 fully connected) for diagnosis purposes [40]. Finally, the most complex custom CNN, proposed by Graham et al. and called MilD-Net+, provides simultaneous gland and lumen segmentation [64].

3.2.2. Popular Architectures with Transfer Learning

The most comfortable way to apply CNNs on imaging problems is the utilization of the machine learning environments, where researchers can easily call already developed architecture. Such architectures gradually became very popular due to their standard implementation as well as their ability to transfer learning from the training in other datasets. According to the concept of transfer learning, it is less computationally expensive to employ a pre-trained deep network instead of a network with randomly generated weights, even if the training set includes images with different characteristics and classes. As a result, in most of the cases, the popular models were trained on the ImageNet dataset, which contained many images of different sources [27]. The most common pre-trained model used for CRC is based on the VGG architectures. Four of the studies, presented by Zhao et al. [95,97], Xu et al. [76] and Jiao et al. [70], employed the VGG-19, while two of the studies employed the VGG-16 [41,101]. Furthermore, two other studies compared different parameters of the general VGG architecture [38,80]. The second and third mostly used CNN for CRC is the Inception.v3 [39,45,53,77,111], the Resnet (ResNet-50 used by Chuang et al. [91], ResNet-18 used by Kiehl et al. [90] and Bilal et al. [78], and ResNet-34 used by Bustos et al. [105] and Bilal et al. [78]), or the combination of them called the InceptionResNet.v2 [100]. These architectures introduced the Inception and the residual blocks, which made the model less sensitive to overfitting. Interesting approaches [67,70,88] were developed using either the U-Net model, where the initial image was encoded to a low resolution and then decoded, providing images with similar characteristics or the ShuffleNet [80,91,103]. Finally, other well-known models were also used, such as AlexNet [57], the YOLO detector [75], the CiFar Model [25], the DenseNet [73], the MobileNet [94], LSTM [71], Xception [51], the DarkNet [48] and EfficientNetB1 [62].

In the category with the pre-trained popular models, all the comparative works could be included. These studies employed either the well-known models referenced above [36,61], or other models such as GoogleNet [99], SqueezeNet [52] and ResNeXT [43]. Finally, two studies utilized [72] or proposed [103] cloud platforms where the user can fine tune several hyper-parameters of popular pre-trained architectures.

3.2.3. Novel Architectures

Many research teams focus on the technical innovation evaluating their proposed methodologies in colorectal image datasets. The studies of these categories are mostly (a) modifications of popular architectures, (b) combinations of techniques into a framework, or (c) ensemble approaches.

Several modified architectures were the HoVer-Net [64] based on the Preact-ResNet-50, the KimiaNet [112] based on the DenseNet, the architecture proposed by Yamashita et al. [104] based on the MobiledNet, and finally, the modification of the loss functions on the ResNet proposed by Medela et al. [113]. Finally, Bian et al. [74] proposed an CNN based on the Inception.v3, adding several residual blocks.

Several studies engaged a CNN architecture with other sophisticated methods and concepts of artificial intelligence. One of the first attempts in the field was developed by Sirinukunwattana et al., proposing a combination of a custom CNN architectures with the Spatial Constrain Regression [84]. A similar concept developed two custom CNN architectures with PMaps approaches [85]. Chen et al. presented a novel deep contour-aware network for the detection and classification of the nuclei [87]. A Deep Belief Network for feature extraction, followed by the Support Vector Machines for classification, was deployed by Sari et al. [69]. A recent work employed a Deep embedding-based Logistic Regression (DELR), which also used active learning for sample selection strategy [60]. In two other studies, the DenseNet was combined with Monte Carlo approaches [46], while the Inception.v3 was cooperated with Adversarial Learning [109]. Finally, Kim et al. [114] combined the InceptionResNet.v2 with Principal Component Analysis and Wavelet Transform.

Some other research teams combined two or more CNNs on a single framework. Two different approaches combined the VGG architectures with the concept of the ResNet [66,92], while the ARA-CNN, proposed by Raczkowski et al. [56], combined the ReSNet with the DarkNet. Lee et al. [107] proposed a framework of an initial custom architecture followed by the Inception.v3. Furthermore, three frameworks based on the ResNet were developed by Zhou et al. [37]. Shaban et al. [68] developed a novel context-aware framework consisting of two stacked CNNs. Finally, another combination between different architectures, which was presented in the literature, is the DeepLab.v2 with ResNet-34 [50].

In recent years, voting systems are increasingly used for classification purposes. These ensemble approaches engage two or more algorithms, where the prediction of the highest performance finally prevails. The first ensemble pipeline was presented by Cao et al. in 2020, which votes according to the likelihood extracted from ResNet-18 [106]. Nguyen et al. [42,110] proposed an ensemble approach with two CNNs (VGG and CapsuleNet), while Kheded et al. deployed an approach with three CNNs as combination backbones: (a) the U-Net with the ResNet, (b) the U-Net with the InceptionResNet.v2 and (c) the DeepLab.v3 with Xception [115]. Another ensemble framework was developed by Skrede et al. [93], with ten CNN models based on the DoMore.v1. The most extended voting systems were presented by Paladini et al. [59], who introduced two ensemble approaches using the ResNet-101, ResNeXt-50, Inception-v3 and DenseNet-161. In the first one, called the Mean-Ensemble-CNN approach, the predicted class of each image was assigned using the average of the predicted probabilities of the four trained models, while in the second one, called the NN-Ensemble-CNN approach, the deep features corresponding to the last FC layer are extracted from the four trained models.

3.2.4. Improving Training with GANs

Apart for the segmentation and classification, DL in CRC has also been applied for the improvement of the training dataset using GANs. There have been three works with GANs' applications presented during the past two years. In the first attempt [108], a Conditional Generative Adversarial Network (CGAN), consisting of six convolution layers for both the generator and the discriminator network, was employed to train the ShuffleNet for the classification. Finally, a very recent study presented a novel GAN architecture, called SAFRON [116], which enabled the generation of images of arbitrarily large sizes after training on relatively small image patches.

Table 1. Deep learning methods on histopathological images for colorectal cancer diagnosis.

Year	First Author	Journal	Aim of Medical Research	Technical Method	Classification Details	Dataset	Performance Metrics
2016	Sirinukunwattana [84]	IEEE Trans Med Imaging	Detection and classification of nuclei	Custom CNN architecture (7-versions) based on the spatially Constrain Regression (a priori)	4-class: epithelial, inflammatory, fibroblast, miscellaneous	>20,000 annotated nuclei from 100 histology images from 10 WSIs	Detection Precision: 0.781, Recall: 0.802, F1 score: 0.802, Classification F1 score: 0.784, AUC: 0.917, Combined detection and classification F1 score: 0.692
	Xu [81]	Neurocomputing	Classification of epithelial and stromal regions	Custom Simple CNN Architecture with 4 Layers (2 × CL and 2 FC) with SVM	Binary (epithelium/stroma)	1376 IHC-stained images of CRC	Classification F1 score: 100%, ACC: 100%, MCC: 100%
	Chen [87]	Med Image Anal	Detection and classification of nuclei	Custom CNN: Novel deep contour-aware network	Binary (bening/malignant)	(1) 2015 MICCAI Gland Segmentation Challenge. Training 85 Images Testing 80, (2) 2015 MICCAI Nuclei Segmentation Challenge: Training 15 Images, Testing 18 images	Detection results (MICCAI Glas): F1 score = 0.887, DICE index 0.868 Hausdorff = 74.731 Segmentation results: D1 and D2 metrics from Challenge
	Popovici [80]	Bioinformatics	Prediction of molecular subtypes	VGG-f (MatConvNet library)	5-class: subtypes (Budinská et al., 2013) Molecular subtypes (denoted A-E)	PETACCURACY:3 clinical trial (Van Cutsem et al., 2009) 300 H/E images	ACC: 0.84, Confusion metrics Precision and Recall per class
	Xu [63]	IEEE Trans Biomed Eng	Classification of Glands	Custom architecture: 3 channel fusions, one based on Faster R-CNN and two based on VGG-16	Binary (bening/malignant)	2015 MICCAI Gland Segmentation Challenge, Training 85 Images Testing 80 Images	Detection results (MICCAI Glas): F1 score (0.893 + 0.843)/2, DICE index (0.908 + 0.833)/2, Hausdorff (44.129 + 116.821)/2
2017	Haj-Hassan [54]	J Pathol Inform	Tumor tissue classification	Custom Simple CNN (2CL and 1FC), with or without initial segmentation	3-class: benign hyperplasia, intraepithelial neoplasia, carcinoma	CHU Nancy Brabois Hospital: 16 multispectral images	Dice and Jaccard with std for segmentation ACC: 99.17%
	Xu [57]	BMC Bioinformatics	Tumor tissue classification	Alexnet—SVM (shared by the Cognitive Vision team at ImageNet LSVRC 2013)	(1) Binary (cancer/not cancer) (2) 6-class: normal (N), ADC, mucinous carcinoma (MC), serrated carcinoma (SC), papillary carcinoma (PC), cribriform comedo-type adenocarcinoma (CCTA)	2014 MICCAI 2014 Brain Tumor Digital Pathology Challenge and CRC image dataset (1) Total 717 H/E Total 693	ACC: (1) Binary: 98% (2) Multiclass: 87.2%
	Jia [41]	IEEE Trans Med Imaging	Diagnosis	3 Stage VGG-16 (publicly available Caffe toolbox)	(1) Binary (Cancer/non cancer) (2) Binary: TMAs (Cancer/non-Cancer)	(1) 330/580 images (CA/NC) (2) 30/30 images (CA/NC)	(2) ODS: 0.447, F-measure: 0.622 (CA), 0.998 (NC)
	Kainz [65]	PeerJ	Classification of Glands	2 × custom CNNs (4 × CL, 2 × FC)	4-class (benign, benign background, malignant, malignant background) add background for each class of the challenge	2015 MICCAI Gland Segmentation Challenge, Training 85 Images (37 benign and 48 malignant). Testing 80 (37/43)	Detection results (MICCAI Glas): F1 score = (0.68 + 0.61)/2, DICE index (0.75 + 0.65)/2, Hausdorff (103.49 + 187.76)/2

Table 1. Cont.

Year	First Author	Journal	Aim of Medical Research	Technical Method	Classification Details	Dataset	Performance Metrics
	Awan [67]	Sci Rep	Grading of CRC	UNET-based architecture	(A) Binary (normal/cancer) (B) 3-class: normal/low grade/high grade	38 WSIs, extracted 139 parts (71 normal, 33 low grade, 35 high grade)	(A) Binary ACC: 97% (B) 3-vlass ACC: 91%
	Wang [58]	Annu Int Conf IEEE Eng Med Biol Soc	Tumor tissue classification	Simple architecture consisting of 1 CL and 1 FC, which is simultaneously operated in both decomposed images	8-class: tumor epithelium, simple stroma, complex stroma, immune cells, debris, normal mucosal glands, adipose tissue, background	University Medical Center Mannheim 1.000 images	ACC: 92.6 ± 1.2
	Bychkov [92]	Sci Rep	Survival	VGG-16 followed by a recurrent ResNet	Binary (low/high risk 5-year disease-specific survival)	Helsinki University Central Hospital, 420 TMAs	Hazard Ratio: 2.3; CI 95%: 1.79–3.03, AUC 0.69
	Eycke [66]	Med Image Anal	Tumor tissue classification/IHC biomarkers quantification	VGG-based architecture including residual units	Binary (bening/malignant)	2015 MICCAI Gland Segmentation Challenge, Training 85 Images Testing 80 (37/43)	Detection results (MICCAI Glas): F1 score = (0.895 + 0.788)/2, DICE index (0.902 + 0.841)/2, Hausdorff (42.943 + 105.926)/2
2018	Weis [83]	Diagn Pathol	Evaluation of tumor budding	Custom architecture consisting of 8 layers	Binary (Tumor bud/no tumor)	HeiData Training dataset 6292 images, 20 IHC pan-cytokeratin WSIs	R2 value: 0.86
	Höfener [85]	Comput Med Imaging Graph	Nuclei detection	2 × Custom CNN architectures based on PMaps approach	No classification, just nuclei detection	Same with Sirinukunwattana et al., >20,000 annotated nuclei from 100 histology images, from 10 WSI	F1 score of 22 different configurations of CNNs Best F1 score: 0.828
	Graham [64]	Med Image Anal	Diagnosis	Custom complex architecture, named Mild-net	Binary (bening/malignant)	(1) MICCAI Gland Segmentation Challenge, (2) same as Awan et al., 2017	(1) F1 socre: (0.914 + 0.844)/2, Dice: (0.913 + 0.836)/2, Hausdorff (41.54 + 105.89)/2 (2) F1 score: 0.825, Dice: 0.875, Hausdorff: 160.14
	Yoon [38]	J Digit Imaging	Diagnosis	6 VGG-based approaches	Binary (normal/Cancer)	Center for CRC, National Cancer Center, Korea, 57 WSIs, 10.280 patches	ACC: 93.48%, SP: 92.76%, SE: 95.1%
2019	Sari [69]	IEEE Trans Med Imaging	Grading of CRC	Feature Extraction from Deep Belief Network and classification employing linear SVM, Comparison with Alexnet, GoogleNet, Inceptionv3, and autoencoders	(1) 3-class: normal (N), Low Grade (LG), High Grade (HG) (2) 5-class: Normal, Low (1), Low (1–2), Low (2), High	(1) 3236 images 1001 N, 1703 LG, 532 HG) (2) 1468 images	(1) mean ACC: 96.13 (2) mean ACC: 79.28

Table 1. Cont.

Year	First Author	Journal	Aim of Medical Research	Technical Method	Classification Details	Dataset	Performance Metrics
	Kather [99]	PLoS Med	Prediction of survival	5 different well-known architectures pre-trained with ImageNet (1) VGG-19, (2) AlexNet, (3) SqueezeNet, (4) GoogleNet, (5) ResNet	9-class: adipose tissue, background, debris, lymphocytes, mucus, smooth muscle, normal colon mucosa, cancer-associated stroma, CRC epithelium/survival predictions	(1) NCT, UMM 86 WSIs (100.000 patches) (2) 25 WSIs DACHS (3) 862 WSIs TCGA WSIs (4) 409 WSIs DACHS	9-class: ACC: 94-99%
	Geessink [98]	Cell Oncocol	Quantification of tumor-stroma ratio (TSR) for prognosis	Custom architecture proposed by Ciombi et al., 2017 (not included by our search)	9-class: tumor, intratumoral stroma, necrosis, muscle, healthy epithelium, fatty tissue, lymphocytes, mucus, erythrocytes	Laboratory for Pathology Eastern Netherlands 74 WSIs	Overall ACC: 94.6%
	Shapcott [26]	Front Bioeng Biotechnol	Classification of nuclei	CNN based on Tensorflow "ciFar" model	4-class: epithelial/inflammatory/fibroblast/other	853 images, 142 TCGA images	Detection ACC: 65% Classification ACC: 76%
	Qaiser [44]	Med Image Anal	Diagnosis	Custom architecture with (4 × CL + ELU), 2FC + Dropout	Binary: tumor/non-tumor	(1) Warwick-UHCW 75 H/E WSIs (112.500 patches), (2) Warwick-Osaka 50 H/E WSIs (75.000 patches)	(A) PHP/CNN: F1 score 0.9243, Precision 0.9267 (B) PHP/CNN: F1 score 0.8273, Precision 0.8311
	Swiderska-Chadaj [75]	Med Image Anal	Detection of lymphocytes	4-different architectures: (1) Custom with 12CL, (2) U-net, (3) YOLLO (based on YOLO detector), (4) LSM (Sirinukunwattana et al. 2016)	3-class: regular lymphocyte distribution/clustered cells/artifacts	28 IHC WSIs	U-Net F1: 0.80 Recall: 0.74 Precision: 0.86
	Graham [86]	Med Image Anal	Classification of nuclei	Novel CNN architecture (named HoVer-Net) based on Preact-ResNet50	4-class: normal, malignant, dysplastic epithelial/inflammatory/miscellaneous/spindle-shaped nuclei (fibroblast, muscle, endothelial)	(1) CoNSeP dataset, 16 WSIs, 41 H/E tiles, (2) Kumar (TCGA) 30 images, (3) CPM-15 (TCGA) 15 images, (4) CPM-17 (TCGA) 32 images, (5) TNBC (Curie Institute) 50 images, (6) CRCHisto 100 images	(1) Dice: 0.853, AJI: 0.571, DQ: 0.702, SQ: 0.778, PQ: 0.547, (2) Dice: 0.826, AJI: 0.618, DQ: 0.770, SQ: 0.773, PQ: 0.597, (4) Dice: 0.869, AJI: 0.705, DQ: 0.854, SQ: 0.814, PQ: 0.697
	Raczkowski [56]	Sci Rep	Tumor tissue classification	Novel architecture (named ARA-CNN), based on ResNet and DarkNet	(A) Binary: tumor/stroma (B) 8-class: tumor epithelium, simple stroma, complex stroma, immune cells, debris, normal mucosal glands, adipose tissue, background	5000 patches (same as Kather et al., 2016)	(1) AUC 0.998 ACC: 99.11 ± 0.97% (2) AUC 0.995 ACC: 92.44 ± 0.81%
	Sena [55]	Oncol Lett	Tumor tissue classification	Custom CNN (4CL, 3FC)	4-class: normal mucosa, preneoplastic lesion, adenoma, cancer	Modena University Hospital, 393 WSIs	ACC: 81.7

Table 1. Cont.

Year	First Author	Journal	Aim of Medical Research	Technical Method	Classification Details	Dataset	Performance Metrics
2020	Iizuka [53]	Sci Rep	Tumor tissue classification	(1) Inception v3, (2) also train an RNN using the features extracted by the Inception	3-class: adenocarcinoma/adenoma/non-neoplastic	Hiroshima University Hospital, Haradoi Hospital, TCGA, 4,036 WSIs	(1) AUC: (ADC: 0.967, Adenoma: 0.99), (2) AUC: (ADC: 0.963, Adenoma: 0.992)
	Shaban [68]	IEEE Trans Med Imaging	Grading of CRC	Novel context-aware framework, consisting of two stacked CNNs	3-Class: Normal, Low Grade, High Grade	Same as Awan et al. 2017 30000 patches	ACC: 95.70
	Holland [52]	J Pathol Inform	Diagnosis	(1) ResNet (Turi Create library framework), (2) SqueezeNet (Turi Create library framework), (3) AlexNet (TensorFlow)	Binary (benign/malignant)	10 slides, 1000 overlapping images	(1) ResNET: ACC: 98%, (2) AlexNet: ACC: 92.1% (3) SqueezeNet: ACC: 80.4%
	Echle [102]	Gastroenterology	MSI prediction	A modified version of Sufflenet (no details)	Binary (MSI/MSS)	TCGA, Darmkrebs: Chancen der Verhütung durch Screening (DACHS), "Quick and Simple and Reliable" trial (QUASAR), Netherlands Cohort Study (NLCS) QUASAR	Cross-validation cohort: mean AUC 0.92, AUPRC of 0.63 Validation cohort: AUROC 0.95 (without image-preprocessing) and AUROC 0.96 (after color normalization)
	Song [50]	BMJ	Diagnosis	A novel architecture based on DeepLab v2 and ResNet-34. Comparison with ResNet-50, DenseNet, Inception.v3, U-Net and DeepLab.v3	Binary (colorectal adenoma/non-neoplasm)	Chinese People's Liberation Army General Hospital, 411 slides CJFH and Cancer Hospital, Chinese Academy of Medical Sciences 168 slides	ACC: 90.4, AUC 0.92
	Zhao [98]	EBioMedicine	Quantification of Tumor–stroma ratio (TSR) for prognosis	VGG-19 pre-trained on the ImageNet using transfer learning with SGDM	9-class: Adipose, Background, Debris, Lymphocyte aggregates, Mucus, Muscle, Normal mucosa, Stroma, Tumor epithelium	TCGA-COAD (461 patients), TCGA-READ (172 patients) Same as Kather et al. 2019	Pearson r (for TSR evaluation between CNN and pathologists): 0.939 ICC evaluation between CNN and pathologists: 0.01 Mean difference in TSR Stroma-high vs. stroma-low patients HR (OS): 1.72 (discovery cohort) and 2.08 (validation study)
	Cao [103]	Theranostics	MSI prediction	An ensemble pipeline for the likelihood of each patch, which is extracted from ResNet-18	Binary (MSI/MSS)	TCGA (429 frozen slides), Tongshu Biotechnology Co. (785 FFPE slides)	(a) TCGA-COAD test set: AUC 0.8848 (b) External Validation set: AUC 0.8504

Table 1. Cont.

Year	First Author	Journal	Aim of Medical Research	Technical Method	Classification Details	Dataset	Performance Metrics
	Xu [39]	J Pathol Inform	Diagnosis	Inception v3 pre-trained on ImageNet	Binary (normal/cancer)	St. Paul's Hospital, 307 H/E images	Median ACC: 99.9% (normal slides), median ACC: 94.8% (cancer slides) Independent dataset: median ACC: 88.1%, AUROC 0.99
	Jang [77]	World J Gastroenterol	Prediction of IHC biomarkers	(A) Simple CNN architecture for the initial binary problem (B) Inception.v3 for the main classification problem	A) Binary (tissue/no-tissue), B) Binary (normal/tumor), C) Binary (APC, KRAS, PIK3CA, SMAD4, TP53) wild-type/mutation	TCGA 629 WSIs (frozen tissue sections 7 FFPE) Seoul St. Mary Hospital (SMH) 142 WSIs	Frozen WSIs: AUC 0.693–0.809 FFPE WSIs: 0.645–0.783
	Medela [113]	J Pathol Inform	Tumor tissue classification	The authors proposed several different functions. For the evaluation, a ResNet backbone was employed, with modified last layer	8-class: tumor epithelium, simple stroma, complex stroma, immune cells, debris and mucus, mucosal glands, adipose tissue, background	University Medical Center Mannheim, 5.000 H/E images	With K = 3: BAC: 85.0 ± 0.6 Silhouette: 0.37 ± 0.02 Davis–Bouldin: 1.41 ± 0.08 With K = 5: BAC: 84.4 ± 0.8 Silhouette: 0.37 ± 0.02 Davis–Bouldin: 1.43 ± 0.09 With K = 7: BAC: 84.5 ± 0.3 Silhouette: 0.37 ± 0.02 Davis-Bouldin: 1.43 ± 0.09
	Skrede [93]	Lancet	Survival	An ensemble approach with ten different CNN models based on DoMorev1	3-class (good/poor prognosis/uncertain)	>12.000.000 image tiles	Uncertain vs. good prognosis HR: 1.89 unadjusted and 1.56 adjusted Poor vs. good prognosis HR: 3.84 unadjusted and 3.04 adjusted Comparison of 3-year cancer-SP: survival of the good prognosis group to the uncertain and poor prognosis groups: SE: 52%, SP: 78%, PDV:19%, NPV: 94%, ACC: 76% Comparison of 3-year cancer-SP: survival of the good and uncertain prognosis groups with the poor prognosis group: SE: 69%, SP: 66%, PDV: 17%, NPV: 96%, ACC: 67%, AUC: 0.713
	Sirinukunwattana [109]	Gut	Consensus molecular subtypes (CMSs) prediction	Inception v3, as well as adversarial learning	4-class: CMS1, CMS2, CMS3, CMS4	(1) FOCUS 510 H/E slides, (2) TCGA 431 H/E slides, (3) GRAMPIAN 265 H/E slides Total: 1.206 slides	(1) AUC 0.88, (2) AUC 0.81, (3) AUC 0.82

Table 1. Cont.

Year	First Author	Journal	Aim of Medical Research	Technical Method	Classification Details	Dataset	Performance Metrics
	Yamashita [104]	Lancet Oncol	MSI prediction	2-stages novel architecture based on a modified MobileNetV2 architecture pre-trained on ImageNet and fine-tuned by transfer learning on the Stanford-CRC dataset	(1) 7-classes: adipose tissue, necrotic debris, lymphocytes, mucin, stroma or smooth muscle, normal colorectal epithelium, and colorectal ADC epithelium (2) Binary (MSI/MSS)	Stanford-CRC dataset (internal); 66,578 tiles from 100 WSIs TCGA (external): 287,543 tiles from 484 WSIs	Internal: AUROC 0.931, External: AUROC 0.779 NPV:93.7%, SE:76.0%, SP:66.6% Reader study Model AUROC 0.865 Pathologist AUROC 0.605
	Zhou [37]	Comput Med Imaging Graph	Tumor tissue classification	A novel 3-framework based on ResNet. Each framework employs different CNN for (a) Image-level binary classification (CA/NC), (b) Cell-level providing the cancer probability in heatmap, (c) Combination framework which merges the output of the previous ones	Binary (cancer/normal)	TCGA 1346 H/E WSIs, First Affiliated Hospital of Zhejiang University, First Affiliated Hospital of Soochow University, Nanjing First Hospital 50 slides	ACC: 0.946 Precision: 0.9636 Recall: 0.9815 F1 score: 0.9725
	Masud [49]	Sensors	Diagnosis	Custom simple CNN architecture with 3 CL, two max pooling 1 batch normalization and 1 dropout	Binary (Colon ADC/colon benign)	LC25000 dataset, James A. Haley Veterans' Hospital, 5.000 images of Colon ADC, 5.000 images of Colon Benign Tissue	Peak classification ACC: 96.33% F-measure score 96.38% for colon and lung cancer identification
	Kwak [88]	Front Oncol	Lymph Node Metastasis (LNM) prediction	U-Net based architecture without (no details)	7-class: normal colon mucosa, stroma, lymphocytes, mucus, adipose tissue, smooth muscle, colon cancer epithelium	TCGA 1000.000 patches	LNM positive group/LNM negative group: OR = 26.654 (PTS score) Ability of PTS score to identify LNM in colon cancer: AUC 0.677
	Krause [108]	J Pathol	MSI prediction	A conditional generative adversarial network (CGAN) for synthetic image generation with 6-CL for both the generator and discriminator network, and a modified ShuffleNet for classification	Binary (MSS/MSI)	TCGA (same as Kather et al., 2019) NLCS cohort (same as Echle et al., 2020)	AUROC 0.742 (patient cohort 1), 0.757 (patient cohort 2), 0.743 (synthetic images), 0.777 (both patient cohorts and synthetic images)

Table 1. Cont.

Year	First Author	Journal	Aim of Medical Research	Technical Method	Classification Details	Dataset	Performance Metrics
	Pai [72]	Histopathology	Tumor microenvironment	CNN developed on the deep learning platform (Aiforia Technologies, Helsinki, Finland) (No details of architecture)	(A) 7-class: carcinoma, tumor budding/poorly differentiated clusters, stroma, necrosis, mucin, smooth muscle, fat (B) 3-class: immature stroma, mature stroma, inflammatory stroma (C) 3-class: low grade carcinoma, high grade carcinoma, signet ring cell carcinoma (D) TILs identification	Stanford University Medical Center (same as Ma et al., 2019) 230 H/E TMAs	MMRD classifying SE: 88% and SP: 73%. ICC between pathologists and model for TB/PDCs, type of stroma, carcinoma grade and TILs: 0.56 to 0.88
	Wang [45]	BMC Med	Diagnosis	AI approach uses Inception.v3 CNN architecture with weights initialized from transfer learning	Binary (cancer/not cancer)	14,234 CRC WSIs and 170,099 patches	ACC: 98.11%, AUC 99.83%, SP: 99.22%, SE: 96.99%
	Riasatian [112]	Med Image Anal	Tumor tissue classification	Proposed a novel architecture (called KimiaNet) based on the DenseNet	8-class: tumor epithelium, simple stroma, complex stroma, immune cells, debris, normal mucosal glands, adipose tissue, background	TCGA 5,000 patches	ACC: 96.38% (KN-I) and 96.80% (KN-IV)
	Jiao [70]	Comput Methods Programs Biomed	Tumor microenvironment	(1) For the foreground, tissue detection employs based on U-NET (2) For 9-class problem, employs the same VGG-19 architecture as Kather et al. and Jhao et al.	9-class: adipose tissue, background, debris, lymphocytes, mucus, smooth muscle, normal colon mucosa, cancer-associated stroma, colorectal ADC epithelium	TCGA 441 H/E images	PFI Stroma HR: 1.665 Necrosis HR: 1.552 Lymphocyte HR: 1.512
	Nearchou [73]	Cancers	Classification of Desmoplastic reaction (DR)	DenseNet neural network, integrated within HALO®	Binary (Immature/other DR type)	528 stage II and III CRC patients treated at the National Defense Medical College Hospital, Japan	Classifier's performance: Dice score: 0.87 for the segmentation of myxoid stroma (test set: 40 patient samples)
	Lee [107]	Int J Cancer	MSI prediction	A framework of an initial CNN architecture based on binary classification of patches, followed by an Inception.v3	(A) Binary (tissue/non-tissue) (B) Binary (normal/tumor) (C) Binary (MSS/MSI-H)	TCGA (COAD, READ) 1,336 frozen slides, 584 FFPE WSIs Seoul St. Mary's Hospital 125 MSS FFPE WSIs, 149 MSI-H FFPE WSIs and 77 MSS FFPE WSIs	TCGA dataset: AUC 0.892 SMH dataset: AUC 0.972
	Wulczyn [94]	NPJ Digit Med	Survival	(1) Tumor segmentation model based on Inception v3, (2) Prognostic model based on Mobile net	Binary (tumor/not tumor)	27,300 slides Validation dataset 1: 9,340 Validation dataset 2: 7,140	Validation dataset 1: AUC 0.70 (95% CI: 0.66–0.73) Validation dataset 2: 0.69 (95% CI: 0.64–0.72)

Table 1. Cont.

Year	First Author	Journal	Aim of Medical Research	Technical Method	Classification Details	Dataset	Performance Metrics
	Shimada [111]	J Gastroenterol	Tumor mutational burden (TMB) prediction	Inception.v3	(A) Binary (neoplastic/non-neoplastic) (B) Binary (TMB-High/TMB-Low)	Japanese cohort TCGA 201 H/E images	AUC 0.910
	Bian [74]	Cancers	Prediction of IHC biomarkers	(1) Modification of Inceptionv3 adding residual block for cellular biomarker distribution prediction and (2) employs Shufflenet.v2 for tumor gene mutation detection	Binary (biomarkers prediction) CD3/CD20, panCK, DAP Binary (tumor mutation genes) APC, TP53, KRAS	Peking University Cancer Hospital and Institute (8697 H/E image patches), TCGA-Colon ADC (COAD) project (50,801 H/E image patches)	Biomarker's prediction: ACC: 90.4% Tumor gene mutation detection: AUC = 0.76 (APC), AUC = 0.77 (KRAS), AUC = 0.79 (TP53)
	Schiele [100]	Cancers	Survival	InceptionResNet.v2 network, pre-trained on images from the ImageNet from Keras	Binary (low/high metastasis risk)	University Hospital Augsburg 291 pT3 and pT4 CRC patients	AUC 0.842, SP: 79.5%, SE: 75.6%, ACC: 75.8%
	Theodosi [101]	Microsc Res Tech	Survival	Pre-trained VGG-16	Binary (5-year survivors/non-survivors)	University Hospital of Patras 162 IHC AIB1 images	ML system: Mean Overall Classification ACC: 87% DL system: Classification ACC: 97%
	Wang [105]	Bioinformatics	MSI prediction	A platform for automated classification where each user can define his own problem. Different popular architectures have been embedded (Inception-V3, ResNet50, Vgg19, MobileNetV2, ShuffleNetV2, and MNASNET)	Binary (MSI/MSS)	TCGA and WSIs	mean ROC (AUC 0.647 ± 0.029)
	Khened [115]	Sci Rep	Slide Image Segmentation and Analysis	A novel ensemble CNN framework with three pre-trained architectures: (a) U-net with DenceNet as the backbone, (b) U-Net with Inception-ResNet.v2 (Inception.v4), (c) Deeplabv3Plus with Xception	(1) Camelyon16: Binary (normal/metastasis), (2) Camelyon17: 4-class: (negative, ITC, Micro and Macro)	DigestPath 660 H/E images (250 with lesions, 410 with no lesions)	Dice: 0.782
	Chuang [91]	Mod Pathol	Detection of nodal micro- and macro-metastasis	ResNet-50	3-class: Micrometastasis/Macrometastasis/Isolated tumor cells	Department of Pathology, Chang Gung Memorial Hospital in Linkou, Taiwan, 3182 H/E WSIs	Slides with >1 lymph node: Macrometastasis: AUC 0.9993, Micrometastasis: AUC 0.9956 Slides with a single lymph node: Macrometastasis: AUC 0.9944, Micrometastasis: AUC 0.9476 Algorithm ACC: 98.50% (95% CI: 97.75–99.25%)

Table 1. Cont.

Year	First Author	Journal	Aim of Medical Research	Technical Method	Classification Details	Dataset	Performance Metrics
	Jones [96]	Histopathology	Survival	No details for DL	7-class: background, necrosis, epithelium, desmoplastic stroma, inflamed stroma, mucin, non-neoplastic mesenchymal components of bowel wall	Oxford Transanal Endoscopic Microsurgery (TEM) database H/E FFPE 150 patients	For desmoplastic to inflamed stroma ratio: AUC: 0.71, SE: 0.92, SP: 0.50, PPV: 0.30, NPV: 0.97 For stroma to immune ratio: AUC: 0.64, SE: 0.92, SP: 0.45, PPV: 0.27, NPV: 0.96
	Pham [71]	Sci Rep	Tumor tissue classification	Time-frequency, time-space, long short-term memory (LSTM) networks	(1) binary (stroma/tumor), (2) 8-class: tumor, simple stroma, complex stroma, immune cells (lymphoid), debris, normal mucosal glands (mucosa), adipose tissue, background	Colorectal cancer data: University Medical Center Mannheim, 625 non-overlapping for each 8 types of tissue images, total 5000 tissue images	(1) ACC: 100, SE: 100, SP: 100, Precision: 100, F1-score: 1 (2) ACC: 99.96%
	Sarker [82]	Cancers	Prediction of IHC biomarker	U-net architecture with, in total, 23 convolutional layers	Binary (ICOS-positive cell/background)	Northern Ireland Biobank (same as Gray et al., 2017)	U-net highest performance: ACC: 98.93%, Dice: 68.84%, AJI = 53.92%, (Backbone: ResNet101, optimizer: Adam, loss function: BCE, batch size: 8)
	Ben Hamida [61]	Comput Biol Med	Tumor tissue classification	(1) Comparison of 4 different architectures Alexnet, VGG-16, ResNet, DenseNet, Inceptionv3, with transfer learning strategy (2) Comparison of SegNet and U-Net for semantic Segmentation	(A) 8-class: tumor, stroma, tissue, necrosis, immune, fat, background, trash (B) Binary (tumor/no-tumor)	(1) AiCOLO (396 H/E slides), (2) NCT Biobank, University Medical Center Mannheim (100,000 H/E patches), (3) CRC-5000 dataset (5,000 images), (4) Warwick (16 H/E)	(1) ResNet On AiCOLO-8: overall ACC: 96.98% On CRC-5000: ACC: 96.77% On NCT-CRC-HE-100k: ACC: 99.76% On merged: ACC: 99.98% (2) On AiCOLO-2 UNet: ACC: 76.18%, SegNet: ACC:81.22%
	Gupta [36]	Diagnostics	Tumor tissue classification	(a) VGG, ResNet, Inception, and IR-v2 for transfer learning, (b) Five types of customized architectures based on Inception-ResNet-v2	Binary (normal/abnormal)	Chang Gung Memorial Hospital, 215 H/E WSIs, 1.303.012 patches	(a) IR-v2 performed better than the others: AUC 0.97, F-score: 0.97 (b) IR-v2 Type 5: AUC 0.99, F-score: 0.99
	Terradillos [51]	J Pathol Inform	Diagnosis	Two-class classifier based on the Xception model architecture	Binary (benign/malignant)	Basurto University Hospital 14.712 images	SE: 0.8228 ± 0.1575 SP: 0.9114 ± 0.0814

Table 1. Cont.

Year	First Author	Journal	Aim of Medical Research	Technical Method	Classification Details	Dataset	Performance Metrics
	Paladini [59]	J Imaging	Tumor tissue classification	2 × Ensemble approach ResNet-101, ResNeXt-50, Inception-v3 and DensNet-161. (1) Mean-Ensemble-CNN approach, the predicted class of each image is assigned using the average of the predicted probabilities of four trained models. (2) In the NN-Ensemble-CNN approach, the deep features corresponding to the last FC layer are extracted from the four trained models	1st database: 8-class (tumor epithelium, simple stroma, complex stroma, immune cells, debris, normal glands, adipose tissue, background) 2nd database: 7-class (tumor, complex stroma, stroma, smooth muscle, benign, inflammatory, debris)	Kather-CRC-2016 Database (5000 CRC images) and CRC-TP Database (280,000 CRC images)	Kather-CRC-2016 Database: Mean-Ensemble-CNN mean ACC: 96.16% NN-Ensemble-CNN mean ACC: 96.14% CRC-TP Database: Mean-Ensemble-CNN ACC: 86.97% Mean-Ensemble-CNN F1-Score: 86.99% NN-Ensemble-CNN ACC: 87.26% NN-Ensemble-CNN F1-Score: 87.27%
	Nguyen [110]	Mod Pathol	Consensus molecular subtypes (CMSs) prediction	A system for tissue detection in WSIs based on an ensemble learning method with two raters, VGG and CapsuleNet	Mucin-to-tumor area ratio quantification and binary classification: high/low mucin tumor	TCGA (871 slides) Bern (775 slides) The Cancer Imaging Archive (TCIA) (373 images)	ICC between pathologists and model for mucin-to-tumor area ratio score: 0.92
	Toğaçar [48]	Comput Biol Med	Diagnosis	DarkNet-19 model based on the YOLO object detection model	Binary (benign/colon ADC)	10,000 images	Colon ADC: ACC: 99.96% Colon benign: ACC: 99.96% Overall ACC: 99.69%
	Zhao [95]	Cancer Immunol Immunother	Lymph Node Metastasis (LNM) prediction	Same CNN as Zhao et al. 2020 (VGG-19 pre-trained on the ImageNet using transfer learning with SGDM)	7-class: tumor epithelium, stroma, mucus, debris, normal mucosa, smooth muscle, lymphocytes, adipose	Training 279 H/E WSIs and Validation 194 H/E WSIs	High CLR density OS in the discovery cohort HR: 0.58 High CLR density OS in the validation cohort HR: 0.45
	Kiehl [89]	EJC	Lymph Node Metastasis (LNM) prediction	ResNet18 pre-trained on H&E-stained slides of the CAMELYON16 challenge	Binary (LNM positive/LNM negative)	DACHS cohort (2,431 patients) TCGA (582 patients)	AUROC on the internal test set: 71% AUROC on the TCGA set: 61.2%
	Xu [76]	Caner Cell Int	Quantification of tumor–stroma ratio (TSR) for prognosis	VGG-19 with or w/o transfer learning	9-class: adipose, background, debris, lymphocytes, mucus, muscle, normal mucosa, stroma, tumor epithelium	283,000 H/E tiles, 154,400 IHC tiles from 243 slides from 121 patients, 22,500 IHC tiles from 114 slides from 57 patients	Test dataset: ACC 0.973, 95% CI 0.971–0.975
	Yu [47]	Nat Commun	Diagnosis	No details for deep learning	Binary (cancer/not cancer)	13.111 WSIs, 62,919 patches	Patch-level diagnosis AUC: 0.980 ± 0.014 Patient-level diagnosis AUC: 0.974 ± 0.013
	Jiao [60]	Comput Methods Programs Biomed	Tumor tissue classification	Deep embedding-based logistic regression (DELR), using active learning for sample selection strategy	8-class: adipose, debris, lymphocytes, mucus, smooth muscle, normal mucosa, stroma, tumor epithelium	180,082 patches	AUC: >0.95

162

Table 1. Cont.

First Author	Journal	Aim of Medical Research	Technical Method	Classification Details	Dataset	Performance Metrics
Brockmoeller [90]	J Pathol	Lymph Nodes Metastasis (LNM) prediction	ShuffleNet with transfer learning for end-to-end prediction	(A) Prediction: Any Lymph Node Metastasis (B) >1 lymph node positive	Koge/Roskilde and Slagelse Hospitals/pT2 cohort (311 H/E sections) Danish Study/pT1 cohort (203 H/E sections)	pT1 CRC >1 LNM AUROC: 0.733 Any LNM AUROC: 0.567 pT2 CRC >1 LNM AUROC: 0.733 Any LNM AUROC: 0.711
Mittal [40]	Cancers	Diagnosis	Custom architecture with 12 CN and 3 FC	Binary (cancer/normal)	15 TMAs	ACC:98%, SP: 98.6%, SE: 98.2%
Kim [114]	Sci Rep	Tumor tissue classification	Combination of InceptionResNet.v2 with PCA and Wavelet transform	5-class: ADC, high-grade adenoma with dysplasia, low-grade adenoma with dysplasia, carcinoid, hyperplastic polyp	Yeouido St. Mary's Hospital 390 WSIs	Dice: 0.804 ± 0.125 ACC: 0.957 ± 0.025 Jac: 0.690 ± 0.174
Tsuneki [62]	Diagnostics	Tumor tissue classification	The authors use the EfficientNetB1 model starting with pre-trained weights on ImageNet	4-class: poorly differentiated ADC, well-to-moderately ADC, adenoma, non-neoplastic	1.799 H/E WSIs	AUC 0.95
Bustos [106]	Biomolecules	Tumor tissue classification/MSI prediction	Resnet-34 pre-trained on ImageNet	(A) 9-class: adipose, background, debris, lymphocytes, mucus, smooth muscle, normal colon epithelium, cancer-associated stroma, colorectal ADC epithelium (B) Binary (MSI-H/MSS)	72 TMAs	(A) Validation test: AUC 0.98 (B) MSI AUC 0.87 ± 0.03
Bilal [78]	Lancet Digit Health	Prediction of molecular pathways and mutations	2 × pre-trained models (1) ResNet-18, (2) adaptive ResNet-34	Binary: (1) High/low mutation density (2) MSI/MSS (3) Chromosomal instability (CIN)/Genomic stability (4) CIMP-high/CIMP-low (5) BRAFmut/BRAFWT (6) TP53mut/TP53WT (7) KRASmut/KRASWT	TCGA (502 slides) Pathology Artificial Intelligence Platform (PAIP) challenge—47 slides (12 microsatellite instable and 35 microsatellite stable)	Mean AUROC Hypermutation: (0.81 [SD 0.03] vs. 0.71), MSI (0.86 [0.04] vs. 0.74), CIN (0.83 [0.02] vs. 0.73), BRAF mutation (0.79 [0.01] vs. 0.66), TP53mut (0.73 [0.02] vs. 0.64), KRAS mutation (0.60 [SD 0.04] vs. 0.60), CIMP-high status 0.79 (SD 0.05)

Table 1. Cont.

Year	First Author	Journal	Aim of Medical Research	Technical Method	Classification Details	Dataset	Performance Metrics
2022	Nguyen [42]	Sci Rep	Diagnosis	Same approach with Nguyen et al., 2021, presented in Mod Pathol	3-class: Tumor/Normal/Other tissue	54 TMA slides	SVEVC: Tumor: Recall:0.938, Precision:0.976, F1-score: 0.957, ACC: 0.939 Normal: Recall: 0.864, Precision: 0.873, F1-score: 0.915, ACC: 0.982 Other tissue: Recall: 0.964, Precision: 0.772, F1-score: 0.858, ACC: 0.947 Overall (average): Recall: 0.922, Precision: 0.907, F1-score: 0.910, ACC: 0.956
	Shen [46]	IEEE/ACM Trans Comput Biol Bioinform	Diagnosis	A DenseNet based architecture of CNN, in an overall framework which employs a Monte Carlo adaptively sampling to localize patches	3-class: loose non-tumor tissue/dense non-tumor tissue/gastrointestinal cancer tissues	(i) TCGA-STAD 432 samples (ii) TCGA-COAD 460 samples (iii) TCGA-READ 171 samples	DP-FTD: AUC 0.779, FROC 0.817 DCRF-FTD: AUC 0.786, FROC 0.821
	Schrammen [79]	J Pathol	Diagnosis/Prediction of IHC biomarkers	Novel method called Slide-Level Assessment Model (SLAM), uses an end-to-end neural network based on ShuffleNet	3-class: Positive tumor slides, Negative tumor slides, Non-tumor slides (A) Binary: BRAF status (mutated or non-mutated) (B) Binary (MSI/MMR) (C) Binary: High grade (grade 3–4)/Low grade (grade 1–2)	(A) Darmkrebs: Chancen der Verhütung durch Screening (DACHS) 2.448 H/E slides B) Yorkshire Cancer Research Bowel Cancer Improvement Program (YCR-BCIP) 889 H/E slides	DACHS cohort Tumor detection AUROC: 0.980 Tumor grading AUROC: 0.751 MSI/MMRD or MSS/MMRP AUROC: 0.909 BRAF status detection AUROC: 0.821 YCR-BCIP cohort MSI/MMRD status detection AUROC: 0.900
	Hosseinzadeh Kassani [43]	Int J Med Inform	Diagnosis	A comparative study between popular architectures (ResNet, VGG, MobileNet, Inceptionv3, InceptionResnetv2, ResNeXt, SE-ResNet, SE-ResNeXt)	Binary (Cancerous/Healthy regions)	DigestPath, 250 H/E WSIs, 1.746 patches	Dice: 82.74% ± 1.77 ACC: 87.07% ± 1.56 F1 score: 82.79% ± 1.79
	Deshpande [116]	Med Image Anal	Diagnosis	Novel GAN architecture, called SAFRON, including loss function which enables generation of images of arbitrarily large sizes after training on relatively small image patches	Binary (benign/malignant)	(A) CRAG (Graham et al., 2019, Awan et al. 2017) 213 colorectal tissue images (B) DigestPath 46 images	ResNet model median classification ACC: 97% with generated images added to the Baseline set, and 93% without

ADC: Adenocarcinoma, ACC: Accuracy, AUC: Area under the ROC Curve, CNN: Convolutional Neural Network, IHC: Immunohistochemistry, SE: Sensitivity, SP: Specificity, TCGA: The Cancer Genome Atlas, SVM: Support Vector Machine, CL: Convolutional layers, FC: Fully-Connected (output) layer, CRC: Colorectal Cancer, TMA: Tissue microarray, WSIs: Whole-slide images, H/E: Hematoxylin and Eosin, MSI: Microsatellite Instability, MMR: Mismatch Repair, MSS: Microsatellite Stable, KRAS: Kirsten rat sarcoma virus, CIN: Chromosomal instability, TP53: Tumor Protein 53, ICOS: Inducible T-cell COStimulator, APC: Adenomatous Polyposis, PIK3CA: Phosphatidylinositol-4,5-Bisphosphate 3-Kinase Catalytic Subunit Alpha.

4. Discussion

A pathology diagnosis focuses on the macroscopic and microscopic examination of human tissues, with the light microscope being the valuable tool for almost two centuries [11]. A meticulous microscopic examination of tissue biopsies is the cornerstone of diagnosis and is a time-consuming procedure. An accurate diagnosis is only the first step for patient treatment. It needs to be complimented with information about grade, stage, and other prognostic and predictive factors [4]. Pathologists' interpretations of tissue lesions become data, guiding decisions for patients' management. A meaningful interpretation is the ultimate challenge. In certain fields, inter- and intra-observer variability are not uncommon [12,13]. In such cases, the interpretation of the visual image can be assisted by objective outputs. Many data have been published over the last 5 years exploring the possibility of moving on to computer-aided diagnosis and the measurement of prognostic and predictive markers for optimal personalized medicine [117,118]. Furthermore, the implementation of AI is now on the horizon. In the last 5 years, extensive research has been conducted to implement AI-based models for the diagnosis of multiple cancer types and, in particular, CRC [14,15,119]. The important aspects in a CRC diagnosis, such as histological type, grade, stromal reaction, immunohistochemical and molecular features have been addressed using breakthrough technologies.

The traditional pathology methods are accompanied by great advantages [120]. The analytical procedures in pathology laboratories are cost-effective and, during recent years, have become automated, eliminating the time and errors of procedures, while maintaining high levels of sensitivity and specificity of techniques, such as IHC [119]. Despite the widespread availability, challenges and limitations of traditional pathology methods remain, such as the differences between laboratories' protocols and techniques, as well as the subjective interpretation between pathologists, resulting in inconsistency in diagnoses [12,13]. Novel imaging systems and WSI scanners promise to upgrade traditional pathology, preserving the code and ethics of practice [119]. The potential of DL algorithms is expanding all over the fields in histopathology. In clinical practice, such algorithms could provide valuable information about the tumor microenvironment quantitative analysis of histological features [76]. Better patient stratification for targeted therapies could be approached by DL-based models predicting mutations, such as MSI status [77,78,107]. More than ever, AI could be of great importance for a pathologist in daily clinical practice. AI is consistently supported by extensive research, which is followed by good performance metrics and potential. Several studies have shown that many DL-based models' predictions did not differ in terms of statistical significance when compared to pathologists' predictions [45,104]. Thus, DL algorithms could provide valuable results for diagnoses in clinical practice, especially when inconsistencies occur. The available scanned histological images can be reviewed and examined by the collaboration of pathologists simultaneously, from different locations [121,122]. For an efficient fully digital workflow, however, the development of technology infrastructure, including computers, scanners, workstations and medical displays is necessary.

Summarizing the presented DL studies from the medical point of view, 17 studies focus on diagnosis, classifying the images as cancer/not cancer, benign/colon ADC or benign/malignant, 17 studies classify tumor tissues, 19 studies investigate the microenvironment of tumors, 14 studies extract histological features related to prognosis, metastasis and survival, and finally, 10 studies detect the microsatellite instability status. The remaining 5 studies that were not described mainly concerned the technical aspects of DL in histological images of CRC. Summarizing the presented DL works from the technical point of view, 80 studies are applications of CNNs, either for image segmentation or classification, and 2 studies employ GANs for the simulation of histological images. The unbalanced distribution between CNN-based and GAN-based studies is an expected result due to the objectives of these two deep learning approaches. CNNs directly classify the images into different categories (e.g., cancer/not cancer). In contrast, GANs just improve the dataset to avoid overtraining and overfitting during the training procedure, without dealing directly with the main medical question. From the CNN-based studies, 10 studies proposed a custom CNN architecture, which was developed from scratch, 42 studies employed already developed architectures, often using transfer learning, and finally, 26 studies implemented novel architectures, such as (a) the modification of those already developed (5 studies), (b) a combination between CNNs or CNNs with other AI techniques (15 studies) and (c) ensemble methods (6 Studies). Finally, two (2) of the studies did not provide any detail about the DL approach.

The application of DL methods in the diagnosis of CRC over the last 5-years seems to be evolving rapidly, faster than other fields of histopathology. However, it seems that there is an expected gradual evolution, starting from the simple techniques of CNNs, then employing transfer learning to the networks, and finally attempting to develop new architectures, focusing on the requirements of the medical question. Additionally, in the last two years, alternative deep learning techniques such as GANs have started to be used. The contribution of such methods will be significant, since DL requires a sufficient size of the training set to perform well and provide generalization. Large data sets may not always be available from the annotations of pathologists and, therefore, need to be enriched with a simulated training set.

It is expected that CNN's application directly in histopathological images will present a better performance compared to traditional techniques. CNNs are advantageous over traditional image processing techniques due to the training procedure, while they are also more robust than the traditional AI techniques because they automatically extract features from the image. In this systematic review, different studies use a variety of performance metrics, while the natures of each classification problem are also different to each other. Therefore, it is not meaningful to calculate the average performance value for all the studies. For this reason, only the accuracy (Acc) and area under the curve (AUC), which were used more than the other metrics, have been used to evaluate each different classification problem. The mean value and Standard Error of Mean have been computed for binary classification problems (Acc = 94.11% $\pm$ 1.3%, AUC = 0.852 $\pm$ 0.066), 3-class classification problems (Acc = 95.5% $\pm$ 1.7%, AUC = 0.931 $\pm$ 0.051), and finally 8-class classification problems (Acc = 94.4% $\pm$ 2.0%, AUC = 0.972 $\pm$ 0.022), which provides sufficient samples of these metrics. The above performance values confirm that DL in colorectal histopathological images can achieve a reliable prediction.

5. Conclusions

When dealing with human disease, particularly cancer, we need in our armamentarium all available resources, and AI is promising to deliver valuable guidance. Specifically for CRC, it appears that the recent exponentially growing relevant research will soon transform the field of tissue-based diagnoses. Preliminary results demonstrate that AI-based models are further applied in clinical cancer research, including CRC, and breast and lung cancer. However, to overcome several limitations, larger numbers of datasets, quality image annotations, as well as external validation cohorts are required to establish the diagnostic accuracy of DL models in clinical practice. Given the available collected data, a part of the current systematic review could be extended to meta-analysis, especially utilizing the data from retrospective studies and survival analysis. The latter could provide us with a comprehensive status for the contribution of DL methods to the diagnosis of CRC.

Author Contributions: Conceptualization, N.G., A.T.T. and A.B.; data curation, A.D., E.B. and T.K.; funding acquisition, N.G. and A.T.T.; methodology, G.N. and A.B.; supervision, N.G., A.T.T. and A.B.; visualization, N.G.; writing—original draft preparation, A.D., E.B., T.K. and N.G.; writing—review and editing, A.D., E.B., T.K., G.N. and A.B. All authors have read and agreed to the published version of the manuscript.

Funding: This research has been co-financed by the European Union and Greek national funds through the Operational Program Competitiveness, Entrepreneurship and Innovation, under the call RESEARCH-CREATE-INNOVATE: T2EDK-03660 (Project: Deep in Biopsies).

Institutional Review Board Statement: Not applicable.

Acknowledgments: Athena Davri is supported by Greece and the European Union—European Regional Development Fund (ERDF) under the Operational Program "Competitiveness Entrepreneurship Innovation" (EPAnEK), NSRF 2014-2020 (MIS 5047236).

Conflicts of Interest: The authors declare no conflict of interest.

References

1. Sung, H.; Ferlay, J.; Siegel, R.L.; Laversanne, M.; Soerjomataram, I.; Jemal, A.; Bray, F. Global Cancer Statistics 2020: GLOBOCAN Estimates of Incidence and Mortality Worldwide for 36 Cancers in 185 Countries. *CA Cancer J. Clin.* **2021**, *71*, 209–249. [CrossRef] [PubMed]
2. Douaiher, J.; Ravipati, A.; Grams, B.; Chowdhury, S.; Alatise, O.; Are, C. Colorectal Cancer-Global Burden, Trends, and Geographical Variations. *J. Surg. Oncol.* **2017**, *115*, 619–630. [CrossRef] [PubMed]
3. Sawicki, T.; Ruszkowska, M.; Danielewicz, A.; Niedźwiedzka, E.; Arłukowicz, T.; Przybyłowicz, K.E. A Review of Colorectal Cancer in Terms of Epidemiology, Risk Factors, Development, Symptoms and Diagnosis. *Cancers* **2021**, *13*, 2025. [CrossRef] [PubMed]
4. Müller, M.F.; Ibrahim, A.E.K.; Arends, M.J. Molecular Pathological Classification of Colorectal Cancer. *Virchows Arch.* **2016**, *469*, 125–134. [CrossRef] [PubMed]
5. Marzouk, O.; Schofield, J. Review of Histopathological and Molecular Prognostic Features in Colorectal Cancer. *Cancers* **2011**, *3*, 2767–2810. [CrossRef] [PubMed]
6. Jass, J.R. Classification of Colorectal Cancer Based on Correlation of Clinical, Morphological and Molecular Features. *Histopathology* **2007**, *50*, 113–130. [CrossRef] [PubMed]
7. Sideris, M.; Papagrigoriadis, S. Molecular Biomarkers and Classification Models in the Evaluation of the Prognosis of Colorectal Cancer. *Anticancer Res.* **2014**, *34*, 2061–2068. [PubMed]
8. Pallag, A.; Roşca, E.; Țiț, D.M.; Muțiu, G.; Bungău, S.G.; Pop, O.L. Monitoring the Effects of Treatment in Colon Cancer Cells Using Immunohistochemical and Histoenzymatic Techniques. *Rom. J. Morphol. Embryol.* **2015**, *56*, 1103–1109. [PubMed]
9. Vogel, J.D.; Eskicioglu, C.; Weiser, M.R.; Feingold, D.L.; Steele, S.R. The American Society of Colon and Rectal Surgeons Clinical Practice Guidelines for the Treatment of Colon Cancer. *Dis. Colon Rectum* **2017**, *60*, 999–1017. [CrossRef] [PubMed]
10. Kelly, M.; Soles, R.; Garcia, E.; Kundu, I. Job Stress, Burnout, Work-Life Balance, Well-Being, and Job Satisfaction among Pathology Residents and Fellows. *Am. J. Clin. Pathol.* **2020**, *153*, 449–469. [CrossRef] [PubMed]
11. Pena, G.P.; Andrade-Filho, J.S. How Does a Pathologist Make a Diagnosis? *Arch. Pathol. Lab. Med.* **2009**, *133*, 124–132. [CrossRef] [PubMed]
12. van Putten, P.G.; Hol, L.; van Dekken, H.; Han van Krieken, J.; van Ballegooijen, M.; Kuipers, E.J.; van Leerdam, M.E. Inter-Observer Variation in the Histological Diagnosis of Polyps in Colorectal Cancer Screening. *Histopathology* **2011**, *58*, 974–981. [CrossRef]
13. Smits, L.J.H.; Vink-Börger, E.; Lijnschoten, G.; Focke-Snieders, I.; Post, R.S.; Tuynman, J.B.; Grieken, N.C.T.; Nagtegaal, I.D. Diagnostic Variability in the Histopathological Assessment of Advanced Colorectal Adenomas and Early Colorectal Cancer in a Screening Population. *Histopathology* **2022**, *80*, 790–798. [CrossRef]
14. Huang, S.; Yang, J.; Fong, S.; Zhao, Q. Artificial Intelligence in Cancer Diagnosis and Prognosis: Opportunities and Challenges. *Cancer Lett.* **2020**, *471*, 61–71. [CrossRef] [PubMed]
15. Thakur, N.; Yoon, H.; Chong, Y. Current Trends of Artificial Intelligence for Colorectal Cancer Pathology Image Analysis: A Systematic Review. *Cancers* **2020**, *12*, 1884. [CrossRef] [PubMed]
16. WHO Classification of Tumours Editorial Board. *WHO Classification of Tumors: Digestive System Tumours*, 5th ed.; International Agency for Research on Cancer: Lyon, France, 2019; ISBN 978-92-832-4499-8.
17. Vilar, E.; Gruber, S.B. Microsatellite Instability in Colorectal Cancer—the Stable Evidence. *Nat. Rev. Clin. Oncol.* **2010**, *7*, 153–162. [CrossRef]
18. Nojadeh, J.N.; Behrouz Sharif, S.; Sakhinia, E. Microsatellite Instability in Colorectal Cancer. *EXCLI J.* **2018**, *17*, 159–168. [CrossRef] [PubMed]
19. Tamura, K.; Kaneda, M.; Futagawa, M.; Takeshita, M.; Kim, S.; Nakama, M.; Kawashita, N.; Tatsumi-Miyajima, J. Genetic and Genomic Basis of the Mismatch Repair System Involved in Lynch Syndrome. *Int. J. Clin. Oncol.* **2019**, *24*, 999–1011. [CrossRef] [PubMed]
20. Boland, C.R.; Goel, A. Microsatellite Instability in Colorectal Cancer. *Gastroenterology* **2010**, *138*, 2073–2087.e3. [CrossRef]
21. Kang, S.; Na, Y.; Joung, S.Y.; Lee, S.I.; Oh, S.C.; Min, B.W. The Significance of Microsatellite Instability in Colorectal Cancer after Controlling for Clinicopathological Factors. *Medicine* **2018**, *97*, e0019. [CrossRef]
22. Arjmand, A.; Tsipouras, M.G.; Tzallas, A.T.; Forlano, R.; Manousou, P.; Giannakeas, N. Quantification of Liver Fibrosis—A Comparative Study. *Appl. Sci.* **2020**, *10*, 447. [CrossRef]
23. Aeffner, F.; Zarella, M.; Buchbinder, N.; Bui, M.; Goodman, M.; Hartman, D.; Lujan, G.; Molani, M.; Parwani, A.; Lillard, K.; et al. Introduction to Digital Image Analysis in Whole-Slide Imaging: A White Paper from the Digital Pathology Association. *J. Pathol. Inform.* **2019**, *10*, 9. [CrossRef]

24. Patel, A.; Balis, U.G.J.; Cheng, J.; Li, Z.; Lujan, G.; McClintock, D.S.; Pantanowitz, L.; Parwani, A. Contemporary Whole Slide Imaging Devices and Their Applications within the Modern Pathology Department: A Selected Hardware Review. *J. Pathol. Inform.* **2021**, *12*, 50. [CrossRef] [PubMed]
25. Jirik, M.; Gruber, I.; Moulisova, V.; Schindler, C.; Cervenkova, L.; Palek, R.; Rosendorf, J.; Arlt, J.; Bolek, L.; Dejmek, J.; et al. Semantic Segmentation of Intralobular and Extralobular Tissue from Liver Scaffold H&E Images. *Sensors* **2020**, *20*, 7063. [CrossRef]
26. Shapcott, M.; Hewitt, K.J.; Rajpoot, N. Deep Learning With Sampling in Colon Cancer Histology. *Front. Bioeng. Biotechnol.* **2019**, *7*, 52. [CrossRef] [PubMed]
27. Deng, J.; Dong, W.; Socher, R.; Li, L.-J.; Li, K.; Fei-Fei, L. ImageNet: A large-scale hierarchical image database. In Proceedings of the 2009 IEEE Conference on Computer Vision and Pattern Recognition, Miami, FL, USA, 20–25 June 2009; Volume 7, pp. 248–255.
28. Graupe, D. *Principles of Artificial Neural Networks, Advanced Series in Circuits and Systems*; World Scientific: London, UK, 2013; Volume 7.
29. Liu, Y.; Gadepalli, K.; Norouzi, M.; Dahl, G.E.; Kohlberger, T.; Boyko, A.; Venugopalan, S.; Timofeev, A.; Nelson, P.Q.; Corrado, G.S.; et al. Detecting Cancer Metastases on Gigapixel Pathology Images. In Proceedings of the 2017 IEEE Conference on Computer Vision and Pattern Recognition (CVPR), Honolulu, HI, USA, 21–26 July 2017.
30. Krizhevsky, A.; Sutskever, I.; Hinton, G.E. ImageNet Classification with Deep Convolutional Neural Networks. *Commun. ACM* **2017**, *60*, 84–90. [CrossRef]
31. Szegedy, C.; Liu, W.; Jia, Y.; Sermanet, P.; Reed, S.; Anguelov, D.; Erhan, D.; Vanhoucke, V.; Rabinovich, A. Going Deeper with Convolutions. In Proceedings of the 2015 IEEE Conference on Computer Vision and Pattern Recognition (CVPR), IEEE, Boston, MA, USA, 7–12 June 2015; pp. 1–9. [CrossRef]
32. Simonyan, K.; Zisserman, A. Very Deep Convolutional Networks for Large-Scale Image Recognition. In Proceedings of the 3rd International Conference on Learning Representations, Conference Track Proceedings, San Diego, CA, USA, 7–9 May 2015. [CrossRef]
33. Huang, G.; Liu, Z.; Van Der Maaten, L.; Weinberger, K.Q. Densely Connected Convolutional Networks. In Proceedings of the 2017 IEEE Conference on Computer Vision and Pattern Recognition (CVPR), Honolulu, HI, USA, 21–26 July 2017; pp. 2261–2269. [CrossRef]
34. Goodfellow, I.J.; Pouget-Abadie, J.; Mirza, M.; Xu, B.; Warde-Farley, D.; Ozair, S.; Courville, A.; Bengio, Y. Generative Adversarial Networks. *Commun. ACM* **2020**, *63*, 139–144. [CrossRef]
35. Page, M.J.; McKenzie, J.E.; Bossuyt, P.M.; Boutron, I.; Hoffmann, T.C.; Mulrow, C.D.; Shamseer, L.; Tetzlaff, J.M.; Akl, E.A.; Brennan, S.E.; et al. The PRISMA 2020 Statement: An Updated Guideline for Reporting Systematic Reviews. *Int. J. Surg.* **2021**, *88*, 105906. [CrossRef] [PubMed]
36. Gupta, P.; Huang, Y.; Sahoo, P.K.; You, J.F.; Chiang, S.F.; Onthoni, D.D.; Chern, Y.J.; Chao, K.Y.; Chiang, J.M.; Yeh, C.Y.; et al. Colon Tissues Classification and Localization in Whole Slide Images Using Deep Learning. *Diagnostics* **2021**, *11*, 1398. [CrossRef]
37. Zhou, C.; Jin, Y.; Chen, Y.; Huang, S.; Huang, R.; Wang, Y.; Zhao, Y.; Chen, Y.; Guo, L.; Liao, J. Histopathology Classification and Localization of Colorectal Cancer Using Global Labels by Weakly Supervised Deep Learning. *Comput. Med. Imaging Graph.* **2021**, *88*, 101861. [CrossRef] [PubMed]
38. Yoon, H.; Lee, J.; Oh, J.E.; Kim, H.R.; Lee, S.; Chang, H.J.; Sohn, D.K. Tumor Identification in Colorectal Histology Images Using a Convolutional Neural Network. *J. Digit. Imaging* **2019**, *32*, 131–140. [CrossRef]
39. Xu, L.; Walker, B.; Liang, P.-I.; Tong, Y.; Xu, C.; Su, Y.; Karsan, A. Colorectal Cancer Detection Based on Deep Learning. *J. Pathol. Inform.* **2020**, *11*, 28. [CrossRef] [PubMed]
40. Mittal, P.; Condina, M.R.; Klingler-Hoffmann, M.; Kaur, G.; Oehler, M.K.; Sieber, O.M.; Palmieri, M.; Kommoss, S.; Brucker, S.; McDonnell, M.D.; et al. Cancer Tissue Classification Using Supervised Machine Learning Applied to Maldi Mass Spectrometry Imaging. *Cancers* **2021**, *13*, 5388. [CrossRef] [PubMed]
41. Jia, Z.; Huang, X.; Chang, E.I.C.; Xu, Y. Constrained Deep Weak Supervision for Histopathology Image Segmentation. *IEEE Trans. Med. Imaging* **2017**, *36*, 2376–2388. [CrossRef] [PubMed]
42. Nguyen, H.-G.; Blank, A.; Dawson, H.E.; Lugli, A.; Zlobec, I. Classification of Colorectal Tissue Images from High Throughput Tissue Microarrays by Ensemble Deep Learning Methods. *Sci. Rep.* **2021**, *11*, 2371. [CrossRef]
43. Hosseinzadeh Kassani, S.; Hosseinzadeh Kassani, P.; Wesolowski, M.J.; Schneider, K.A.; Deters, R. Deep Transfer Learning Based Model for Colorectal Cancer Histopathology Segmentation: A Comparative Study of Deep Pre-Trained Models. *Int. J. Med. Inform.* **2022**, *159*, 104669. [CrossRef] [PubMed]
44. Qaiser, T.; Tsang, Y.-W.; Taniyama, D.; Sakamoto, N.; Nakane, K.; Epstein, D.; Rajpoot, N. Fast and Accurate Tumor Segmentation of Histology Images Using Persistent Homology and Deep Convolutional Features. *Med. Image Anal.* **2019**, *55*, 1–14. [CrossRef] [PubMed]
45. Wang, K.S.; Yu, G.; Xu, C.; Meng, X.H.; Zhou, J.; Zheng, C.; Deng, Z.; Shang, L.; Liu, R.; Su, S.; et al. Accurate Diagnosis of Colorectal Cancer Based on Histopathology Images Using Artificial Intelligence. *BMC Med.* **2021**, *19*, 76. [CrossRef] [PubMed]
46. Shen, Y.; Ke, J. Sampling Based Tumor Recognition in Whole-Slide Histology Image with Deep Learning Approaches. *IEEE/ACM Trans. Comput. Biol. Bioinform.* **2021**, *14*, 1. [CrossRef]
47. Yu, G.; Sun, K.; Xu, C.; Shi, X.-H.; Wu, C.; Xie, T.; Meng, R.-Q.; Meng, X.-H.; Wang, K.-S.; Xiao, H.-M.; et al. Accurate Recognition of Colorectal Cancer with Semi-Supervised Deep Learning on Pathological Images. *Nat. Commun.* **2021**, *12*, 6311. [CrossRef]

48. Toğaçar, M. Disease Type Detection in Lung and Colon Cancer Images Using the Complement Approach of Inefficient Sets. *Comput. Biol. Med.* **2021**, *137*, 104827. [CrossRef]
49. Masud, M.; Sikder, N.; Nahid, A.-A.; Bairagi, A.K.; AlZain, M.A. A Machine Learning Approach to Diagnosing Lung and Colon Cancer Using a Deep Learning-Based Classification Framework. *Sensors* **2021**, *21*, 748. [CrossRef] [PubMed]
50. Song, Z.; Yu, C.; Zou, S.; Wang, W.; Huang, Y.; Ding, X.; Liu, J.; Shao, L.; Yuan, J.; Gou, X.; et al. Automatic Deep Learning-Based Colorectal Adenoma Detection System and Its Similarities with Pathologists. *BMJ Open* **2020**, *10*, e036423. [CrossRef]
51. Terradillos, E.; Saratxaga, C.; Mattana, S.; Cicchi, R.; Pavone, F.; Andraka, N.; Glover, B.; Arbide, N.; Velasco, J.; Etxezarraga, M.; et al. Analysis on the Characterization of Multiphoton Microscopy Images for Malignant Neoplastic Colon Lesion Detection under Deep Learning Methods. *J. Pathol. Inform.* **2021**, *12*, 27. [CrossRef]
52. Holland, L.; Wei, D.; Olson, K.; Mitra, A.; Graff, J.; Jones, A.; Durbin-Johnson, B.; Mitra, A.; Rashidi, H. Limited Number of Cases May Yield Generalizable Models, a Proof of Concept in Deep Learning for Colon Histology. *J. Pathol. Inform.* **2020**, *11*, 5. [CrossRef] [PubMed]
53. Iizuka, O.; Kanavati, F.; Kato, K.; Rambeau, M.; Arihiro, K.; Tsuneki, M. Deep Learning Models for Histopathological Classification of Gastric and Colonic Epithelial Tumours. *Sci. Rep.* **2020**, *10*, 1504. [CrossRef]
54. Haj-Hassan, H.; Chaddad, A.; Harkouss, Y.; Desrosiers, C.; Toews, M.; Tanougast, C. Classifications of Multispectral Colorectal Cancer Tissues Using Convolution Neural Network. *J. Pathol. Inform.* **2017**, *8*, 1. [CrossRef]
55. Sena, P.; Fioresi, R.; Faglioni, F.; Losi, L.; Faglioni, G.; Roncucci, L. Deep Learning Techniques for Detecting Preneoplastic and Neoplastic Lesions in Human Colorectal Histological Images. *Oncol. Lett.* **2019**, *18*, 6101–6107. [CrossRef]
56. Rączkowski, Ł.; Możejko, M.; Zambonelli, J.; Szczurek, E. ARA: Accurate, Reliable and Active Histopathological Image Classification Framework with Bayesian Deep Learning. *Sci. Rep.* **2019**, *9*, 14347. [CrossRef] [PubMed]
57. Xu, Y.; Jia, Z.; Wang, L.B.; Ai, Y.; Zhang, F.; Lai, M.; Chang, E.I.C. Large Scale Tissue Histopathology Image Classification, Segmentation, and Visualization via Deep Convolutional Activation Features. *BMC Bioinform.* **2017**, *18*, 281. [CrossRef] [PubMed]
58. Wang, C.; Shi, J.; Zhang, Q.; Ying, S. Histopathological Image Classification with Bilinear Convolutional Neural Networks. *Proc. Annu. Int. Conf. IEEE Eng. Med. Biol. Soc. EMBS* **2017**, *2017*, 4050–4053. [CrossRef]
59. Paladini, E.; Vantaggiato, E.; Bougourzi, F.; Distante, C.; Hadid, A.; Taleb-Ahmed, A. Two Ensemble-CNN Approaches for Colorectal Cancer Tissue Type Classification. *J. Imaging* **2021**, *7*, 51. [CrossRef]
60. Jiao, Y.; Yuan, J.; Qiang, Y.; Fei, S. Deep Embeddings and Logistic Regression for Rapid Active Learning in Histopathological Images. *Comput. Methods Programs Biomed.* **2021**, *212*, 106464. [CrossRef] [PubMed]
61. Ben Hamida, A.; Devanne, M.; Weber, J.; Truntzer, C.; Derangère, V.; Ghiringhelli, F.; Forestier, G.; Wemmert, C. Deep Learning for Colon Cancer Histopathological Images Analysis. *Comput. Biol. Med.* **2021**, *136*, 104730. [CrossRef] [PubMed]
62. Tsuneki, M.; Kanavati, F. Deep Learning Models for Poorly Differentiated Colorectal Adenocarcinoma Classification in Whole Slide Images Using Transfer Learning. *Diagnostics* **2021**, *11*, 2074. [CrossRef]
63. Xu, Y.; Li, Y.; Wang, Y.; Liu, M.; Fan, Y.; Lai, M.; Chang, E.I.C. Gland Instance Segmentation Using Deep Multichannel Neural Networks. *IEEE Trans. Biomed. Eng.* **2017**, *64*, 2901–2912. [CrossRef] [PubMed]
64. Graham, S.; Chen, H.; Gamper, J.; Dou, Q.; Heng, P.A.; Snead, D.; Tsang, Y.W.; Rajpoot, N. MILD-Net: Minimal Information Loss Dilated Network for Gland Instance Segmentation in Colon Histology Images. *Med. Image Anal.* **2019**, *52*, 199–211. [CrossRef] [PubMed]
65. Kainz, P.; Pfeiffer, M.; Urschler, M. Segmentation and Classification of Colon Glands with Deep Convolutional Neural Networks and Total Variation Regularization. *PeerJ* **2017**, *2017*, e3874. [CrossRef]
66. Van Eycke, Y.R.; Balsat, C.; Verset, L.; Debeir, O.; Salmon, I.; Decaestecker, C. Segmentation of Glandular Epithelium in Colorectal Tumours to Automatically Compartmentalise IHC Biomarker Quantification: A Deep Learning Approach. *Med. Image Anal.* **2018**, *49*, 35–45. [CrossRef] [PubMed]
67. Awan, R.; Sirinukunwattana, K.; Epstein, D.; Jefferyes, S.; Qidwai, U.; Aftab, Z.; Mujeeb, I.; Snead, D.; Rajpoot, N. Glandular Morphometrics for Objective Grading of Colorectal Adenocarcinoma Histology Images. *Sci. Rep.* **2017**, *7*, 2220–2243. [CrossRef] [PubMed]
68. Shaban, M.; Awan, R.; Fraz, M.M.; Azam, A.; Tsang, Y.W.; Snead, D.; Rajpoot, N.M. Context-Aware Convolutional Neural Network for Grading of Colorectal Cancer Histology Images. *IEEE Trans. Med. Imaging* **2020**, *39*, 2395–2405. [CrossRef] [PubMed]
69. Sari, C.T.; Gunduz-Demir, C. Unsupervised Feature Extraction via Deep Learning for Histopathological Classification of Colon Tissue Images. *IEEE Trans. Med. Imaging* **2019**, *38*, 1139–1149. [CrossRef] [PubMed]
70. Jiao, Y.; Li, J.; Qian, C.; Fei, S. Deep Learning-Based Tumor Microenvironment Analysis in Colon Adenocarcinoma Histopathological Whole-Slide Images. *Comput. Methods Programs Biomed.* **2021**, *204*, 106047. [CrossRef] [PubMed]
71. Pham, T.D. Time-Frequency Time-Space Long Short-Term Memory Networks for Image Classification of Histopathological Tissue. *Sci. Rep.* **2021**, *11*, 13703. [CrossRef] [PubMed]
72. Pai, R.K.; Hartman, D.; Schaeffer, D.F.; Rosty, C.; Shivji, S.; Kirsch, R.; Pai, R.K. Development and Initial Validation of a Deep Learning Algorithm to Quantify Histological Features in Colorectal Carcinoma Including Tumour Budding/Poorly Differentiated Clusters. *Histopathology* **2021**, *79*, 391–405. [CrossRef] [PubMed]
73. Nearchou, I.P.; Ueno, H.; Kajiwara, Y.; Lillard, K.; Mochizuki, S.; Takeuchi, K.; Harrison, D.J.; Caie, P.D. Automated Detection and Classification of Desmoplastic Reaction at the Colorectal Tumour Front Using Deep Learning. *Cancers* **2021**, *13*, 1615. [CrossRef] [PubMed]

74. Bian, C.; Wang, Y.; Lu, Z.; An, Y.; Wang, H.; Kong, L.; Du, Y.; Tian, J. Immunoaizer: A Deep Learning-based Computational Framework to Characterize Cell Distribution and Gene Mutation in Tumor Microenvironment. *Cancers* **2021**, *13*, 1659. [CrossRef] [PubMed]
75. Swiderska-Chadaj, Z.; Pinckaers, H.; van Rijthoven, M.; Balkenhol, M.; Melnikova, M.; Geessink, O.; Manson, Q.; Sherman, M.; Polonia, A.; Parry, J.; et al. Learning to Detect Lymphocytes in Immunohistochemistry with Deep Learning. *Med. Image Anal.* **2019**, *58*, 101547. [CrossRef] [PubMed]
76. Xu, Z.; Li, Y.; Wang, Y.; Zhang, S.; Huang, Y.; Yao, S.; Han, C.; Pan, X.; Shi, Z.; Mao, Y.; et al. A Deep Learning Quantified Stroma-Immune Score to Predict Survival of Patients with Stage II–III Colorectal Cancer. *Cancer Cell Int.* **2021**, *21*, 585. [CrossRef]
77. Jang, H.J.; Lee, A.; Kang, J.; Song, I.H.; Lee, S.H. Prediction of Clinically Actionable Genetic Alterations from Colorectal Cancer Histopathology Images Using Deep Learning. *World J. Gastroenterol.* **2020**, *26*, 6207–6223. [CrossRef]
78. Bilal, M.; Raza, S.E.A.; Azam, A.; Graham, S.; Ilyas, M.; Cree, I.A.; Snead, D.; Minhas, F.; Rajpoot, N.M. Development and Validation of a Weakly Supervised Deep Learning Framework to Predict the Status of Molecular Pathways and Key Mutations in Colorectal Cancer from Routine Histology Images: A Retrospective Study. *Lancet Digit. Health* **2021**, *3*, e763–e772. [CrossRef]
79. Schrammen, P.L.; Ghaffari Laleh, N.; Echle, A.; Truhn, D.; Schulz, V.; Brinker, T.J.; Brenner, H.; Chang-Claude, J.; Alwers, E.; Brobeil, A.; et al. Weakly Supervised Annotation-Free Cancer Detection and Prediction of Genotype in Routine Histopathology. *J. Pathol.* **2022**, *256*, 50–60. [CrossRef] [PubMed]
80. Popovici, V.; Budinská, E.; Dušek, L.; Kozubek, M.; Bosman, F. Image-Based Surrogate Biomarkers for Molecular Subtypes of Colorectal Cancer. *Bioinformatics* **2017**, *33*, 2002–2009. [CrossRef]
81. Xu, J.; Luo, X.; Wang, G.; Gilmore, H.; Madabhushi, A. A Deep Convolutional Neural Network for Segmenting and Classifying Epithelial and Stromal Regions in Histopathological Images. *Neurocomputing* **2016**, *191*, 214–223. [CrossRef] [PubMed]
82. Sarker, M.M.K.; Makhlouf, Y.; Craig, S.G.; Humphries, M.P.; Loughrey, M.; James, J.A.; Salto-tellez, M.; O'Reilly, P.; Maxwell, P. A Means of Assessing Deep Learning-based Detection of ICOS Protein Expression in Colon Cancer. *Cancers* **2021**, *13*, 3825. [CrossRef] [PubMed]
83. Weis, C.A.; Kather, J.N.; Melchers, S.; Al-ahmdi, H.; Pollheimer, M.J.; Langner, C.; Gaiser, T. Automatic Evaluation of Tumor Budding in Immunohistochemically Stained Colorectal Carcinomas and Correlation to Clinical Outcome. *Diagn. Pathol.* **2018**, *13*, 64. [CrossRef] [PubMed]
84. Sirinukunwattana, K.; Raza, S.E.A.; Tsang, Y.W.; Snead, D.R.J.; Cree, I.A.; Rajpoot, N.M. Locality Sensitive Deep Learning for Detection and Classification of Nuclei in Routine Colon Cancer Histology Images. *IEEE Trans. Med. Imaging* **2016**, *35*, 1196–1206. [CrossRef] [PubMed]
85. Höfener, H.; Homeyer, A.; Weiss, N.; Molin, J.; Lundström, C.F.; Hahn, H.K. Deep Learning Nuclei Detection: A Simple Approach Can Deliver State-of-the-Art Results. *Comput. Med. Imaging Graph.* **2018**, *70*, 43–52. [CrossRef] [PubMed]
86. Graham, S.; Vu, Q.D.; Raza, S.E.A.; Azam, A.; Tsang, Y.W.; Kwak, J.T.; Rajpoot, N. Hover-Net: Simultaneous Segmentation and Classification of Nuclei in Multi-Tissue Histology Images. *Med. Image Anal.* **2019**, *58*, 101563. [CrossRef] [PubMed]
87. Chen, H.; Qi, X.; Yu, L.; Dou, Q.; Qin, J.; Heng, P.A. DCAN: Deep Contour-Aware Networks for Object Instance Segmentation from Histology Images. *Med. Image Anal.* **2017**, *36*, 135–146. [CrossRef]
88. Kwak, M.S.; Lee, H.H.; Yang, J.M.; Cha, J.M.; Jeon, J.W.; Yoon, J.Y.; Kim, H.I. Deep Convolutional Neural Network-Based Lymph Node Metastasis Prediction for Colon Cancer Using Histopathological Images. *Front. Oncol.* **2021**, *10*, 1–9. [CrossRef] [PubMed]
89. Kiehl, L.; Kuntz, S.; Höhn, J.; Jutzi, T.; Krieghoff-Henning, E.; Kather, J.N.; Holland-Letz, T.; Kopp-Schneider, A.; Chang-Claude, J.; Brobeil, A.; et al. Deep Learning Can Predict Lymph Node Status Directly from Histology in Colorectal Cancer. *Eur. J. Cancer* **2021**, *157*, 464–473. [CrossRef] [PubMed]
90. Brockmoeller, S.; Echle, A.; Ghaffari Laleh, N.; Eiholm, S.; Malmstrøm, M.L.; Plato Kuhlmann, T.; Levic, K.; Grabsch, H.I.; West, N.P.; Saldanha, O.L.; et al. Deep Learning Identifies Inflamed Fat as a Risk Factor for Lymph Node Metastasis in Early Colorectal Cancer. *J. Pathol.* **2022**, *256*, 269–281. [CrossRef] [PubMed]
91. Chuang, W.Y.; Chen, C.C.; Yu, W.H.; Yeh, C.J.; Chang, S.H.; Ueng, S.H.; Wang, T.H.; Hsueh, C.; Kuo, C.F.; Yeh, C.Y. Identification of Nodal Micrometastasis in Colorectal Cancer Using Deep Learning on Annotation-Free Whole-Slide Images. *Mod. Pathol.* **2021**, *34*, 1901–1911. [CrossRef]
92. Bychkov, D.; Linder, N.; Turkki, R.; Nordling, S.; Kovanen, P.E.; Verrill, C.; Walliander, M.; Lundin, M.; Haglund, C.; Lundin, J. Deep Learning Based Tissue Analysis Predicts Outcome in Colorectal Cancer. *Sci. Rep.* **2018**, *8*, 3395. [CrossRef] [PubMed]
93. Skrede, O.J.; De Raedt, S.; Kleppe, A.; Hveem, T.S.; Liestøl, K.; Maddison, J.; Askautrud, H.A.; Pradhan, M.; Nesheim, J.A.; Albregtsen, F.; et al. Deep Learning for Prediction of Colorectal Cancer Outcome: A Discovery and Validation Study. *Lancet* **2020**, *395*, 350–360. [CrossRef]
94. Wulczyn, E.; Steiner, D.F.; Moran, M.; Plass, M.; Reihs, R.; Tan, F.; Flament-Auvigne, I.; Brown, T.; Regitnig, P.; Chen, P.H.C.; et al. Interpretable Survival Prediction for Colorectal Cancer Using Deep Learning. *Npj Digit. Med.* **2021**, *4*, 71. [CrossRef] [PubMed]
95. Zhao, M.; Yao, S.; Li, Z.; Wu, L.; Xu, Z.; Pan, X.; Lin, H.; Xu, Y.; Yang, S.; Zhang, S.; et al. The Crohn's-like Lymphoid Reaction Density: A New Artificial Intelligence Quantified Prognostic Immune Index in Colon Cancer. *Cancer Immunol. Immunother.* **2021**. [CrossRef] [PubMed]
96. Jones, H.J.S.; Cunningham, C.; Askautrud, H.A.; Danielsen, H.E.; Kerr, D.J.; Domingo, E.; Maughan, T.; Leedham, S.J.; Koelzer, V.H. Stromal Composition Predicts Recurrence of Early Rectal Cancer after Local Excision. *Histopathology* **2021**, *79*, 947–956. [CrossRef]

97. Geessink, O.G.F.; Baidoshvili, A.; Klaase, J.M.; Ehteshami Bejnordi, B.; Litjens, G.J.S.; van Pelt, G.W.; Mesker, W.E.; Nagtegaal, I.D.; Ciompi, F.; van der Laak, J.A.W.M. Computer Aided Quantification of Intratumoral Stroma Yields an Independent Prognosticator in Rectal Cancer. *Cell. Oncol.* **2019**, *42*, 331–341. [CrossRef] [PubMed]
98. Zhao, K.; Li, Z.; Yao, S.; Wang, Y.; Wu, X.; Xu, Z.; Wu, L.; Huang, Y.; Liang, C.; Liu, Z. Artificial Intelligence Quantified Tumour-Stroma Ratio Is an Independent Predictor for Overall Survival in Resectable Colorectal Cancer. *EBioMedicine* **2020**, *61*, 103054. [CrossRef]
99. Kather, J.N.; Krisam, J.; Charoentong, P.; Luedde, T.; Herpel, E.; Weis, C.A.; Gaiser, T.; Marx, A.; Valous, N.A.; Ferber, D.; et al. Predicting Survival from Colorectal Cancer Histology Slides Using Deep Learning: A Retrospective Multicenter Study. *PLoS Med.* **2019**, *16*, e1002730. [CrossRef] [PubMed]
100. Schiele, S.; Arndt, T.T.; Martin, B.; Miller, S.; Bauer, S.; Banner, B.M.; Brendel, E.M.; Schenkirsch, G.; Anthuber, M.; Huss, R.; et al. Deep Learning Prediction of Metastasis in Locally Advanced Colon Cancer Using Binary Histologic Tumor Images. *Cancers* **2021**, *13*, 2074. [CrossRef]
101. Theodosi, A.; Ouzounis, S.; Kostopoulos, S.; Glotsos, D.; Kalatzis, I.; Asvestas, P.; Tzelepi, V.; Ravazoula, P.; Cavouras, D.; Sakellaropoulos, G. Employing Machine Learning and Microscopy Images of AIB1-Stained Biopsy Material to Assess the 5-Year Survival of Patients with Colorectal Cancer. *Microsc. Res. Tech.* **2021**, *84*, 2421–2433. [CrossRef] [PubMed]
102. Echle, A.; Grabsch, H.I.; Quirke, P.; van den Brandt, P.A.; West, N.P.; Hutchins, G.G.A.; Heij, L.R.; Tan, X.; Richman, S.D.; Krause, J.; et al. Clinical-Grade Detection of Microsatellite Instability in Colorectal Tumors by Deep Learning. *Gastroenterology* **2020**, *159*, 1406–1416.e11. [CrossRef] [PubMed]
103. Cao, R.; Yang, F.; Ma, S.C.; Liu, L.; Zhao, Y.; Li, Y.; Wu, D.H.; Wang, T.; Lu, W.J.; Cai, W.J.; et al. Development and Interpretation of a Pathomics-Based Model for the Prediction of Microsatellite Instability in Colorectal Cancer. *Theranostics* **2020**, *10*, 11080–11091. [CrossRef] [PubMed]
104. Yamashita, R.; Long, J.; Longacre, T.; Peng, L.; Berry, G.; Martin, B.; Higgins, J.; Rubin, D.L.; Shen, J. Deep Learning Model for the Prediction of Microsatellite Instability in Colorectal Cancer: A Diagnostic Study. *Lancet Oncol.* **2021**, *22*, 132–141. [CrossRef]
105. Wang, Y.; Coudray, N.; Zhao, Y.; Li, F.; Hu, C.; Zhang, Y.-Z.; Imoto, S.; Tsirigos, A.; Webb, G.I.; Daly, R.J.; et al. HEAL: An Automated Deep Learning Framework for Cancer Histopathology Image Analysis. *Bioinformatics* **2021**, *37*, 4291–4295. [CrossRef] [PubMed]
106. Bustos, A.; Payá, A.; Torrubia, A.; Jover, R.; Llor, X.; Bessa, X.; Castells, A.; Carracedo, Á.; Alenda, C. XDEEP-MSI: Explainable Bias-Rejecting Microsatellite Instability Deep Learning System in Colorectal Cancer. *Biomolecules* **2021**, *11*, 1786. [CrossRef]
107. Lee, S.H.; Song, I.H.; Jang, H.J. Feasibility of Deep Learning-Based Fully Automated Classification of Microsatellite Instability in Tissue Slides of Colorectal Cancer. *Int. J. Cancer* **2021**, *149*, 728–740. [CrossRef]
108. Krause, J.; Grabsch, H.I.; Kloor, M.; Jendrusch, M.; Echle, A.; Buelow, R.D.; Boor, P.; Luedde, T.; Brinker, T.J.; Trautwein, C.; et al. Deep Learning Detects Genetic Alterations in Cancer Histology Generated by Adversarial Networks. *J. Pathol.* **2021**, *254*, 70–79. [CrossRef] [PubMed]
109. Sirinukunwattana, K.; Domingo, E.; Richman, S.D.; Redmond, K.L.; Blake, A.; Verrill, C.; Leedham, S.J.; Chatzipli, A.; Hardy, C.; Whalley, C.M.; et al. Image-Based Consensus Molecular Subtype (ImCMS) Classification of Colorectal Cancer Using Deep Learning. *Gut* **2021**, *70*, 544–554. [CrossRef] [PubMed]
110. Nguyen, H.G.; Lundström, O.; Blank, A.; Dawson, H.; Lugli, A.; Anisimova, M.; Zlobec, I. Image-Based Assessment of Extracellular Mucin-to-Tumor Area Predicts Consensus Molecular Subtypes (CMS) in Colorectal Cancer. *Mod. Pathol.* **2022**, *35*, 240–248. [CrossRef]
111. Shimada, Y.; Okuda, S.; Watanabe, Y.; Tajima, Y.; Nagahashi, M.; Ichikawa, H.; Nakano, M.; Sakata, J.; Takii, Y.; Kawasaki, T.; et al. Histopathological Characteristics and Artificial Intelligence for Predicting Tumor Mutational Burden-High Colorectal Cancer. *J. Gastroenterol.* **2021**, *56*, 547–559. [CrossRef]
112. Riasatian, A.; Babaie, M.; Maleki, D.; Kalra, S.; Valipour, M.; Hemati, S.; Zaveri, M.; Safarpoor, A.; Shafiei, S.; Afshari, M.; et al. Fine-Tuning and Training of Densenet for Histopathology Image Representation Using TCGA Diagnostic Slides. *Med. Image Anal.* **2021**, *70*, 102032. [CrossRef] [PubMed]
113. Medela, A.; Picon, A. Constellation Loss: Improving the Efficiency of Deep Metric Learning Loss Functions for the Optimal Embedding of Histopathological Images. *J. Pathol. Inform.* **2020**, *11*, 38. [CrossRef] [PubMed]
114. Kim, H.; Yoon, H.; Thakur, N.; Hwang, G.; Lee, E.J.; Kim, C.; Chong, Y. Deep Learning-Based Histopathological Segmentation for Whole Slide Images of Colorectal Cancer in a Compressed Domain. *Sci. Rep.* **2021**, *11*, 6047. [CrossRef]
115. Khened, M.; Kori, A.; Rajkumar, H.; Krishnamurthi, G.; Srinivasan, B. A Generalized Deep Learning Framework for Whole-Slide Image Segmentation and Analysis. *Sci. Rep.* **2021**, *11*, 11579. [CrossRef]
116. Deshpande, S.; Minhas, F.; Graham, S.; Rajpoot, N. SAFRON: Stitching Across the Frontier Network for Generating Colorectal Cancer Histology Images. *Med. Image Anal.* **2022**, *77*, 102337. [CrossRef] [PubMed]
117. van der Laak, J.; Litjens, G.; Ciompi, F. Deep Learning in Histopathology: The Path to the Clinic. *Nat. Med.* **2021**, *27*, 775–784. [CrossRef]
118. Wang, Y.; He, X.; Nie, H.; Zhou, J.; Cao, P.; Ou, C. Application of Artificial Intelligence to the Diagnosis and Therapy of Colorectal Cancer. *Am. J. Cancer Res.* **2020**, *10*, 3575–3598. [PubMed]
119. Montezuma, D.; Monteiro, A.; Fraga, J.; Ribeiro, L.; Gonçalves, S.; Tavares, A.; Monteiro, J.; Macedo-Pinto, I. Digital Pathology Implementation in Private Practice: Specific Challenges and Opportunities. *Diagnostics* **2022**, *12*, 529. [CrossRef]

120. Baxi, V.; Edwards, R.; Montalto, M.; Saha, S. Digital Pathology and Artificial Intelligence in Translational Medicine and Clinical Practice. *Mod. Pathol.* **2022**, *35*, 23–32. [CrossRef] [PubMed]
121. Oliveira, S.P.; Neto, P.C.; Fraga, J.; Montezuma, D.; Monteiro, A.; Monteiro, J.; Ribeiro, L.; Gonçalves, S.; Pinto, I.M.; Cardoso, J.S. CAD Systems for Colorectal Cancer from WSI Are Still Not Ready for Clinical Acceptance. *Sci. Rep.* **2021**, *11*, 14358. [CrossRef] [PubMed]
122. Yoshida, H.; Kiyuna, T. Requirements for Implementation of Artificial Intelligence in the Practice of Gastrointestinal Pathology. *World J. Gastroenterol.* **2021**, *27*, 2818–2833. [CrossRef] [PubMed]

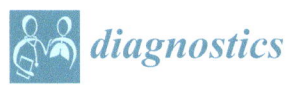

Guidelines

Best Practice Recommendations for the Implementation of a Digital Pathology Workflow in the Anatomic Pathology Laboratory by the European Society of Digital and Integrative Pathology (ESDIP)

Filippo Fraggetta [1,2], Vincenzo L'Imperio [1,3], David Ameisen [1,4], Rita Carvalho [1,5], Sabine Leh [1,6,7], Tim-Rasmus Kiehl [1,5], Mircea Serbanescu [1,8], Daniel Racoceanu [1,9], Vincenzo Della Mea [1,10], Antonio Polonia [1,11,12], Norman Zerbe [1,5] and Catarina Eloy [1,11,12,]*

1. European Society of Digital and Integrative Pathology (ESDIP), Rua da Constituição n°668, 1° Esq/Traseiras, 4200-194 Porto, Portugal; filippofra@hotmail.com (F.F.); vincenzo.limperio@gmail.com (V.L.); david.ameisen@gmail.com (D.A.); rita.carvalho@charite.de (R.C.); sabine.leh@helse-bergen.no (S.L.); rasmus.kiehl@charite.de (T.-R.K.); mircea_serbanescu@yahoo.com (M.S.); daniel.racoceanu@sorbonne-universite.fr (D.R.); vincenzo.dellamea@uniud.it (V.D.M.); apolonia@ipatimup.pt (A.P.); norman.zerbe@charite.de (N.Z.)
2. Pathology Unit, "Gravina" Hospital, Caltagirone, ASP Catania, Via Portosalvo 1, 95041 Caltagirone, Italy
3. Department of Medicine and Surgery, Pathology, ASST Monza, San Gerardo Hospital, University of Milano-Bicocca, 20900 Monza, Italy
4. Imginit SAS, 152 Boulevard du Montparnasse, 75014 Paris, France
5. Charité–Universitätsmedizin Berlin, Corporate Member of Freie Universität Berlin and Humboldt-Universität zu Berlin, Institute of Pathology, Charitéplatz 1, 10117 Berlin, Germany
6. Department of Pathology, Haukeland University Hospital, Jonas Lies Vei 65, 5021 Bergen, Norway
7. Department of Clinical Medicine, University of Bergen, Jonas Lies Vei 87, 5021 Bergen, Norway
8. Department of Medical Informatics and Biostatistics, University of Medicine and Pharmacy of Craiova, 200349 Craiova, Romania
9. Sorbonne Université, Institut du Cerveau—Paris Brain Institute—ICM, Inserm, CNRS, APHP, Inria Team "Aramis", Hôpital de la Pitié Salpêtrière, 75013 Paris, France
10. Department of Mathematics, Computer Science and Physics, University of Udine, 33100 Udine, Italy
11. Ipatimup Diagnostics, Institute of Molecular Pathology and Immunology of Porto University (Ipatimup), 4200-804 Porto, Portugal
12. Medical Faculty, University of Porto, 4200-319 Porto, Portugal
* Correspondence: celoy@ipatimup.pt

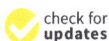

Abstract: The interest in implementing digital pathology (DP) workflows to obtain whole slide image (WSI) files for diagnostic purposes has increased in the last few years. The increasing performance of technical components and the Food and Drug Administration (FDA) approval of systems for primary diagnosis led to increased interest in applying DP workflows. However, despite this revolutionary transition, real world data suggest that a fully digital approach to the histological workflow has been implemented in only a minority of pathology laboratories. The objective of this study is to facilitate the implementation of DP workflows in pathology laboratories, helping those involved in this process of transformation to identify: (a) the scope and the boundaries of the DP transformation; (b) how to introduce automation to reduce errors; (c) how to introduce appropriate quality control to guarantee the safety of the process and (d) the hardware and software needed to implement DP systems inside the pathology laboratory. The European Society of Digital and Integrative Pathology (ESDIP) provided consensus-based recommendations developed through discussion among members of the Scientific Committee. The recommendations are thus based on the expertise of the panel members and on the agreement obtained after virtual meetings. Prior to publication, the recommendations were reviewed by members of the ESDIP Board. The recommendations comprehensively cover every step of the implementation of the digital workflow in the anatomic pathology department, emphasizing the importance of interoperability, automation and tracking of the entire process before the introduction of a scanning facility. Compared to the available national and international guidelines, the present document represents a practical, handy reference for the correct implementation of the digital workflow in Europe.

Keywords: digital pathology; anatomic pathology workflow; whole slide imaging; laboratory information system

1. Introduction

The interest in implementing digital pathology (DP) workflows to obtain whole slide image (WSI) files for diagnostic purposes has increased in the last few years. This is due to the opportunities offered by WSI, e.g., telepathology and image analysis, including computational pathology tools based on artificial intelligence [AI] methods. The increasing performance of technical components and the Food and Drug Administration (FDA) approval of systems for primary diagnosis [1] led to increased interest in applying DP workflows. Moreover, in the last few years, several studies evaluating performance demonstrated the non-inferiority of WSI compared to conventional light microscopy [2–4] for primary histological diagnosis. This may help to alleviate concerns about the possible risk of DP-related diagnostic errors [5]. Indeed, the restrictions suffered during the COVID-19 pandemic, the reduction in the number of pathologists and the increase in workload, with rising number and complexity of cases, also raised the interest in DP. Several definitions for DP have been proposed so far [6,7], a common opinion being that DP encompasses the photographic documentation of the macroscopy of the specimens ("gross pathology"), the digitization of glass slides (virtual microscopy) and telepathology. By some definitions, DP involves merely the digitization of glass slides. In this study, "DP" is significantly distanced from the reductive paradigm of only glass slide digitization, moving towards a more integrative approach that comprises interventions in all stations of work in the pathology laboratory, introducing and supporting innovation. DP implicitly consists of all the associated technologies to allow improvements and innovations in workflow, including, for instance, laboratory management systems (LIS), digital dictation, dashboards and workflow management, electronic specimen labelling and tracking, and synoptic reporting tools. The objective of this study is to facilitate the implementation of DP workflows in pathology laboratories, helping those involved in this process of transformation to: (a) identify the scope and the boundaries of the DP transformation; (b) introduce automation to reduce errors; (c) introduce appropriate quality control to guarantee the safety of the process and (d) implement the hardware and software needed to implement DP systems inside the pathology laboratory. Since several recommendations and guidelines have already been proposed, primarily focusing on the validation of WSI for clinical purposes or on the technical environment, this paper mainly covers DP implementation and all the prerequisites for a pathology laboratory to change from an analogue to a digital workflow [8]. Considering all that has been reported about DP workflow implementation and its associated benefits, it is anticipated that this new methodology has many advantages that should be attractive and convenient for all pathology laboratories worldwide, independently of their dimension, workload, number of pathologists or type of activity (academic/nonacademic, private/public) [6,7,9–11].

So far, there are several possibilities to transit and to manage "images" in a digital workflow: an LIS-based approach [12,13], a scanner vendor approach [7] or an intermediate software approach (e.g., Linköping University [14]). Independently of the type of strategy chosen to switch towards a digital visualization of images (LIS-centric, vendor based or third-party software), the new system should be able to integrate every possible instrument (e.g., one or more scanners from same or different vendors with the possibility to manage different images from a variety of sources), preferably associated with a tracking system because of automation and innovation. The cost-effectiveness of DP has already been documented in implementation models that discuss the scope of investment, the potential return on investment, and cost-savings of DP, as well as any proposed income deriving from the adoption of WSIs [15]. Moreover, the adequate adaptation of a routine clinical workflow can finally lead to an optimization of resources (e.g., space, time, personnel, and equipment).

These are intended as recommendations and suggestions for the implementation of the full DP workflow in the routine clinical practice of anatomic pathology laboratories. The introduction of a DP workflow even allows the implementation of computational pathology tools, i.e., artificial intelligence (AI). The following sections explain, point-by-point, the steps needed for the progressive, secure, and efficient transition into a DP workflow. Regarding cytopathology, there are several barriers that still need to be overcome for routine cytopathology to go digital and support wider adoption and sustainability. Therefore, the present study mainly focuses on histopathology and its transition to the DP workflow Box 1.

Box 1. Digital pathology workflow implementation—Step by Step.

Summary
Digital pathology is pathology—A holistic approach that comprehends interventions in all stations of work at the pathology laboratory, introducing innovation.
Digital pathology is attractive and convenient for pathology laboratories worldwide.
Digital pathology represents a safer and more efficient way of working and should be considered the new standard in pathology.
Implementation of a digital pathology workflow is the milestone to fully benefit from the potential of WSI and a prerequisite for the application of AI in routine diagnostics.

---

2. Involvement of the Team in the Digital Pathology Transformation of the Laboratory

The implementation of digital pathology requires a multidisciplinary approach from the very beginning. The leading team should involve in-house participants (pathologists, laboratory technicians, administrative staff) and the hospital's IT and technical services [6]. IT services might be organized in different ways depending on the size of the department and depending on local or national policies. For example, the IT services may be provided by individuals, by a separate department or by a subcontractor. The most important thing is that these groups work together and that they form a team. Subsequently, close collaboration with companies providing the digital pathology system and the laboratory information system will become necessary. Especially in larger departments, digital transformation will usually be organized as a project that includes a project manager, a steering group and different working groups. There are several ways of introducing the topic and designing the appropriate options for the laboratory at hand, and it might be useful to visit pathology departments with digital workflows to learn from their successes and failures. There are a couple of papers that share experiences and provide valuable information [6,7]. Describing user scenarios is another method to understand the needs of one's own laboratory and communicate these to the IT and technical departments and possible suppliers. In addition, before starting a tender, it is helpful to gather information about suppliers and products. To obtain a successful implementation of the "DP" and to avoid deficiencies, the multidisciplinary team that is going to lead the "digital revolution" in each department should follow some crucial steps, as previously reported. In particular, for the correct and rapid implementation of DP in every department, it is advisable to create awareness, participation, appropriate work conditions, communication among the team members, and monitor the outcomes of this revolution. This approach could help in facing the heterogeneous patterns of reactions that different actors of the team could express, including the "enthusiasts", the "sceptics", and the "undecideds". All the possible measures to increase the trust and involvement of pathologists should be applied to all staff members. To establish a successful DP workflow, a thorough stakeholder analysis should be carried out, and a communication strategy should be established based on this analysis. The team must ensure that all internal stakeholders (pathologists, laboratory personnel and administrative staff) are continuously informed from the beginning. In this setting, sharing the vision of DP with laboratory and administrative personnel, encouraging them to provide feedback, expressing potential concerns and suggestions (e.g., using frequent meetings on-site) and providing appropriate discussion during all phases of the deployment will facilitate a safe and effective implementation. The team must be aware that DP should be perceived as an integral part of the laboratory workflow rather than an "add-on" [6]. The contingent situation due to the COVID-19 pandemic can be further leveraged to boost the implementation of DP in the laboratories, stressing the need to maintain pathology services by making it possible for pathologists to work from home [16]. Implementing DP as the standard laboratory practice requires learning new technical skills to capture all the advantages of this technology. Just as significant as the internal stakeholders is the involvement of IT services. IT will be crucial in many aspects of the project (LIS adaptations, integrations, storage, testing etc.). The involvement should start in the early phases. For example, consider a laboratory office tour to establish communication with the other components of the project in clear language, understand what is expected and what is potentially achievable from your deployment, and what each professional group will be expected to contribute in terms of time and staff. Explain your ideas for future digital workflows and see what potential dependencies and solutions your IT colleagues can generate.

3. Optimization of Resources in the DP Workflow

In a fully digital laboratory, the processes and records are electronic file-based, the environment is paperless, with glass slides being substituted at the end of the workflow by WSIs. The optimization of resources, namely time, space, people and instruments, creates conditions for increased efficiency and, consequently, decreased costs. The LEAN approach represents a valuable strategy to optimize the workflow, leading to a more logical distribution of the spaces to minimize staff and sample traffic inside the laboratory. It also allows for a more harmonic and well-planned articulation between human resources and available instruments, which results in time and cost-effectiveness. Although it is not a strict prerequisite for adopting DP, it could further allow for better allocation of resources [17]. This can start from a more rational disposition of the spaces/offices inside the pathology laboratory. An inefficient arrangement of the physical spaces, typical of the old, "analogue" workflow, can partly impair the smooth crosstalk among the different components of the process. Previous experiences in implementation models stress the need to analyze the pre-existing workflow before implementing DP [6,7]. A careful analysis of the pre-existing analogic workflow before the transition should consider the flow of the samples (workstation location) in the laboratory and time intervals (hands-on and waiting times) for each workstation, verifying the information technology support and establishment of adequate quality control checkpoints. The lack of structural organization of some pathology laboratories, including the physical placement of the different workstations, may contribute negatively to the desirable, efficient crosstalk between workstations. The reorganization of such a laboratory structure with the intent to decrease unnecessary movements of the staff, and time loss, can be useful for every laboratory, independently of DP implementation. For instance, the scanning workstation should be located near the staining and mounting instruments, accelerating the production line but far from the microtome area to avoid the interference of paraffin with the scanning mechanisms. After this retrospective analysis and reorganization of the structure, the optimal choices for the automation of each workstation must be made, namely by the introduction of a reliable tracking system, and different instruments would preferably work in a coordinated fashion, connected (mono-or bi-directionally) to the LIS (or LIMS).

4. The Role and Potentialities of Laboratory Information (Management) System (LIS/LIMS) and Informatics Resources

Independently of the system employed to manage the WSI (LIS, scanner or third party), pathology laboratories mainly depend on laboratory information systems (LISs) to support their operations and, ultimately, carry out their patient care mission. For these reasons, one of the crucial points is to ensure the full integration of the systems involved in the digital transition. Although many LISs have evolved with sophisticated and more user-friendly software over the past few decades, supporting a broader range of functions, many others have not evolved, thus preventing possible integration with other technologies deployed in the laboratories. Modern LISs play different roles in all phases of patient testing, including specimen and test order entry, specimen processing and tracking. They track and organize the laboratory's workflow, mainly through event logs and histology protocols. The maintenance of such logs can follow the default configurations of the system or can be customized by each laboratory to display the most useful information. A typical example of the system's default configuration for a log (e.g., routine histology) includes accession number, timestamp, patient and specimen data, histology protocol(s) ordered, other stains ordered and comments about the specimen or the request. LISs now incorporate multiple features that, until recently, were either unavailable or required a significant customization effort to be obtained. The Association for Pathology Informatics produced a comprehensive list of basic and advanced LIS features that may be used to evaluate LIS capabilities [18]. Moreover, the next generation LIS should be able to link digital images to the respective cases appropriately. With the rising use of whole slide imaging (WSI) for clinical purposes, a consensual increase in capabilities to connect and integrate WSI systems and LIS is to be expected (e.g., open WSI from the LIS, log the viewed areas/magnification on all WSI or even apply image analysis and store result data). Further advances in the development of LISs are expected in the future, starting from the integration of more sophisticated tools to support data mining and the analysis of pathology and clinical data sets. The LIS may evolve into a multimodality "pathologist cockpit" that not only provides LIS functions but also displays pathology imaging and other medical imaging, supplies analytical tools, provides access to clinical data (e.g., Electronic Health Record [EHR]) [19] as well as other data sources [20]. A more recent guideline paper [21] underlined the importance of digital pathology interoperability, with a LIS being able to connect all the instruments present in the laboratory to support critical DP use cases. Moreover, increasing requests for molecular and genetic tests on pathology specimens (e.g., next-generation sequencing) impose further innovation in LISs to integrate and optimize these data with the traditional pathology report for optimal patient management [22] in an integrative model. Finally, the transition will allow information integration from grossing, enable collaborative work and incorporate quality control results.

5. Automation of Workflow and Tracking System

Automation and using a robust tracking system can significantly reduce errors related to handwriting transcription and misspelling that can cause samples to be dissociated from a particular patient ("mismatching"). Automation is a "strong recommendation" emanating from these recommendations, as it can benefit both pathology laboratories using DP and those using glass slides for diagnosis. Besides the introduction of a suitable LIS/LIMS that can help monitor the instruments' performance connected to each sample, further automation can be introduced in the workstations. This includes the reagents used and tracking all the staff that were at any point involved in sample processing by differential log-ins or scanning of individual ID codes at all workstations. The possible automation of workstations obviously depends on budget, existing instruments, and the experience of the technical staff. Devices such as a robotic stainer and a cover-slipper will bring consistent slide quality, avoiding frequent re-staining and ongoing readjustments to scanning protocols. The same is true for the automation of embedding and cutting processes, for which available systems on the market appear promising. However, these are not yet widely used in practice [23]. The goals of a tracking system are to keep the sample automatically, correctly, and permanently labelled during the time that it circulates in the laboratory. The identification of the sample, using labels on the containers, printed in the cassettes/paraffin blocks, printed on the glass slides and then present in the WSI files, is a best practice rule that is recommended to be adopted for the use of the WSI. In this setting, the perfect compatibility (interoperability) of the instrumentation used to label and to process the samples within the AP laboratory, and with the other laboratories in the same institution, is crucial to avoid possible issues (e.g., blurring or shading of the labels during subsequent processing of specimens/slides). The sample identifiers, of which there are usually several (see Section 5), should be managed automatically and electronically connected to the patient's LIS entry. The integration between the tracking system and LIS with an electronic interface between the LIS and the printers is essential to maintaining continuity of identification. The link established between the asset (tissue container/cassette/block) and the LIS will help reduce errors and can be achieved by printing different data types on the assets, such as barcodes or 2D (QR) codes. These can be linked to different types of data in the LIS. Eventually, other systems with code reader compatibility will be able to read them [24]. The introduction of radiofrequency identification (RFID) technologies is a promising method to track the assets, although cost and system integration barriers still limit their implementation [25,26]. In the case of pathology laboratories, introducing at least one barcode reader per workstation is recommended. Tracking an individual sample with the combined use of printers and code readers accelerates the work at the microtome stations, helping histotechnologists track each block and slide, ensuring the adequate identification and concordance between the individual block and slide labels [27]. The LISs typically offer the laboratories some capability to customize the format and content of their slide labels. As will be further explained in the subsequent sections of the document, the employment of unequivocal 2D barcodes can have a multitude of applications in the proposed digital workflow, significantly reducing the operations time and error rates. The impact of such implementation can be noted starting from the accessioning phases, where the sample is assigned its unequivocal code that will be used later during the processing and reporting steps. This can further help in the creation of tissue cassettes, in the production of tissue glass slides, in the automatic request of additional histochemical and immunohistochemical (IHC) stains, as well as in the double check that should be carried out at every checkpoint to ensure correspondence among received material, grossed specimen, embedded sample and cut sections. This is facilitated by the additional use of barcode readers and by the implementation of newly introduced instruments to capture the cut surface directly from the paraffin block [28], which is at this point essential to guarantee a sustainable and reliable quality control process (see Section 5).

As will be further explained in the following sections of this paper, the use of unequivocal 2D barcodes can have many applications in the proposed digital workflow, significantly reducing the operations time and error rates. The impact of such implementation can be noted starting from the accessioning phases, where the sample is assigned its unequivocal code that will be used later during the processing and reporting steps. This can further help in the creation of tissue cassettes, the production of glass slides, automatic requests for additional histologic and IHC stains, as well as in the double-check that should be carried out at every checkpoint to ensure the correspondence among arrived material, grossed specimen, embedded sample and cut sections. This is facilitated by the additional use of barcode readers and by implementing instruments capable of capturing the cut surface directly from the paraffin block (see Section 5).

6. Quality Control Program and Definition of Checkpoints

Quality control of products from a pathology laboratory is essential to guarantee that a patient receives a correct diagnosis. In Europe, the certification and accreditation of laboratories are not equally and uniformly performed across the territory. Instead, many laboratories design their own quality control program, more or less simplified, often involving only segments of sample processing adequate to their intent. Although adopting a quality management system is not strictly required in all countries as a prerequisite for implementing DP workflow, laboratories with a robust system of quality management may find the DP workflow easier to implement as they are already aware of the critical control checkpoints through the analogue workflow. To support those laboratories that are not yet familiar with quality control programs, a detailed description of some suggested checkpoints suitable for adaptation to each laboratory are provided. The checkpoints described here derive from the need to control the performance of a new instrument in the pipeline—the scanner. They also originate from introducing new standard operative procedures (SOPs), tools/instruments and quality control of the processes (Figure 1).

Simultaneously, per each workstation, some technical modifications are discussed to facilitate the scanning process and increase the quality of the WSI. We highlight that time loss within the laboratory is frequently motivated by a mismatch of samples and poor sample quality (either due to a pre-analytical or analytical factor). Investing in a workflow with a good quality of samples that are easy to track decreases the time lost, considering that this loss is very difficult to estimate because it is not generally recorded.

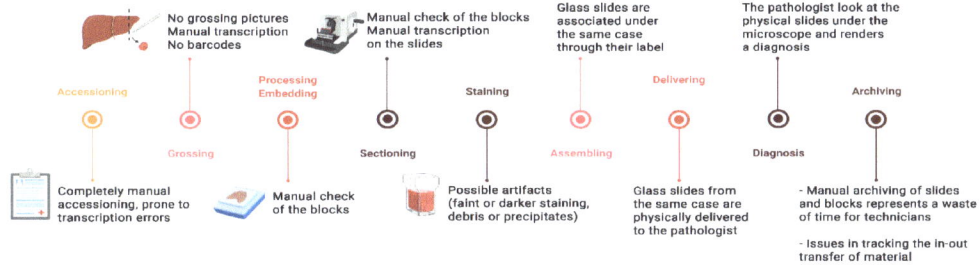

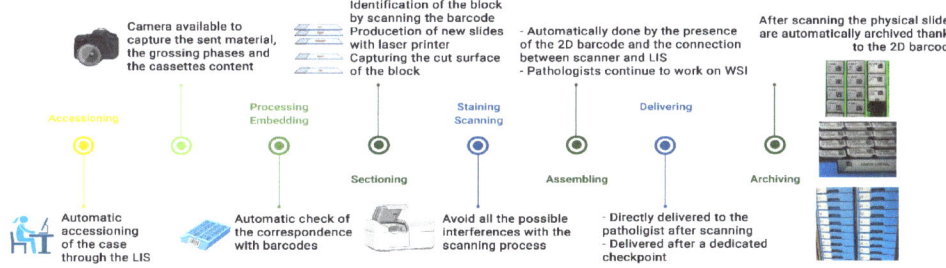

Figure 1. Differences among analog and the digital workflows. Credit: created with BioRender.

6.1. Accessioning Checkpoints

During the accessioning phase, samples that arrive at the pathology laboratory are registered in the LIS and given a case number. Analyzing the classical analog accessioning procedures allows for a critical evaluation of the potential issues that can and do happen. Mistakes can occur in the compilation of paper requests from the submitting department or outside hospital (for internal and external cases, respectively). The staff responsible for the accessioning phase can miss discrepancies between the sample/slide and the request or even mismatch this pair. The manual insertion of the specimen/patient data into the LIS can impair the link with the patient profile present in the hospital information system (HIS), generally due to an inappropriate transcription of a patient's identification data, eventually causing a duplication of patients' profile, and consuming time. In a laboratory with a DP workflow, laboratory personnel have the possibility of completing these accessioning tasks automatically to minimize the risk of errors. The different identification codes (IDs) used in the various subsequent steps play a crucial role here. Similar to a pyramid or hierarchy, different types of IDs are attributed to the patient, and everything associated with this accessioning event, as follows:

- Patient ID

- C ID
- Specimen container ID (entry lab)
- Sample IDs
- Block IDs
- Slide IDs

For DP, a mechanism is needed to get the following types of required case information to the administrative and the pathologist: patient ID and demographic information, description of the specimen, clinical history and questions or requests for the pathologist. In the digital pathology laboratory, the accessioning is modified and may include some or all of the following (Table 1):

- Sample/slides arrive in the pathology laboratory with a label containing a code (entry lab, preferentially 2D type) associated with patient and case data.
- By scanning the code on the label of the case, the administrative is able to open the digital request on pathology LIS automatically, allowing the automatic synchronization of the information from the hospital system or creating the specific page for cases/patients coming from outside.
- A case ID for the sample is generated.
- The case ID is then used in all sorts of assets generated for that case (cassettes, new slides, special stains, digital slides).
- The administrator can take pictures of both the container and the specimen, and these photos will be attached to the case file.
- All of the documents received together with the specimen are scanned and attached to the case file or directly transmitted to the LIS digitally (Optical Character Recognition, OCR).

Table 1. Suggested checkpoints at the accessioning workstation.

	Accessioning Checkpoints
1.	Samples/slides are accessioned, using an order entry system, after the scanning of a code that identifies the patient/case, imports all the necessary information from the integrated HIS and opens the digital request: a procedure that introduces automation and consequent reduction of transcription errors.
2.	A number and the respective identification code are generated for each sample, and the identification code is used for various assets generated for that case: procedure that allows the tracking of the sample while it is circulating in the laboratory.
3.	Dedicated personnel take a picture of the container and of the specimen, and those photos are attached to the case file: procedure that documents the product entering the laboratory as well as the respective identification; this may represent an important medico-legal registry.
4.	The documents that may be received with the specimen are scanned and attached to the case file or directly transmitted digitally (OCR): a procedure that facilitates access to relevant information that is prevented from being lost in a workstation.

6.2. Grossing Checkpoints

After accessioning, cases are ready to be macroscopically analyzed, described and grossed by the pathologist or trained technical staff. As this happens in accessioning, the grossing workstation may be a source of human errors. These errors may include some of the following: wrong assignment of the macroscopic description and grossing of one patient in the paperwork of another patient, loss of manual transcription of specimen descriptions, deterioration of the numbers on the cassettes and incongruences among the sample received, grossed and subsequently processed in the absence of step-by-step picture documentation.

As in the other workstations, through automation the DP workflow can help reduce to a minimum the human interference needed in the grossing phase. The previously described process would be as follows (Table 2):

- The grossing operator (e.g., pathologist/resident/pathologist's assistant) can access the case/patient file by directly scanning the code on the sample container.
- Pictures are taken of the sample before it is described and grossed, as well as during grossing, and finally of all tissue cassettes with slices; those images are directly linked to the case using the software integration paths between the LIS and the image capture instrument.
- The grossing operator performs a macroscopic description of the sample through automated speech recognition systems that report the text in the appropriate section of the case/patient file using the software integrations paths between the LIS and the dictation system instrument.
- The operator can produce cassettes by using a specific printer (preferably laser printer) to assign an identification code corresponding to the particular case, as established during the accessioning and using the software integration paths between the LIS and the printer. The cassettes and marker media should be appropriately tested to demonstrate the indelibility or impossibility of washing away or removing the identification code. The suggested code is 2D (e.g., QR code), which can include a greater character count (higher data density), require a smaller footprint, and have fewer scan and printer failures than 1D codes.
- An image of the cassette with the grossed specimen should be obtained at the bench, allowing retrieval of this at the following steps.

Table 2. Suggested checkpoints at the grossing workstation.

	Grossing Checkpoints
1.	Scanning the identification code on the sample container allows for automatic access to the patient/case data, preventing transcription errors.
2.	The photographic documentation of the sample as it is in the container, during grossing and within the cassettes (for comparison to what is arrived at the embedding station) guarantees the preservation of the case features and identification. The automatic introduction of the photographs into the patient/case file at the LIS prevents mismatches and time loss.
3.	The macroscopic description of the sample is dictated and converted to text through voice recognition functions of the LIS or of an instrument connected to the LIS preventing transcription errors and time loss.
4.	Cassettes are printed with the identification code of the sample to be tracked in subsequent workstations.
5.	The material inserted in the cassette during grossing can be captured to obtain retrievable pictures at the following steps.

6.3. Grossing-to-Processing and Processing Checkpoints

After the grossing phase, cassettes containing the specimens are ready to be processed. At this stage, further checkpoints may be needed to verify that all the cassettes generated at the grossing workstation are present in the rack to be processed. This double-check is still routinely and primarily done manually in most pathology laboratories. In a DP workflow, this task may be carried out by scanning the codes printed in the cassettes of the rack before they are processed and checking if all the produced cassettes are submitted to the subsequent phase, integrating the information in the LIS. During the processing phase, both the instruments and programs used should be preferentially recorded through the employment of an appropriately integrated LIS, allowing for tracking the specimens/cases at this workstation. This system can be further deployed to track the usage of reagents for processing, helping in the safe disposal of these reagents. Moreover, the integration with the LIS can further help aggregate specimens and cassettes in different racks based on their processing time and scanner time/protocol requirements (e.g., fast vs. standard processing), or even separate specimens processed in different instruments.

6.4. Embedding Checkpoints

Once the processed specimen inside the cassettes have arrived at the embedding room, operators (technicians) should be able to access the pictures taken during the grossing phase by simply scanning the barcode (Table 2). This will allow them to compare them with the content of cassettes after processing, checking their correspondence to rule out the loss of biological material. Correct embedding may prevent the creation of poor-quality virtual slides. One of the possible issues during the scanning phase is represented by the presence of large fragments, which are more prone to be hydrated during the processing steps and thus more complicated to be captured by the scanner. To address this problem, the fragments should be reduced during the grossing phase, and the embedding checkpoint is essential to control this point. Similarly, tissue fragments well oriented, levelled, and close to each other in paraffin, may constitute good substrates for better-quality glass slides. If the sample to be analyzed is too large to be fitted in a regular glass slide, the recent introduction of dedicated scanners for "macro" glass slides provides the possibility of this solution directly from the grossing room [29].

6.5. Sectioning Checkpoints

The sectioning workstation is a time-consuming phase of the laboratory flow where errors are frequent. Here, the automation can facilitate the technician's work bringing increased control, fewer errors, and resulting in less time spent. The sectioning workstation is complex and requires the rapid manipulation of specimens and instruments in a consecutive way. The introduction of a slide printer, a code reader, a desktop interface, and similar devices can be initially perceived as a further complication of this step. Checkpoints can be installed at this workstation depending on the laboratory's needs and may prevent important errors (Table 3). Moreover, the employment of a slide printer (e.g., laser) at the sectioning station connected to the tracking system should be preferred on the "classic" handwritten or printed labels to reduce the risk of mismatches. The LIS should also be the source of all the information regarding the types of stains to be performed (i.e., IHC or "special" tinctorial stains) from a specific block. Moreover, the introduction of dedicated instruments to capture the cut surface of each paraffin block [28] could represent an additional checkpoint, helping to further reduce tissue inconsistencies among the blocks and the final glass/virtual slides. The sectioning process should follow the highest operative standards to minimize errors and poor quality in the subsequent scanning phase. Indeed, the irregular thickness of a tissue section, and the presence of holes or scratches and debris erroneously collected from the bath can impair the correct scan of the final glass slide product. The same is true for sections located at the edges of the slides, which may pass undetected by the scanner. Thus, the sections should be thin enough during the cutting phase and preferentially located in the middle of the physical glass slides to ensure the most appropriate scanning quality. Automatic microtomes may contribute to decreased tissue thickness variations.

Table 3. Suggested checkpoint at the sectioning workstation.

Sectioning Checkpoints
1. The code printed on the paraffin block may be scanned to open the case file through the integrated LIS preventing transcription errors.
2. The technician can check how many and which kinds of slides are needed for each block directly on the LIS.
3. For each paraffin block, one or more printed glass slides are then generated through a dedicated printer, with all the slides having a unique identifier.
4. After sectioning, each paraffin block may be photographed to assess whether all the material emerged on the glass slide/WSI.
5. The sectioning phase should follow high operative standards, reducing the risk of artifacts that can impair the scanning phase.

6.6. Staining and Mounting Checkpoints

Once in the staining workstation, the slides produced in the digital workflow are identified through their code to define which staining protocol they should follow, as per internal LIS prerecorded indications, using automated staining platforms. As in the previous step, the staining process should follow the highest qualitative standards to reduce possible modifications that can interfere with the scanning phase (faint or darker staining, debris/precipitates). For this purpose, implementing an internal checkpoint with daily controls and/or external quality control can help assess the quality of stained slides [30]. Automating the staining may contribute to a stable result, allowing the design of a scanning protocol applicable to most of the slides, avoiding restaining and rescanning slides. The production of consistent staining with a clean background is relevant because it decreases the size of the produced digital slides. A final word is needed to address the mounting process and respective automation. To minimize the interference of the mounting medium in the scanning process, the laboratory must select the mounter, the coverslip type, and respective mounting medium to be used in all sorts of glass slides so that the scanner can be calibrated accordingly. Before the scanning phase, it is of paramount importance to check whether the slide is in an adequate state for scanning. After the staining/cover-slipping phase, it should be dry to prevent scanning problems (e.g., stitching, blurring, out of focus areas). Moreover, the scanning phase can be either affected by the different positions of the coverslips, leading to a misalignment of the slides in the rack. Differences in the type of coverslip can be responsible for a high rate of WSIs being out of focus. The use of automatic mounters obviates variations in the quality of the mounting and prevents errors if an adequate revision of the mounter is provided.

6.7. Correct Assigning of the WSI to the Case Checkpoints

Please refer to Section 7 of the present document.

6.8. Archiving Checkpoints

After the sectioning and scanning phases, blocks and slides can be appropriately archived to be retrieved whenever is necessary. This task has been historically performed manually by operators (technicians or laboratory assistants), leading to loss and misplacement of blocks/slides, with obvious medico-legal consequences. Moreover, the wide practice of consulting archival material by all the laboratory workers, including residents and students for didactic purposes, can further complicate the correct positioning of these specimens. Based on these observations, the full integration with the LIS and the presence of unique identifiers, both on the blocks and glass slides, allow an automated archiving of all the biological material, as well as its safe and unbiased retrieval if needed (e.g., request of external consultation). For archiving of the WSI, please refer to the data retention policy (Section 8 of the present document).

7. Scanner for Slide Digitization

This section contains some considerations and recommendations for selecting and managing the most appropriate digital slide scanner (Table 4). As in other medical specialties, which have been dramatically changed by the introduction of a wide variety of digital devices for the routine daily work [31], it is not the focus of the present recommendations to draw a meticulous review of the technical characteristics of a scanner, since several studies have already been published on this subject [32,33].

Table 4. Recommendations for the scanning phase.

Scanning Checkpoints
1. At any given time, two scanners digitise twice the number of slides compared to a single scanner, and three scanners triple this (e.g., for a caseload of 300 slides per day, employing three scanners with 100-slide capacity could be better than using a single scanner with a 300-slide capacity).
2. It is advisable to scan during the daytime, with the lab personnel present to solve unexpected problems.
3. Scanning sessions during the night might be problematic in some already established workflows; thus, if there are problems with the scanning process, it might be better to avoid scanning after working hours.
4. A single-scanner approach is not recommended when contemplating a daily routine diagnostic workflow.
5. Consider the possibility of a continuous loading and eventual prioritisation of a batch of slides.

The most appropriate scanner should be selected based on the needs of the specific laboratory (e.g., primary diagnosis, consultation, education, and research). The following section focuses on the possible impact of such a choice on DP workflow implementation. According to the LEAN approach, as previously stated in chapter 2, the positioning of the scanners should follow the logic of an automated workflow and thus be placed as close as possible to the staining and cover-slipping stations, making their implementation in the entire process easier and smooth [6,7]. The transition to digital pathology also includes choosing the most appropriate types and numbers of scanners for the lab. Although it is highly dependent on the needs of each specific laboratory, one way to estimate the number of scanners is to review previous DP experiences [6,7]. In this context, each department should be aware of the expected application of the scanners, the total time required for the scanning process, and the time that can be dedicated to this part of the workflow. Some formulas to calculate the numbers of scanners needed in the lab have been proposed [6,7]. However, many variables must be considered when calculating the number of scanners required to digitize the entire slide volume within the same workday, thus not interfering with the TAT. These variables are limited by the technical specifications of the scanners and the informatics networks (including bandwidth and switches), type and location of storage, together with the existing workflow within the lab (i.e., availability of the personnel 24/7). One of the possible pitfalls in calculating the actual scanning time per slide/batch, and thus the number of scanners required per lab, could be represented by the reported scanning times by each vendor, generally calculated on a sample tissue of 1.5 cm $\times$ 1.5 cm in size and with a local storage solution. However, this is far away from the routine practice of an anatomic pathology laboratory that must accommodate very small pieces of tissue (e.g., biopsies) as well as large surgical samples, and that may even have the possibility of storing the WSI remotely or in the cloud. Moreover, since the implementation of scanners should not impact the existing workflow and eventually lead to its improvement, there is a need to evaluate a continuous loading capability to preserve the same or similar workloads over time compared to the conventional analogue counterpart. This should be coupled with the possibility of prioritizing a specific batch of slides.

However, a few comments are needed. Overall, scanning during working hours should be preferred for practical and logistical reasons. If there are problems with the scanning process, it might be better to avoid scanning after working hours. For example, it has been reported that the mean scanning time in a routine environment is about 6 min for scanning a slide at an equivalent of 40 $\times$ magnification [34]. Therefore, it takes about 4 h for one rack of 40 slides and up to 40 h to digitize all of the slides that fit inside the scanner (using an AT2, Leica Biosystems, Nussloch, Germany). However, it is well known that the scanning process may stop for several reasons, including sticky glass, connection problems or software and hardware problems. The result may be an incomplete digitization of slides, with consequent interruption of routine workflow in the subsequent morning. Based on the previous observations, and since the scanning process should be a continuous workflow in the lab, scanning during the day should be preferred to the overnight approach. This could enable lab personnel to react to the possible technical issues mentioned above. This could even lead to modifications in other parts of the pathology workflow to adapt routine specimen processing to the loading schedules required by the scanners. In this setting, the laboratory can choose to switch from bulk production of slides at the end of the day to a more continuous production of samples. Once the number of scanners needed and the required scanning time has been defined, the laboratory should verify whether the number of working operators employed in the department is sufficient to run the instruments for the specified length of time. Otherwise, the calculation of the necessary personnel is required, considering both:

1. The scanning process.
2. Virtual slide quality control.

The first part mainly consists of loading/unloading slides in the scanner and taking snapshots to ensure that the instrument captures all the material on the glass. On the other hand, the quality control phase is equally important and may be time-consuming, encompassing all the quality check procedures of the final WSI and related data. The points discussed above pertain to "regular" scanners for bright field microscopy. Other "special" scanners exist, e.g., those for dark field microscopy (immunofluorescence and fluorescence in-situ hybridization, FISH), as well as those for whole mount slides (macro slides). Because of their highly specific fields of application [35], they are not the object of these recommendations.

8. Validation of WSI for Clinical Use

Several validation studies for WSI have been published, and most show broad concordance between the conventional microscope and the digital diagnosis [3,36]. Regarding staining and sample types applicable to WSI-based diagnosis, most basic tissue slides stained with hematoxylin and eosin (H&E), as well as most special stains and IHC stains, are expected to be usable. However, they require appropriate validation studies, followed by trial periods until the users have reached an adequate learning level. The recommended validation period for the clinical use of WSI should allow each pathologist to follow a training phase with parallel access to glass and digital slides for each case, with different wash-out intervals of time proposed.

This path for the implementation of WSI for primary diagnosis has been followed by different laboratories worldwide [8,37,38]. Some pathologists' professional societies (e.g., College of American Pathologists) have proposed detailed guidelines for this validation process [32,39]. These have recently been updated, although they are mainly centered on validating WSIs in the diagnostic setting, not considering all the preanalytical phases of the digital workflow [40]. Here we discuss further critical points that have recently emerged as impactful in the implementation and validation of WSI. They include the most appropriate visualization devices, assessment of scan quality, tissue coverage of the block, glass slide and virtual slide and the proper assignment of the WSI to the case and/or the patient.

8.1. The Visualization Chain: The Most Appropriate Monitor and Display. The Pathologist Workstation

The typical pathologist workstation is composed of one computer and two monitors. One monitor displays the LIS showing patient data and different dashboards with the possibility to access the patient's documents or slides. The other monitor is dedicated to the visualization of the WSIs or other images. Several documents have already described all of the features needed to implement the visualization instruments in DP, namely, monitor quality, brightness and contrast, color depth, fidelity and profiles [32,41]. Many pathology departments already operate with workstations equipped with high-contrast (e.g., minimum contrast ratio of 1000:1), high–resolution (e.g., 16:10, 27″ diagonal matrix, 2560 × 1600), and bright displays (e.g., a maximum brightness of 300 cd/m^2). Some FDA-approved built-in solutions for digital pathology employ medical-grade displays. However, the minimum requirements for DP monitors are still debated, and there is no consensus on how to assess their quality. External sources of variability further complicate this matter, such as the distance from the monitor and the illumination conditions of the room, which makes unbiased comparisons among the different devices available more difficult. This heterogeneity, and the large variety of supply in the digital market, has been recently reviewed [41], stressing the need for appropriate information of pathologists on this topic due to the complexity of the available technologies, which are changing at a fast pace. Alternatively, an easy-to-access and point-of-use quality assessment tool has been proposed, which tests color accuracy and may be a valuable indicator of the suitability of a particular screen for digital pathology diagnostics. Further validation is needed for its definitive employment in this setting [42]. Many comments could be made to identify the minimum computer technical requirement at the pathologist's workstation. Dedicated random access memory (RAM) allows pathologists to visualize the WSI correctly. However, there is no standard in selecting CPU or RAM, as the management of WSIs may be affected by several parameters (i.e., network connection, switches etc.). A recent mid-range gaming computer will undoubtedly exceed the technical requirements to approach DP.

8.2. Scan Quality Assessment

After digitization, the produced WSI should be checked to ensure appropriate image quality to avoid any technical interference with the final diagnosis. Although most of the routine slides (about 90%), if properly processed, should not present scanning problems, some special slides (e.g., IHC or FISH) would benefit from dedicated scanning protocols and could be affected by more digitization issues. On the other hand, a minority of the "routine" slides (about 10%) could still be affected by scanning issues, stressing the need to adopt alternative protocols to obtain WSI from these challenging samples. This is based mainly on the assessment of focus quality, which can be partly assisted by the automated metric implemented in some available scan systems but should be performed on every slide to decide whether to rescan the sample. This can be done systematically by the lab personnel (e.g., technicians) for every scanning set before assigning the case to a pathologist. Alternatively, the pathologist can perform this check once after case review, requesting a rescan of a glass slide similar to the way that an additional recut or a special stain is ordered in the LIS. However, under real-life conditions, the entire manual check could be rather time-consuming and troublesome, especially in light of the need for subsequent deployment of image analysis algorithms. For this reason, automation of this phase is highly recommended. It can further speed up the digital transition process, ensuring an adequate quality of the scanned slide for potential subsequent AI analyses [43]. Suppose pathologists review a slide with blurry areas. In that case, it is up to their judgment to decide whether these artefacts will interfere with their safe diagnosis of the image, and order rescans as necessary. However, even in this case, it can be challenging for the human naked eye to unmask potential slight imperfections of the scanned slides that can impair the employment of AI algorithms. Even in these cases, the introduction of focus quality assessment [44] and quality control computational tools have been developed. In this setting, further validations are needed to implement such algorithms in routine practice [43,45].

8.3. Tissue Coverage

A critical assumption with using WSI in clinical settings is that scanned slides are completely accurate digital representations of glass slides. Therefore, it is of paramount importance that all tissue fragments present on glass slides be recognized and captured for review on the resulting digital slides.

Typically, two main different images are generated during the digitization process:

- The overview (rendering the macro/slide label files) that is a low-resolution snapshot of the entire glass slide.
- The "digital image" of the glass slide generated by a microscope camera (rendering baseline tiled image, thumbnail and multiple intermediate tiled images stacked in a pyramid) often acquired at the chosen magnification.

Many WSI devices include systems to detect tissue samples on a slide to limit scanning to relevant tissue-containing areas. For example, some scanners are programmed to omit the blank areas on the slide during the scanning process, where tissue is presumed to be absent, to speed up the process and generate files of smaller size. However, sometimes the tissue detection mechanism can fail to identify small or pale pieces of tissue automatically (e.g., label them as blank areas), or the user may not appropriately select the region containing the entire tissue analyzable. This may lead to potential errors that can cause serious discrepancies between the tissue present on the glass slide and the WSI. In this setting, overview images can help avoid such errors and represent a valuable tool for quality assessment purposes [46]. The macro image provides a low-magnification overview of all the tissue pieces and empty space on the glass slide. It serves mainly to guide the scanner's tissue detection system, focus-point selection, and subsequent high-resolution digitization of tissue recognized and/or manually selected by an operator. However, the macro image is not necessarily displayed by default by all WSI vendors. Pathologists and laboratory personnel should be adequately trained on how to find and use the macro image as part of essential quality control. An alternative way to ensure that all the available tissue is present on the WSI is to compare the obtained digital slide with the original glass slide. However, this process could be time-consuming and represent a continuing additional workload for the lab personnel (e.g., histotechnologists), avoidable with the proposed double-check practice with the macro images made by each pathologist when the virtual cases are assigned [46].

Other possible sources of tissue coverage errors can result from inappropriate placement of tissue sections on the glass slide (e.g., below the label or on the external frame of the slide), which can fall outside the area recognized by the scanner. To address this issue, it is also essential to check the technical specifications of the scanner, specifically regarding the predefined detectable area that could be insufficient to cover the entirety of the physical glass slide containing tissue. These issues can be addressed by following the point-by-point indications reported above on the sectioning and cover-slipping checkpoints. Finally, very few cases with concordant WSI and macro images can still hide discrepancy issues with the entire amount of tissue sent for the analysis in the lab. This could be addressed by the manual, analog comparison of the tissue block with the macro images and the WSI, as suggested in the relative checkpoint in Section 5. However, the use of appropriate instruments to take a picture of the cut surface of the block can represent a valuable digital cost-effective alternative to reduce the error rate further. The pathologist can then readily check the three-way concordance among digitized cut surface of the block, macro images and WSI for every assigned case, reducing the error rate close to zero.

8.4. Assignment of Images to the Correct Case/Patient File

At the end of the scanning process, one of the most important steps is correctly assigning the digitized slides to the appropriate case/patient. As already mentioned, during the scanning phase a macro image is generated representing a snapshot of the entire glass slide that usually includes the slide label with identifiers (e.g., case accession number, barcode, text showing a patient name, and slide level or stain details). As per other steps mentioned in Section 5, a 2D barcode is crucial here as well to allow the scanning system, adequately integrated with the LIS, to link the scanned slides to specific specimens and patients. In some cases, according to institute policies, the dedicated personnel can perform a double-check after the automatic assignment of slides. It has been reported that errors in recognizing the printed barcode on the slide (or barcodes printed in the label) may occur, thus preventing the WSI to be matched with the corresponding case. This is due mainly to the poor quality of the printed barcode (or because it is missing a part of the barcode). This ultimately results in a case that is not ready to be reported, with a consequent delay in diagnosis. A checkpoint should be performed at this step to verify that all the stained slides have been digitized and assigned to the correct cases. Usually, scanner vendors create specific folders of "unassigned" (or barcode-less) slides for this purpose.

9. Open Topics (Not Fully Addressed in This Document)

9.1. Data Retention Policies and Image Storage Solutions

Data retention policies and image storage solutions for WSIs still represent open and debated topics, and no strict recommendations have been provided yet, although some suggestions and indications can be found in different documents and guidelines [32]. General recommendations, including those from the College of American Pathologists (CAP), currently advise retaining glass slides for at least ten years [47], with suggested periods of retaining digital pathology storage for a period ranging from a few years up to several years [48]. However, regulation on the retention of virtual slides, when used for primary diagnosis, is still lacking. Some documents suggest applying the same indications used for glass slides for WSIs, too [31]. Other recommendations are to keep the digital image for a period of two laboratory inspection cycles in case of any need to review it (e.g., for audits, quality control, medico-legal reasons) [32]. However strict and precise European guidelines are still needed to define the minimum period of time for WSI storage. Until then, pathology departments should determine an appropriate retention policy for the digital images [49].

Closely related to the retention policy is the appropriate storage of the images: where, how, and which slides must be stored is still an unresolved issue with multiple possibilities that can be adapted to each laboratory's needs. Regarding the solutions available on the actual storage of the WSIs, organized and redundant storage solutions (e.g., Network Attached Storage, NAS, or Redundant Array of Independent Disks, RAID) are preferred to simple external/internal hard drives, considered negligent by some authors [31]. The possibility of multiple backup copies and disaster recovery procedures should also be kept in consideration [48]. Moreover, the issue related to the file extension of the WSIs that should be employed during the back-up is still unsolved. One of the essential requirements is represented by the capability of ensuring the changelessness, the guaranteed future and future-proofing of the data (e.g., the unity of patient or case data and the actual image content), as well as the easy accessibility of the WSIs, even after years. This can be obtained by the use of a DICOM-capable archive, although the eventual loss of quality related to the compression/conversion from one image extension to another is still a matter of debate. Finally, identifying the amount and type of storage needed is important, as it is one of the highest costs when implementing DP and needs to be adapted to the calculated yearly needs of each laboratory [15].

It has to be underlined that digital pathology storages need to be built to be interoperable and useful. This requires high-quality datasets, seamless communication across IT systems and standard data formats [50]. Interoperability is of paramount importance for achieving the full potential of digitization in healthcare and medicine to avoid the risk of having data difficult to exchange, process and interpret. Interoperability should be technical, syntactic, semantic and organizational [50]. In this line, it has been suggested that enterprise Vendor Neutral Archiving, composed of hardware and software, could be used to accumulate images directly from various image acquisition sources with the possibility to manage images and other end-user applications such as electronic health records, laboratory information systems, and other health-related information systems and databases [51].

9.2. Evaluation of the Results Obtained with the Digital Transition

The process of DP implementation has designs and consequences that are distinct in each pathology laboratory. Monitoring the effects of the digital transformation of the laboratory is good practice. It may include an analysis of the following parameters before and after the implementation: results of quality control, turn-around time, workload for technicians and pathologists, ergonomics of each workstation, and the general satisfaction of the staff. For validation and quality control of the implemented digital workflow, we direct the reader to the recommendations already in use [32,33,40].

9.3. Preparing for the Subsequent Steps after Implementing the Digital Workflow

Having a digital repository that contains clinical and histological information can lay the foundation for using numerous computational pathology tools. The application of image analysis algorithms can allow the identification of specific cell or tissue compartments (e.g., nuclei, mitosis, glands, stroma, among others) for quantification (e.g., cell or mitosis counting) as well as for classification purposes (e.g., grading) [52]. Some practical applications of these tools range from helping in the more rigorous scoring of some IHC-stained sections (e.g., programmed death-ligand 1 [PD-L1] and human epidermal growth factor receptor 2 (HER2) scoring) to the quantification of the proliferation index (Ki-67) in many neoplasms (e.g., breast, lymphomas and neuroendocrine tumours) [53,54]. Moreover, the recent introduction of more sophisticated elaboration algorithms allows further information starting from the digitized images and integrating the clinical, laboratory and radiological data to obtain diagnostic, classification and prognostic hints through the application of the so-called artificial intelligence (AI) [55,56]. Further simplifications in the work of pathologists are possible in the future, such as the automation of time-consuming repetitive tasks and the extraction of more data from the tissue to support precision medicine.

10. Closing Remarks

The present recommendations represent a European guidance for transitioning from a classic, "analogue" to a completely digital workflow in every anatomic pathology department. Ten basic principles (Table 5) resulted from the discussion among international experts after implementing the available updated national guidelines. Based on the present document, the anatomic pathology societies of every European country should be able to direct the departments towards DP transition. Updates in the future will provide dedicated indications on the adoption of computer-aided diagnosis and AI tools.

Table 5. Summary of the recommendations for the implementation of the digital workflow.

	Principles	Type of Action
1.	The transformation of a laboratory toward Digital Pathology requires a multidisciplinary approach (pathologists, technicians, IT).	Recommendation
2.	Involve all the team in the transition process toward Digital Pathology (Educational phase).	Recommendation
3.	Spare valuable resources (e.g., spaces, time and people) employing the LEAN approach to optimize the process.	Suggestion
4.	Analyze the potentialities of the laboratory information (management) system (LIS/LIMS) and be aware of the information resources.	Recommendation
5.	Start the automation of all the possible processes, implementing a tracking system and defining the appropriate checkpoints for every phase.	Recommendation
6.	Design a quality control program mapping the necessary quality control steps.	Recommendation
7.	Choose an appropriate scanner.	Suggestion
8.	Validate WSI for clinical use.	Recommendation
9.	Evaluate the impact and results of the digital transformation and other members of the team to perform the same analysis.	Recommendation
10.	Prepare the next steps for digital pathology implementation after the workflow is well established.	Recommendation

Author Contributions: Conceptualization, F.F. and C.E.; methodology, V.L.; writing—original draft preparation, F.F. and V.L.; writing—review and editing, D.A., R.C., S.L., T.-R.K., M.S., D.R., V.D.M., A.P., N.Z.; supervision, F.F. and C.E. All authors have read and agreed to the published version of the manuscript.

Funding: This research received no external funding.

Institutional Review Board Statement: Not applicable.

Informed Consent Statement: Not applicable.

Data Availability Statement: All the data used are present within the manuscript.

Acknowledgments: We would like to thank Umberto Malapelle and Pasquale Pisapia from the University of Naples Federico II for their support in the creation of the iconography of this manuscript.

Conflicts of Interest: Filippo Fraggetta holds a US Patent App. 16/688,613, 2020 Sample imaging and imagery archiving for imagery comparison. David Ameisen is a partner at imginIT, SAS.

References

1. Evans, A.J.; Bauer, T.W.; Bui, M.M.; Cornish, T.C.; Duncan, H.; Glassy, E.F.; Hipp, J.; McGee, R.S.; Murphy, D.; Myers, C.; et al. US Food and Drug Administration Approval of Whole Slide Imaging for Primary Diagnosis: A Key Milestone Is Reached and New Questions Are Raised. *Arch. Pathol. Lab. Med.* **2018**, *142*, 1383–1387. [CrossRef]
2. Snead, D.R.J.; Tsang, Y.-W.; Meskiri, A.; Kimani, P.K.; Crossman, R.; Rajpoot, N.M.; Blessing, E.; Chen, K.; Gopalakrishnan, K.; Matthews, P.; et al. Validation of Digital Pathology Imaging for Primary Histopathological Diagnosis. *Histopathology* **2016**, *68*, 1063–1072. [CrossRef]
3. Goacher, E.; Randell, R.; Williams, B.; Treanor, D. The Diagnostic Concordance of Whole Slide Imaging and Light Microscopy: A Systematic Review. *Arch. Pathol. Lab. Med.* **2017**, *141*, 151–161. [CrossRef]
4. Mukhopadhyay, S.; Feldman, M.D.; Abels, E.; Ashfaq, R.; Beltaifa, S.; Cacciabeve, N.G.; Cathro, H.P.; Cheng, L.; Cooper, K.; Dickey, G.E.; et al. Whole Slide Imaging Versus Microscopy for Primary Diagnosis in Surgical Pathology. *Am. J. Surg. Pathol.* **2018**, *42*, 39–52. [CrossRef]
5. Evans, A.J.; Salama, M.E.; Henricks, W.H.; Pantanowitz, L. Implementation of Whole Slide Imaging for Clinical Purposes: Issues to Consider from the Perspective of Early Adopters. *Arch. Pathol. Lab. Med.* **2017**, *141*, 944–959. [CrossRef]
6. Available online: https://www.virtualpathology.leeds.ac.uk/research/clinical/docs/2018/pdfs/18778_Leeds%20Guide%20to%20Digital%20Pathology_Brochure_A4_final_hi.pdf (accessed on 10 November 2021).
7. Available online: https://www.usa.philips.com/c-dam/b2bhc/us/landing-pages/pdxus/how-to-go-digital-in-pathology.pdf (accessed on 10 November 2021).
8. Retamero, J.A.; Aneiros-Fernandez, J.; del Moral, R.G. Complete Digital Pathology for Routine Histopathology Diagnosis in a Multicenter Hospital Network. *Arch. Pathol. Lab. Med.* **2020**, *144*, 221–228. [CrossRef]
9. Fraggetta, F.; Garozzo, S.; Zannoni, G.F.; Pantanowitz, L.; Rossi, E.D. Routine Digital Pathology Workflow: The Catania Experience. *J. Pathol. Inform.* **2017**, *8*, 51.
10. Fraggetta, F.; Caputo, A.; Guglielmino, R.; Pellegrino, M.G.; Runza, G.; L'Imperio, V. A Survival Guide for the Rapid Transition to a Fully Digital Workflow: The "Caltagirone Example". *Diagnostics* **2021**, *11*, 1916. [CrossRef]
11. Eloy, C.; Vale, J.; Curado, M.; Polónia, A.; Campelos, S.; Caramelo, A.; Sousa, R.; Sobrinho-Simões, M. Digital Pathology Workflow Implementation at IPATIMUP. *Diagnostics* **2021**, *11*, 2111. [CrossRef]
12. Sinard, J.H.; Castellani, W.J.; Wilkerson, M.L.; Henricks, W.H. Stand-Alone Laboratory Information Systems versus Laboratory Modules Incorporated in the Electronic Health Record. *Arch. Pathol. Lab. Med.* **2015**, *139*, 311–318. [CrossRef]
13. Sepulveda, J.L.; Young, D.S. The Ideal Laboratory Information System. *Arch. Pathol. Lab. Med.* **2013**, *137*, 1129–1140. [CrossRef]
14. Pantanowitz, L.; Asa, S.; Bodén, A.; Treanor, D.; Jarkman, S.; Lundström, C. 2020 Vision of Digital Pathology in Action. *J. Pathol. Inform.* **2019**, *10*, 27. [CrossRef]
15. Quigley, J.; Lujan, G.; Hartman, D.; Parwani, A.; Roehmholdt, B.; Meter, B.; Ardon, O.; Hanna, M.; Kelly, D.; Sowards, C.; et al. Dissecting the Business Case for Adoption and Implementation of Digital Pathology: A White Paper from the Digital Pathology Association. *J. Pathol. Inform.* **2021**, *12*, 17. [CrossRef]
16. Hanna, M.G.; Reuter, V.E.; Ardon, O.; Kim, D.; Sirintrapun, S.J.; Schüffler, P.J.; Busam, K.J.; Sauter, J.L.; Brogi, E.; Tan, L.K.; et al. Validation of a Digital Pathology System Including Remote Review during the COVID-19 Pandemic. *Mod. Pathol.* **2020**, *33*, 2115–2127. [CrossRef]
17. Zarbo, R.J. Creating and Sustaining a Lean Culture of Continuous Process Improvement. *Am. J. Clin. Pathol.* **2012**, *138*, 321–326. [CrossRef]
18. Tuthill, J.; Friedman, B.; Splitz, A.; Balis, U. The Laboratory Information System Functionality Assessment Tool: Ensuring Optimal Software Support for Your Laboratory. *J. Pathol. Inform.* **2014**, *5*, 7. [CrossRef]

19. Petrides, A.K.; Bixho, I.; Goonan, E.M.; Bates, D.W.; Shaykevich, S.; Lipsitz, S.R.; Landman, A.B.; Tanasijevic, M.J.; Melanson, S.E.F. The Benefits and Challenges of an Interfaced Electronic Health Record and Laboratory Information System: Effects on Laboratory Processes. *Arch. Pathol. Lab. Med.* **2017**, *141*, 410–417. [CrossRef]
20. Krupinski, E.A. Optimizing the Pathology Workstation "Cockpit": Challenges and Solutions. *J. Pathol. Inform.* **2010**, *1*, 19. [CrossRef]
21. Dash, R.C.; Jones, N.; Merrick, R.; Haroske, G.; Harrison, J.; Sayers, C.; Haarselhorst, N.; Wintell, M.; Herrmann, M.D.; Macary, F. Integrating the Health-Care Enterprise Pathology and Laboratory Medicine Guideline for Digital Pathology Interoperability. *J. Pathol. Inform.* **2021**, *12*, 16. [CrossRef]
22. Roy, S.; Pfeifer, J.D.; LaFramboise, W.A.; Pantanowitz, L. Molecular Digital Pathology: Progress and Potential of Exchanging Molecular Data. *Expert Rev. Mol. Diagn.* **2016**, *16*, 941–947. [CrossRef]
23. Phelan, S.M. Impact of the Introduction of a Novel Automated Embedding System on Quality in a University Hospital Histopathology Department. *J. Histol. Histopathol.* **2014**, *1*, 3. [CrossRef]
24. Hanna, M.G.; Pantanowitz, L. Bar Coding and Tracking in Pathology. *Clin. Lab. Med.* **2016**, *36*, 13–30. [CrossRef] [PubMed]
25. Bostwick, D.G. Radiofrequency Identification Specimen Tracking in Anatomical Pathology: Pilot Study of 1067 Consecutive Prostate Biopsies. *Ann. Diagn. Pathol.* **2013**, *17*, 391–402. [CrossRef] [PubMed]
26. Lou, J.J.; Andrechak, G.; Riben, M.; Yong, W.H. A Review of Radio Frequency Identification Technology for the Anatomic Pathology or Biorepository Laboratory: Much Promise, Some Progress, and More Work Needed. *J. Pathol. Inform.* **2011**, *2*, 34. [PubMed]
27. Snyder, S.R.; Favoretto, A.M.; Derzon, J.H.; Christenson, R.H.; Kahn, S.E.; Shaw, C.S.; Baetz, R.A.; Mass, D.; Fantz, C.R.; Raab, S.S.; et al. Effectiveness of Barcoding for Reducing Patient Specimen and Laboratory Testing Identification Errors: A Laboratory Medicine Best Practices Systematic Review and Meta-Analysis. *Clin. Biochem.* **2012**, *45*, 988–998. [CrossRef]
28. L'Imperio, V.; Gibilisco, F.; Fraggetta, F. What Is Essential Is (No More) Invisible to the Eyes: The Introduction of Blocdoc in the Digital Pathology Workflow. *J. Pathol. Inform.* **2021**, *12*, 32.
29. Pantanowitz, L.; Farahani, N.; Parwani, A. Whole Slide Imaging in Pathology: Advantages, Limitations, and Emerging Perspectives. *Pathol. Lab. Med. Int.* **2015**, *23*, 23–33. [CrossRef]
30. Janowczyk, A.; Zuo, R.; Gilmore, H.; Feldman, M.; Madabhushi, A. HistoQC: An Open-Source Quality Control Tool for Digital Pathology Slides. *JCO Clin. Cancer Inform.* **2019**, *3*, 1–7. [CrossRef]
31. Ferrini, F.; Sannino, G.; Chiola, C.; Capparé, P.; Gastaldi, G.; Gherlone, E. Influence of Intra-Oral Scanner (I.O.S.) on The Marginal Accuracy of CAD/CAM Single Crowns. *Int. J. Environ. Res. Public Health* **2019**, *16*, 544. [CrossRef]
32. Hufnagl, P.; Zwönitzer, R.; Haroske, G. Guidelines Digital Pathology for Diagnosis on (and Reports Of) Digital Images Version 1.0 Bundesverband Deutscher Pathologen e.V. (Federal Association of German Pathologist). *Diagn. Pathol.* **2018**, *4*, 266. [CrossRef]
33. Available online: https://www.rcpath.org/uploads/assets/f465d1b3-797b-4297-b7fedc00b4d77e51/Best-practice-recommendations-for-implementing-digital-pathology.pdf (accessed on 10 November 2021).
34. Hanna, M.G.; Reuter, V.E.; Hameed, M.R.; Tan, L.K.; Chiang, S.; Sigel, C.; Hollmann, T.; Giri, D.; Samboy, J.; Moradel, C.; et al. Whole Slide Imaging Equivalency and Efficiency Study: Experience at a Large Academic Center. *Mod. Pathol.* **2019**, *32*, 916–928. [CrossRef]
35. L'Imperio, V.; Brambilla, V.; Cazzaniga, G.; Ferrario, F.; Nebuloni, M.; Pagni, F. Digital Pathology for the Routine Diagnosis of Renal Diseases: A Standard Model. *J. Nephrol.* **2021**, *34*, 681–688. [CrossRef]
36. Azam, A.S.; Miligy, I.M.; Kimani, P.K.-U.; Maqbool, H.; Hewitt, K.; Rajpoot, N.M.; Snead, D.R.J. Diagnostic Concordance and Discordance in Digital Pathology: A Systematic Review and Meta-Analysis. *J. Clin. Pathol.* **2021**, *74*, 448–455. [CrossRef]
37. Thorstenson, S.; Molin, J.; Lundström, C. Implementation of Large-Scale Routine Diagnostics Using Whole Slide Imaging in Sweden: Digital Pathology Experiences 2006–2013. *J. Pathol. Inform.* **2014**, *5*, 14.
38. Williams, B.J.; Treanor, D. Practical Guide to Training and Validation for Primary Diagnosis with Digital Pathology. *J. Clin. Pathol.* **2020**, *73*, 418–422. [CrossRef]
39. Pantanowitz, L.; Sinard, J.H.; Henricks, W.H.; Fatheree, L.A.; Carter, A.B.; Contis, L.; Beckwith, B.A.; Evans, A.J.; Lal, A.; Parwani, A.V.; et al. Validating Whole Slide Imaging for Diagnostic Purposes in Pathology: Guideline from the College of American Pathologists Pathology and Laboratory Quality Center. *Arch. Pathol. Lab. Med.* **2013**, *137*, 1710–1722. [CrossRef]
40. Evans, A.J.; Brown, R.W.; Bui, M.M.; Chlipala, E.A.; Lacchetti, C.; Milner, D.A.; Pantanowitz, L.; Parwani, A.V.; Reid, K.; Riben, M.W.; et al. Validating Whole Slide Imaging Systems for Diagnostic Purposes in Pathology: Guideline Update from the College of American Pathologists in Collaboration with the American Society for Clinical Pathology and the Association for Pathology Informatics. *Arch. Pathol. Lab. Med.* **2021**, online ahead of print. [CrossRef]
41. McClintock, D.; Abel, J.; Ouillette, P.; Williams, C.; Blau, J.; Cheng, J.; Yao, K.; Lee, W.; Cornish, T.; Balis, U.J. Display Characteristics and Their Impact on Digital Pathology: A Current Review of Pathologists' Future "microscope". *J. Pathol. Inform.* **2020**, *11*, 23. [CrossRef] [PubMed]
42. Point of Use QA Pathology. Available online: https://www.virtualpathology.leeds.ac.uk/research/systems/pouqa/pathology/ (accessed on 10 November 2021).
43. Kohlberger, T.; Liu, Y.; Moran, M.; Chen, P.-H.C.; Brown, T.; Hipp, J.D.; Mermel, C.H.; Stumpe, M.C. Whole-Slide Image Focus Quality: Automatic Assessment and Impact on AI Cancer Detection. *J. Pathol. Inform.* **2019**, *10*, 39. [CrossRef] [PubMed]

44. Senaras, C.; Niazi, M.K.K.; Lozanski, G.; Gurcan, M.N. DeepFocus: Detection of out-of-Focus Regions in Whole Slide Digital Images Using Deep Learning. *PLoS ONE* **2018**, *13*, e0205387. [CrossRef] [PubMed]
45. Hosseini, M.S.; Brawley-Hayes, J.A.Z.; Zhang, Y.; Chan, L.; Plataniotis, K.; Damaskinos, S. Focus Quality Assessment of High-Throughput Whole Slide Imaging in Digital Pathology. *IEEE Trans. Med. Imaging* **2020**, *39*, 62–74. [CrossRef]
46. Fraggetta, F.; Yagi, Y.; Garcia-Rojo, M.; Evans, A.; Tuthill, J.; Baidoshvili, A.; Hartman, D.; Fukuoka, J.; Pantanowitz, L. The Importance of eSlide Macro Images for Primary Diagnosis with Whole Slide Imaging. *J. Pathol. Inform.* **2018**, *9*, 46. [CrossRef] [PubMed]
47. Available online: https://elss.cap.org/elss/ShowProperty?nodePath=/UCMCON/Contribution%20Folders/WebApplications/pdf/retention-laboratory-records-and-materials.pdf (accessed on 10 November 2021).
48. Available online: https://digitalpathologyassociation.org/_data/cms_files/files/Archival_and_Retrieval_in_Digital_Pathology_Systems.pdf (accessed on 13 November 2021).
49. Stathonikos, N.; Nguyen, T.Q.; van Diest, P.J. Rocky Road to Digital Diagnostics: Implementation Issues and Exhilarating Experiences. *J. Clin. Pathol.* **2021**, *74*, 415–420. [CrossRef] [PubMed]
50. Lehne, M.; Sass, J.; Essenwanger, A.; Schepers, J.; Thun, S. Why Digital Medicine Depends on Interoperability. *NPJ Digit. Med.* **2019**, *2*, 79. [CrossRef] [PubMed]
51. Pantanowitz, L.; Sharma, A.; Carter, A.B.; Kurc, T.; Sussman, A.; Saltz, J. Twenty Years of Digital Pathology: An Overview of the Road Travelled, What Is on the Horizon, and the Emergence of Vendor-Neutral Archives. *J. Pathol. Inform.* **2018**, *9*, 40. [CrossRef]
52. Janowczyk, A.; Madabhushi, A. Deep Learning for Digital Pathology Image Analysis: A Comprehensive Tutorial with Selected Use Cases. *J. Pathol. Inform.* **2016**, *7*, 29. [CrossRef] [PubMed]
53. Aeffner, F.; Zarella, M.; Buchbinder, N.; Bui, M.; Goodman, M.; Hartman, D.; Lujan, G.; Molani, M.; Parwani, A.; Lillard, K.; et al. Introduction to Digital Image Analysis in Whole-Slide Imaging: A White Paper from the Digital Pathology Association. *J. Pathol. Inform.* **2019**, *10*, 9. [CrossRef] [PubMed]
54. Racoceanu, D.; Capron, F. Towards Semantic-Driven High-Content Image Analysis: An Operational Instantiation for Mitosis Detection in Digital Histopathology. *Comput. Med. Imaging Graph.* **2015**, *42*, 2–15. [CrossRef]
55. Cui, M.; Zhang, D.Y. Artificial Intelligence and Computational Pathology. *Lab. Investig.* **2021**, *101*, 412–422. [CrossRef]
56. Racoceanu, D.; Capron, F. Semantic Integrative Digital Pathology: Insights into Microsemiological Semantics and Image Analysis Scalability. *Pathobiology* **2016**, *83*, 148–155. [CrossRef]

MDPI AG
Grosspeteranlage 5
4052 Basel
Switzerland
Tel.: +41 61 683 77 34

Diagnostics Editorial Office
E-mail: diagnostics@mdpi.com
www.mdpi.com/journal/diagnostics

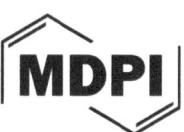

Disclaimer/Publisher's Note: The title and front matter of this reprint are at the discretion of the . The publisher is not responsible for their content or any associated concerns. The statements, opinions and data contained in all individual articles are solely those of the individual Editor and contributors and not of MDPI. MDPI disclaims responsibility for any injury to people or property resulting from any ideas, methods, instructions or products referred to in the content.

www.ingramcontent.com/pod-product-compliance
Lightning Source LLC
LaVergne TN
LVHW072344090526
838202LV00019B/2476